Martin Keuchel

Friedrich Hagenmüller

David E. Fleischer

Editors

Atlas of Video Capsule Endoscopy

Martin Keuchel

Friedrich Hagenmüller

David E. Fleischer

Editors

Atlas of Video Capsule Endoscopy

With 990 Color Figures

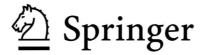

Martin Keuchel, M.D.
Medical Department I, Asklepios Klinik Altona
Paul-Ehrlich-Str. 1, 22763 Hamburg, Germany

Friedrich Hagenmüller, M.D.
Professor of Medicine
Medical Department I, Asklepios Klinik Altona
Paul-Ehrlich-Str. 1, 22763 Hamburg, Germany

David E. Fleischer, M.D.
Professor of Medicine, Mayo Clinic College of Medicine
Chair, Division of Gastroenterology and Hepatology, Mayo Clinic
13400 East Shea Boulevard, Scottsdale, AZ 82529, USA

Library of Congress Control Number: 2006925850

ISBN-10 3-540-23128-5   Springer Medizin Verlag Heidelberg
ISBN-13 978-3-540-23128-5   Springer Medizin Verlag Heidelberg

Springer Medizin Verlag
Springer.com
© Springer Medizin Verlag Heidelberg 2006
Printed in Germany

Editor: Hinrich Küster, Heidelberg, Germany
Project Manager: Meike Seeker, Heidelberg, Germany
Copyediting: Susan M. Peters, Hamburg, Germany
Design: deblik Berlin

SPIN 11018117
Typesetting: Michaela Baumann, Fotosatz-Service Köhler GmbH, Würzburg, Germany
Printing: Stürtz GmbH, Würzburg, Germany

Printed on acid-free paper   2126SM – 5 4 3 2 1 0

Foreword

Wireless capsule endoscopy represents a revolutionary advance in noninvasive imaging of the digestive tract, particularly the small bowel. Well over 300,000 examinations have been performed in a relatively short time, testifying to the enormous unmet need to conquer the last bastion in digestive endoscopy. Capsule technology was developed to assist in the evaluation of diseases of the entire digestive tract, from the esophagus to the colon, but especially of the small bowel where it facilitates discovery of diseases that are often not detectable with other modalities.

Potential clinical indications and applications are constantly expanding. Currently, evaluation of obscure gastrointestinal bleeding is the foremost important indication for capsule endoscopy, occasionally followed by push enteroscopy or double-balloon endoscopy. The mean diagnostic value of capsule endoscopy for finding the cause of obscure bleeding is approximately 60%. The clinical utility of capsule endoscopy in the diagnosis of Crohn's disease continues to evolve. Capsule endoscopy appears particularly useful in patients, including children, who have symptoms and signs suggestive of Crohn's disease, when conventional diagnostic modalities remain negative. Other novel indications abound such as villous atrophy in celiac disease, lymphangiectasia, nodular lymphoid hyperplasia, drug-induced mucosal injury, radiation damage etc. Before introduction of the capsule, it was not readily possible to establish the extent of small bowel involvement in celiac disease. The strength of the capsule seems to lie in its ideal ability to diagnose, monitor, and assess complications in the latter disease. A modified capsule (PillCam) appears useful in screening patients with esophageal diseases, such as suspected columnar metaplasia or varices.

This atlas, the first commercially available in the field and now appearing in the English language for expanded usefulness, testifies to all the above indications and applications. Through meticulously selected examples from their extensive databank, the authors teach the reader the spectrum of abnormalities and phenomena that one can encounter in patients examined with capsule endoscopy. Spread out through the atlas are »pearls« of intriguing findings and clinical correlates. The astute reader readily becomes acquainted with the wealth of variety of capsule images, the limitations of the technique, and possibilities for improvement, e.g., through prior purgative administration, motility modulation, application of the »Patency Capsule« in suspected stenosis, esophageal capsule endoscopy etc. Overall failures are rare and mainly related to incomplete small bowel examination.

Obviously the overall usefulness and applicability of capsule endoscopy needs to be evaluated in the light of all other novel imaging modalities such as virtual CT/MR enteroscopy, 3D reconstructions etc., but one can confidently predict that capsule technology is here to stay. Further improvements and sophisticated innovations are on the horizon such as longer battery life span, perhaps possibilities for re-energizing batteries with extracorporal electromagnetic energy, improved image quality, real-time imaging, steering capabilities, control of movement direction and velocity, autonomous radio-controlled robotic capsular endoscopy, and ultimately possibilities for therapeutic action.

The authors of this superb atlas, which was first published in the German language and has now been reformatted and updated in an English version, are truly to be congratulated. Drs. Keuchel, Hagenmüller, and Fleischer together with more than 50 renowned experts from all over the world deserve our esteem. Early on they recognized and accepted the potential of this novel dimension of automated intestinal imaging. They had the vision and conviction that producing a teaching atlas of high educational quality would be immensely helpful in increasing awareness and gaining experience, if not expertise, with this novel imaging possibility. I hope and wish that this first English version of the first atlas of capsule endoscopy will be greatly appreciated by the gastrointestinal community worldwide. May its success stimulate the authors to continue their dedicated work through further in-depth study of the clinical applicability of this novel imaging modality.

Prof. Emer. GNJ Tytgat
Past President of the World Gastroenterology Organisation

Preface

Since its introduction in 2001, video capsule endoscopy has developed at an explosive pace. The ability to examine the entire small bowel noninvasively has shined a light into the »black box« of endoscopy. At the same time, many of the findings in this new modality are still unclear in terms of their classification and clinical relevance.

A major goal of this atlas is to help the reader interpret a capsule endoscopy examination. It does this by relating the images to corresponding histologic, endoscopic, radiologic, surgical, and clinical reference findings. For this international atlas, a board of world-renowned experts could be won as authors, guaranteeing a state-of-the-art presentation of the different aspects of capsule endoscopy, which is gratefully appreciated. A correlative task of this magnitude could be accomplished only through the generous help of numerous colleagues, who provided us with their own images and video capsule findings. They are all listed in the Appendix, and we gratefully acknowledge their contributions.

The support of the teams at Asklepios Klinik Altona and Mayo Clinic Scottsdale is gratefully acknowledged. Renate Höhne, MD, Ernst Malzfeldt, MD, and Mr. Wolfgang Frier contributed to the success of this atlas by preparing and processing numerous images, and Mrs. Karin Ahmadi did the same through her extensive research of the literature.

We thank Mr. Hinrich Küster of Springer Publishers for his outstanding services in the creation of this atlas, and we thank Ms. Susan M. Peters, Ms. Michaela Baumann and Ms. Meike Seeker for their skillful editing and production work. Last but not least we thank our families for their support and understanding during the time of preparing this book.

Hamburg/Scottsdale
February 2006

Martin Keuchel
Friedrich Hagenmüller
David E. Fleischer

Table of Contents

List of Contributors

Adler, Samuel N., M.D.
Clinical Associate Professor
Divison of Gastroenterology, Bikur-Cholim
Hospital, 5 Straus Street, Jerusalem, Israel

Appleyard, Mark, M.D.
Gastroenterology Department, Royal Brisbane
and Women´s Hospital, Butterfield Street,
Herston, Queensland 4029, Australia

Barkin, Jamie S., M.D., F.A.C.P, M.A.C.G.
Professor of Medicine, University of Miami School
of Medicine
Division of Gastroenterology, Mount Sinai
Medical Center, 4300 Alton Road, Miami Beach,
FL 33140, USA

Barth, Eberhard, M.D.
Clinic for Gastroenterology and Rheumatology,
Mittelweg 123, 20148 Hamburg, Germany

Bjarnason, Ingvar, M.D., Ph.D.
Professor of Medicine
Department of Medicine, King's College
Hospital, Denmark Hill, London SE5 9RS, UK

Burke, Carol A., M.D.
Center for Colon Polyp and Cancer Prevention,
Department of Gastroenterology,
The Cleveland Clinic Foundation, Cleveland,
OH 44195, USA

Caselitz, Jörg, M.D.
Professor of Medicine
Department of Pathology, Asklepios Klinik
Altona, Paul-Ehrlich-Str. 1, 22763 Hamburg,
Germany

Cave, David R., M.D., Ph.D.
Professor of Medicine
Clinical Gastroenterology Research, University
of Massachusetts Memorial Medical Center,
55 Lake Avenue North, Worcester, MA 01655, USA

Cheng, Michael W., M.D.
Division of Gastroenterology, Mount Sinai
Medical Center, 4300 Alton Road, Miami Beach,
FL 33140, USA

Costamagna, Guido, M.D.
Professor of Medicine
Digestive Endoscopy Unit, Catholic University,
Largo A. Gemelli 8, 00168 Rome, Italy

Costea, Florin, M.D.
GI Department, Montreal General Hospital,
1650 Cedar Avenue, Montreal, Quebec,
H3G 1A4, Canada

de' Angelis, Gian Luigi, M.D.
Professor of Medicine
University of Parma, Università degli Studi
di Parma, Via A. Gramsci 14, 43100 Parma, Italy

De Franchis, Roberto, M.D.
Professor of Medicine
Department of Internal Medicine, University
of Milan, IRCCS Ospedale Policlinico, Via Pace 9,
20122 Milano, Italy

Delvaux, Michel, M.D., Ph.D.
Professor of Medicine
Department of Internal Medicine and Digestive
Pathology, Centre Hospitalier Universitaire
de Nancy, Hôpitaux de Brabois, Allée de Morvan,
54511 Vandoeuvre Les Nancy, France

Dirks, Martha H., M.D., C.M., F.R.C.P.C.
Assistant Professor of Pediatrics,
University of Montreal
Division of Gastroenterology, Hepatology
and Nutrition, Hôpital Sainte-Justine,
3175 Chemin de la Côte Sainte-Catherine,
Montreal, Quebec, H2T 1C5, Canada

Dulai, Gareth S., M.D.
Associate Professor, David Geffen School
of Medicine, University of California
Gastroenterology, Kaiser Permanente,
9400 East Rosecrans Avenue, Bellflower,
CA 90706, USA

Eliakim, Rami, M.D.
Professor of Medicine, Bruce Rappaport
School of Medicine, Haifa
Department of Gastroenterology, Rambam
Medical Center, Bruce Rappaport School
of Medicine, Bar Galim, 31096 Haifa, Israel

Ell, Christian, M.D.
Professor of Medicine
Department of Internal Medicine II,
Dr. Horst-Schmidt Kliniken, Wiesbaden,
Ludwig-Erhard-Str. 100, 65199 Wiesbaden,
Germany

Fennerty, M. Brian, M.D.
Professor of Medicine and Section Chief
Division of Gastroenterology, Oregon Health
and Science University, 3181 SW Sam Jackson
Park Road, PV-310, Portland, OR 97201-3098,
USA

Fleischer, David E., M.D.
Professor of Medicine, Mayo Clinic College
of Medicine
Chair, Division of Gastroenterology and
Hepatology, Mayo Clinic Arizona,
13400 East Shea Boulevard, Scottsdale,
AZ 85259, USA

Fry, Lucia C., M.D.
Division of Gastroenterology, Hepatology
and Infectious Diseases,
Otto-von-Guericke University, Leipzigerstr. 44,
39120 Magdeburg, Germany

Gay, Gérard, M.D.
Professor of Medicine
Department of Internal Medicine and Digestive
Pathology , Centre Hospitalier Universitaire
de Nancy, Hôpitaux de Brabois, Allée de Morvan,
54511 Vandoeuvre Les Nancy, France

Hagenmüller, Friedrich, M.D.
Professor of Medicine
Medical Department I, Asklepios Klinik Altona,
Paul-Ehrlich-Str. 1, 22763 Hamburg, Germany

Hara, Amy K., M.D.
Assistant Professor of Medicine,
Mayo Clinic College of Medicine
Department of Diagnostic Radiology,
Mayo Clinic, 13400 East Shea Boulevard,
Scottsdale, AZ 85259, USA

Hartmann, Dirk, M.D.
Department of Gastroenterology,
Klinikum Ludwigshafen, Bremserstr. 79,
67063 Ludwigshafen, Germany

Iddan, Gavriel J., D.Sc.
44 A, Einstein Street Haifa, 34602, Israel

Jensen, Dennis M., M.D.
Professor of Medicine, David Geffen School
of Medicine, University of California
VA Greater Los Angeles Healthcare Center,
CURE, 11301 Wilshire Boulevard, Los Angeles,
CA 90073-1003, USA

Keuchel, Martin, M.D.
Medical Department I, Asklepios Klinik Altona,
Paul-Ehrlich-Str. 1, 22763 Hamburg, Germany

Kita, Hiroto, M.D.
Department of Gastroenterology, Jichi Medical
School, 3311-1 Yakushiji, Minamikawachi,
Kawachi, Tochigi, 329-0498, Japan

Korman, Louis Y., M.D.
Associate Clinical Professor of Medicine,
George Washington University School
of Medicine
Division of Gastroenterology, Department
of Veterans Affairs Medical Center,
50 Irving Street NW, Washington, DC 20422, USA

Kornbluth, Asher, M.D.
Associate Clinical Professor of Medicine,
Mount Sinai School of Medicine
The Henry D. Janowitz Division
of Gastroenterology, Mt. Sinai,
1751 York Avenue, New York, NY 10128, USA

Legnani, Peter E., M.D.
The Henry D. Janowitz Division
of Gastroenterology, Mt. Sinai,
1751 York Avenue, New York, NY 10128, USA

Leighton, Jonathan A., M.D.
Associate Professor of Medicine, Mayo Clinic
College of Medicin
Division of Gastroenterology and Hepatology,
Mayo Clinic, 13400 East Shea Boulevard,
Scottsdale, AZ 85259, USA

Lewis, Blair S., M.D.
Associate Clinical Professor of Medicine,
Mont Sinai School of Medicine
1067 Fifth Avenue, New York, NY 10128, USA

Maiden, Laurence, M.D., B.Sc., M.R.C.P.
King's College Hospital, Denmark Hill,
London SE5 9RS, UK

Malzfeldt, Ernst-Joachim, M.D.
Department of Diagnostic Radiology and
Nuclear Medicine, Asklepios Klinik Altona,
Paul-Ehrlich-Str. 1, 22763 Hamburg, Germany

Maunoury, Vincent, M.D., Ph.D.
Department of Gastroenterology,
Hôpital Claude Huriez, University Hospital,
59037 Lille Cedex, France

May, Andrea, M.D.
Professor of Medicine
Department of Internal Medicine II,
Dr. Horst-Schmidt Kliniken, Wiesbaden,
Ludwig-Erhard-Str. 100, 65199 Wiesbaden,
Germany

Murray, Joseph A., M.D.
Professor of Medicine, Mayo Clinic College
of Medicine
Division of Gastroenterology, Mayo Clinic,
200 1st Street SW, Rochester, MN 55905-0001,
USA

Pennazio, Marco, M.D.
Gastroenterology Unit 2, Department
of Gastroenterology and Clinical Nutrition,
San Giovanni A.S. Hospital, Via Cavour 31,
10123 Torino, Italy

Reddy, D. Nageshwar, M.D., D.M., F.A.M.S.,
F.R.C.P.
Asian Institute of Gastroenterology, 6-3-661,
Somajiguda, Hyderabad - 500 082, India

Riccioni, Maria Elena, M.D.
Digestive Endoscopy Unit, Catholic University,
Largo A. Gemelli 8, 00168 Rome, Italy

Riemann, Jürgen F., M.D.
Professor of Medicine
Department of Gastroenterology,
Klinikum Ludwigshafen, Bremserstr. 79,
67063 Ludwigshafen, Germany

Rösch, Thomas, M.D.
Professor of Medicine
Medical Clinic – Hepatology and
Gastroenterology, Charité Campus
Virchow-Klinikum, Augustenburger Platz 1,
13353 Berlin, Germany

Sachdev, Ritu, M.D.
Division of Gastroenterology,
Caritas St. Elizabeth's Medical Center,
736 Cambridge Streem Boston, MA 02135, USA

Sant'Anna, Ana Maria Guilhon de Araújo, M.D.
Assistant Professor of Pediatrics
Division of Pediatric Gastroenterology,
McMaster University, 1200 Main Street W,
Hamilton, Ontario, L8N 3Z5, Canada

Schmiegel, Wolff, M.D.
Professor of Medicine
Department of Medicine, Knappschafts-
krankenhaus, Ruhr-University Bochum,
In der Schornau 23–25, 44892 Bochum,
Germany

Schulmann, Karsten, M.D.
Department of Medicine, Knappschaftskranken-
haus, Ruhr-University Bochum,
In der Schornau 23–25, 44892 Bochum, Germany

Schulz, Hans-Joachim, M.D.
Professor of Medicine
Clinic for Internal Medicine I, Paritätisches
Krankenhaus Lichtenberg, Fanningerstr. 32,
10365 Berlin, Germany

Schuppan, Detlef, M.D., Ph.D.
Professor of Medicine
Division of Gastroenterology, Beth Israel
Deaconess Medical Center, Harvard University,
330 Brookline Avenue, Boston, MA 02215, USA

Seidman, Ernest G., M.D.
Professor of Medicine, University of Montreal
Division of Gastroenterology, McGill University
Health Centre, 1650 Cedar Avenue, Montreal,
Quebec, H3G 1A4, Canada

Selby, Warwick A., M.D.
Clinical Associate Professor of Medicine,
University of Sydney
AW Morrow Gastroenterology and Liver Centre,
Royal Prince Alfred Hospital, Camperdown,
NSW 2050, Sydney, Australia

Sharma, Virender K., M.D.
Associate Professor of Medicine,
Mayo Clinic College of Medicine
Esophageal Clinic, Mayo Clinic, 13400 East Shea
Boulevard, Scottsdale, AZ 85259, USA

Soares, Jose, M.D.
Hospital General de Santo Antonio, Largo da
Escola Medica, 4099-001 Porto, Portugal

Swain, C. Paul, M.D.
Professor of Medicine
Department of Surgical Oncology
and Technology, Imperial College and
St Mary's Hospital, 41 Willow Road,
London NW3 1TN, UK

Teichmann, Wolfgang, M.D.
Professor of Medicine
Surgical Department I, Asklepios Klinik Altona,
Paul-Ehrlich-Str. 1, 22763 Hamburg, Germany

Thomson, Mike, M.D.
Centre for Pediatric Gastroenterology,
Sheffield Children's Hospital, Western Bank,
Sheffield S10 2TH, UK

Tóth, Ervin, M.D., Ph.D.
Professor of Medicine
Department of Medicine, Malmö University
Hospital, 20502 Malmö, Sweden

Van Gossum, André, M.D.
Professor of Medicine
Department of Gastroenterology and
Hepatopancreatology, Hôpital Erasme,
Université Libre de Bruxelles,
Route de Lennik 808, 1070 Brussels, Belgium

Voderholzer, Winfried, M.D.
Department of Hepatology and
Gastroenterology, Charité Hospital,
Campus Mitte, Schumannstr. 20/21,
10117 Berlin, Germany

von Herbay, Axel, M.D.
Professor of Medicine
Gastrointestinal Pathology, St Mark´s Hospital,
Northwick Park, Watford Road, Harrow,
HA1 3UJ, UK

Wegener, Otto-Henning, M.D.
Professor of Medicine
Department of Diagnostic Radiology and
Nuclear Medicine, Asklepios Klinik Altona,
Paul-Ehrlich-Str. 1, 22763 Hamburg, Germany

Yamamoto, Hironori, M.D., Ph.D.
Professor of Medicine
Department of Gastroenterology, Jichi Medical
University, 3311-1 Yakushiji, Shimotsuke,
Tochigi, 329-0498, Japan

Abbreviations

aGI GVHD	Acute gastrointestinal graft-versus-host disease
AIDS	Acquired immunodeficiency syndrome
Allo-SCT	Allogeneic stem cell transplantation
ANCA	Antineutrophil cytoplasmic antibodies
5-ASA	5-Aminosalicylic acid
ASCA	Anti-*Saccharomyces cerevisiae* antibodies
CARD15	Caspase recruitment domain 15
CCD	Charge-coupled device
CD	Crohn's disease
CD4	Cluster of differentiation 4 (T-helper lymphocytes)
CD8	Cluster of differentiation 8 (T suppressor lymphocytes)
CD 34	Cluster of differentiation 34 (vascular marker)
CD117	Cluster of differentiation 117 (c-kit)
CE	Capsule endoscope
CE Mark	European Conformity (Communauté Européene)
CEST	Capsule Endoscopy Structured Terminology
CMOS	Complementary metal oxide semiconductor
CMV	Cytomegalovirus
CNS	Central nervous system
COL	Colonoscopy
COX	Cyclooxygenases
CREST	Calcinosis, Raynaud's phenomenon, esophageal dysfunction, sclerodactyly, telangiectasia
CRP	C-reactive protein
CT	Computed tomography
CTE	Computed tomography enterography/enteroclysis
CVID	Common variable immunodeficiency syndrome
EATL	Enteropathy-associated T-cell lymphoma
EBV	Epstein-Barr virus
ECG	Electrocardiogram
EDP	Electronic data processing
EGD	Esophagogastroduodenoscopy
EMA	Endomysial antibodies
EMR	Endoscopic mucosal resection
ENT	Ear, nose, and throat
ESR	Erythrocyte sedimentation rate
FAP	Familial adenomatous polyposis
FDA	Food and Drug Administration
Fe	Iron
FJP	Familial juvenile polyposis
GAVE	Gastric antral vascular ectasia
GI	Gastrointestinal
GIST	Gastrointestinal stromal tumor
GVHD	Graft-versus-host disease
H&E	Hematoxylin and eosin stain
HHT	Hereditary hemorrhagic telangiectasia
HIV	Human immunodeficiency virus
HLA	Human leukocyte antigen
HNPCC	Hereditary nonpolyposis colon cancer
IBD	Inflammatory bowel disease
IBS	Irritable bowel syndrome
ICCE	International Conference on Capsule Endoscopy
ICU	Intensive care unit
IgA	Immunoglobulin A
IgE	Immunoglobulin E
IgM	Immunoglobulin M
IL-5	Interleukin 5
IOE	Intraoperative enteroscopy
IPSID	Immunoproliferative disease of the small intestine
JPL	Jet Propulsion Laboratory
JPS	Juvenile polyposis syndrome
LDL	Low-density lipoproteins
LED	Light-emitting diode
MAI	*Mycobacterium avium intracellulare*
MALT	Mucosa-associated lymphatic tissue
MHz	Megahertz
6-MP	6-Mercaptopurine
MRCP	Magnetic resonance cholangiopancreatography
MRE	Magnet resonance enterography/enteroclysis
MRI	Magnetic resonance imaging
MST	Minimal Standard Terminology
NK	Natural killer cells
NOD2	Nucleotide oligodimerization domain 2
NPV	Negative predictive value
NSAIDs	Nonsteroidal anti-inflammatory drugs
OGIB	Obscure gastrointestinal bleeding
OMED	Organisation Mondiale d'Endoscopie Digestive
PAS	Periodic acid–Schiff
PCR	Polymerase chain reaction
PE	Push enteroscopy
PEG	Polyethylene glycol
PJS	Peutz-Jeghers syndrome
PPV	Positive predictive value
SB	Small bowel
SBFT	Small bowel follow through
SBI	Suspected Blood Indicator
SD	Standard deviation
SI	Small intestine
Si	Silicon
SLE	Systemic lupus erythematosus
Tc	Technetium
Th2	T-helper 2 cells
TNF	Tumor necrosis factor
tTG	Tissue transglutaminase
USB	Universal serial bus
VCE	Video capsule endoscopy
VCR	Videocassette recorder
VIP	Vasoactive intestinal peptide
VLDL	Very low-density lipoproteins
WG	Wegener's granulomatosis

Video Capsule Endoscopy

1

1.1 A Short History of the Gastrointestinal Capsule

G.J. Iddan

The origin of the work on the capsule can be traced back to the year1981. I was at that time on a sabbatical leave from my work as an electro-optical engineer at Rafael (government defense lab) working during that sabbatical for a medical instrument company in Boston (USA). A gastroenterologist friend (Prof. Eitan Scapa) explained to me some of the shortcomings of the fiber bundle endoscope, emphasizing the inability to view the small intestine and its rigidity. At that time I did not have any clue as to how to solve these intriguing and interesting problems.

In the meantime small CCD (charge-coupled device) imagers had been developed and made available mainly in Japan for use in handheld video cameras. The endoscope manufacturers were quick to incorporate them into the endoscope, thus replacing the fiber bundle that was used for image transmission and making the device much more flexible.

Viewing the small intestine remained however without a satisfactory solution.

The gastroenterologist friend of mine kept querying me about ways to solve the problem all along, and while I was on another sabbatical in1991 I started to think about the possibility of separating the CCD head of the endoscope leaving it connected to the endoscope via an umbilical cable. It was explained to me that this would be impossible since the required cable length of about 5 m would be too long to safely pull it out and the process might last a few hours during which the endoscope would have to stay inside the patient.

My intuitive response at that point was: why not cut the CCD head from the endoscope and attach a mini-transmitter to the head, thus letting the »head« move free of any physical connection.

At that point the chance of solving the riddle seemed more realistic and in 1992 I started spending more time on the new idea. I realized however that the task I was facing was very far from having a solution.

Consultation with a CCD expert was very discouraging since simple calculations indicated that a CCD camera head would only be able to operate for about 10 min on miniature batteries.

A list of the problems facing the design included:

- Shortage of energy for the CCD, illumination and transmission
- Contamination of the optical window in the intestine
- Long hours of viewing time for the doctor

In addition it was explained to me that there are not too many pathologies to be found in the small intestine and hence such a device would have only limited demand.

I decided to continue my interest in the problem since it seemed very interesting and challenging – I was sure that the miniaturization would be solved in due time – and decided to focus on the three major problems that were mentioned.

First I figured that to avoid window contamination and obscuration, the optics would have to be designed in a way that would guarantee constant rubbing of the tissue on an ogive-shaped window to facilitate contact imaging and ensure self-wiping of the transparent window. A talented optical designer came up with a fine solution and a prototype was built (1993) shown in ◻ Fig. 1.1-1; a ¼″ conventional CCD was used

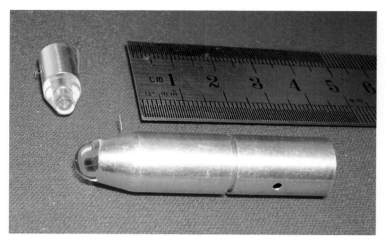

◻ **Fig. 1.1-1.** Early **noningestible** wired devices with a ¼″ CCD used for testing the optics and the illumination

to test the optics and the results were good. Encouraged, the next problem of long viewing hours was solved by separating the system into three components: ***capsule*** containing imager and transmitter, ***recorder*** containing antenna array receiver and recording medium, and ***workstation*** incorporating reader, processing software, and monitor. Simultaneously we performed experiments to find the proper wavelength and power level required for wireless transmission of video via biological tissue; the experiments were done on a defrosted chicken bought in a nearby supermarket. It seemed that we were on the right track but for one major obstacle—power required by the CCD.

While casually reading one of the photonics magazines I came upon an article written by Eric Fossum, a scientist from Jet Propulsion Laboratory (JPL), describing a new type of imager active pixel sensor (APS) that can be integrated on a single Si chip, but even more interesting it claimed to consume only 1% of the power required by an equivalent CCD imager. This was exactly what I was hoping for and light appeared at the end of the tunnel.

At this point the decision was made to apply for a patent which was submitted on 17 January 1994.

It was now the time (1994) to search for investment funds and start full-time work on the project; in reality we were facing difficulties in finding support since investors considered it »science fiction, an Asimov-type adventure.« During my search for investment I came in 1995 upon a small company making miniature CCD cameras for medical applications and tried to interest its manager in the new video pill; the manager, Mr. Gavriel Meron, became excited and tried to raise money from his board but was refused.

At the same time I succeeded in getting some funds for the establishment of a new start-up in the area of 3D imaging from a new investment body, RDC Ltd. It was an indication that the high-tech market was on the rise. While working at 3DV on the imaging start-up we were awarded in 1997 the first patent on a video capsule: USP 5,604,531 »in vivo camera system.« The patent approval triggered action by RDC and Mr. Meron joined RDC and incorporated a new start-up, Given Imaging Ltd. I served simultaneously as a VP at the 3D imaging start-up and as a consultant at Given Imaging. With initial funds available, expert workers were hired and capsule development went on at full steam. Mr. Meron was able to attract more investors in Israel and abroad.

It was during a Gastro Conference in 1997 that Mr. Meron first met Prof. Paul Swain from London and they were both surprised to find that they were working independently on related subjects. Professor Swain

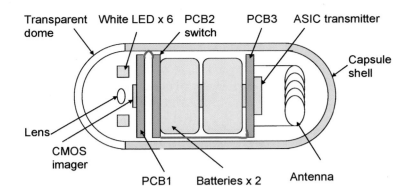

Transparent dome · White LED x 6 · PCB2 switch · PCB3 · ASIC transmitter · Capsule shell · Lens · CMOS imager · PCB1 · Batteries x 2 · Antenna

Fig. 1.1-2. A schematic view of the capsule and its components

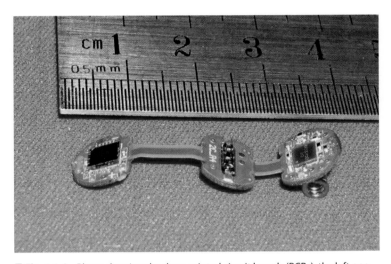

Fig. 1.1-3. Photo showing the three printed circuit boards (PCBs): the left one holds the CMOS imager, the central one holds the reed switch, and the right one holds the application-specific integrated circuit (ASIC) transmitter on the top and the antenna on the bottom

and his team were aiming at a wireless gastric camera. An agreement of cooperation resulted and Professor Swain joined the Given team and contributed extensively to the development and to the animal and clinical experiments. Professor Swain described his group's efforts in the historical review published in our article in *Gastrointestinal Endoscopy Clinics of North America* (Iddan and Swain 2004).

Work progressed rapidly under the supervision of Dr. Arkady Glukhovsky who was at that time the research and development manager. A CMOS (complementary metal oxide semiconductor) camera chip was designed by Eric Fossum to specifications written by Mr. Dov Avni, our video expert, and it was manufactured at Tower Semiconductors (Figs. 1.1-2 and 1.1-3). In October 1999 at the private clinic of Prof. E. Scapa near Tel Aviv, the first real capsule was swallowed by Professor Swain who insisted on being the first person to swallow the capsule and after some initial difficulties clear images were received. A bottle of wine was opened and the video capsule turned into reality.

As a result of our initial success more funds become available and work accelerated resulting in May 2000 in an article published in *Nature* (Iddan et al. 2000) describing the new capsule. Experiments on consenting patients started in Israel, Europe, and the United States of America with encouraging results. Given was now ready for initial public offering (IPO) on the NASDAQ stock market in August 2001, but then the Twin Towers were hit and all action came to a halt. A couple of weeks later, Given was issued to the public as the first issue after the tower disaster. I personally continued working toward new capsules that would be capable of imaging the stomach and the colon.

Given Imaging has by now opened subsidiaries in North America, Europe, and the Far East and sells about 10 thousand capsules per month. Letters of gratitude from doctors and patients who were helped by the capsule are often received at the company's headquarters.

Internet

www.givenimaging.com: Given Imaging Ltd. Yoqneam, Israel

References

Iddan G, Meron G, Glukhovsky A, Swain P (2000) Wireless capsule endoscopy. Nature 405:417

Iddan GJ, Swain CP (2004) History and development of capsule endoscopy. Gastrointest Endosc Clin N Am 14:1–9

1.2   Fields of Application

F. Hagenmüller, M. Keuchel, D.E. Fleischer

The list of potential applications for VCE of the small intestine increases steadily. Some have been established in several prospective studies, some are based on small series, retrospective analyses or case reports, and others are only suggested according to theoretical considerations. Guidelines on the indication for VCE vary in restrictiveness (Rey et al. 2004; Rösch and Ell 2004). In this chapter, »fields of application« are discussed rather than »indications« as the term is frequently associated with issues of reimbursement. Regulations governing reimbursement have been implemented worldwide, but still vary from country to country.

Obscure Gastrointestinal Bleeding

Obscure gastrointestinal (GI) bleeding was the first application of VCE and is still the most important indication. The most frequent findings in patients with obscure GI bleeding are angiectasias, ulcers, tumors, and diverticula. However, almost every disease leading to morphologic alteration of the small intestine may cause bleeding (◻ Fig. 1.2-1).

Several prospective studies have documented the efficacy of VCE in identifying a source of previously unexplained bleeding in the small intestine. These studies found a higher diagnostic yield with VCE than with push enteroscopy (Chap. 12).

In a meta-analysis by Triester et al. (2005) including 14 prospective studies, VCE had a diagnostic yield of 66% compared with 34% for push enteroscopy (p<0.0001, 375 patients). When comparing VCE with radiologic tests, the diagnostic yield was 68% for VCE vs only 8% for radiology (p<0.001, 88 patients).

Analysis of details, however, did not result in such coherent findings. Observations from the Italian multicenter study show a diagnostic yield for VCE of 92% in persisting overt obscure bleeding and 44% in occult bleeding. However, in patients with a history of previous overt bleeding, the diagnostic yield was only 13% (Pennazio et al. 2004). Selby (2004) found a similar diagnostic yield for Australian patients with occult vs overt bleeding and in patients undergoing single or multiple upper and lower endoscopies prior to VCE. Both studies suggest that VCE should be used early in the work-up of obscure gastrointestinal bleeding after

negative upper and lower GI endoscopy. Nevertheless, a substantial amount of relevant gastric or colonic findings by VCE (Kitiyakara and Selby 2005) may lead to repeat upper and lower GI endoscopy prior to VCE in referral centers (Rösch and Ell, 2004).

Whereas the French multicenter trial documented a negative predictive value of 100% for a normal VCE study (Delvaux et al. 2004), groups from Israel (Bar-Meir et al. 2004) and from the United States (Jones et al. 2005) found lesions at a repeated VCE in a significant percentage of patients with an initially normal examination.

The role of VCE for the investigation of iron deficiency anemia with no clinical bleeding is being studied.

Crohn's Disease

Studies on VCE in patients with suspected Crohn's disease are less homogeneous than the studies on obscure bleeding. However, VCE is clearly superior in detecting mucosal lesions (◻ Fig. 1.2-2) compared to radiological tests (Chap. 6.1 and Chap. 12). A meta-analysis (Triester et al. 2006) found a diagnostic yield for lesions typical for Crohn's disease for VCE of 62% vs 27% for small bowel radiography (10 studies, 226 patients, p<0.0001) and of 73% for VCE vs 41% for CT enterography (3 studies, 70 patients, p<0.0001).

The application of VCE in patients with clinically suspected Crohn's disease but a negative conventional imaging examination is now widely accepted. Suggestions from the International Conference on Capsule Endoscopy (ICCE) consensus panel (Kornbluth et al. 2005) were to use the presence of two or more of the following symptoms or signs to define the clinical suspicion of Crohn's disease in future studies: abdominal pain or diarrhea; iron deficiency anemia; elevated erythrocyte sedimentation rate (ESR) or C-reactive protein (CRP); hypoalbuminemia; extraintestinal manifestations; family history of IBD; abnormal serologies. Validation of this approach is pending.

Also in patients with established Crohn's disease, VCE had a higher detection rate for mucosal lesions than CT enteroclysis. However, 27% of the patients had to be excluded from VCE because of stenosis seen at CT enteroclysis (Voderholzer et al. 2005).

VCE can be of potential value in the evaluation of indeterminate colitis (diagnosis changed to probable Crohn's disease in 12 of 22 patients with isolated colitis; Mow et al. 2004).

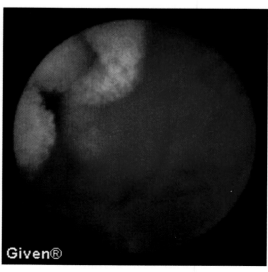

◻ **Fig. 1.2-1.** Active bleeding in the jejunum

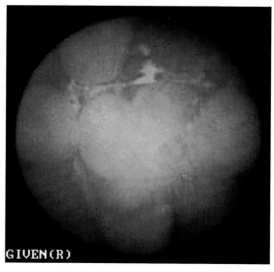

◻ **Fig. 1.2-2.** Crohn's disease

Complicated Celiac Sprue

Patients with long-standing celiac disease have an increased risk of complications, mainly erosions with bleeding and iron deficiency anemia, intussusception but also carcinoma and lymphoma. The US study by Culliford et al. (2005) and the European multicenter study (Krauss et al. 2005) have demonstrated persisting typical mucosal changes in most patients with complicated celiac disease. Additionally, a high percentage of patients with recurring complaints in spite of a gluten-free diet had unexpected findings (■ Fig. 1.2-3). These findings were mainly erosions, but also single cases of malignant tumor. Thus, surveillance by VCE of symptomatic patients adhering to a gluten-free diet to exclude complications is an increasingly accepted indication.

VCE findings in celiac sprue have shown a good correlation with histology in a small number of patients (Petroniene et al. 2005). At present, antibody tests and duodenoscopy with histology are still considered the gold standard for the diagnosis of suspected celiac sprue. A consensus panel (Cellier et al. 2005) has proposed seropositive (endomysial or anti-tissue transglutaminase antibodies) patients either unwilling or unable to undergo upper GI endoscopy as well as seropositive patients with negative histology as possible candidates for VCE. However, this approach will have to be substantiated by prospective studies.

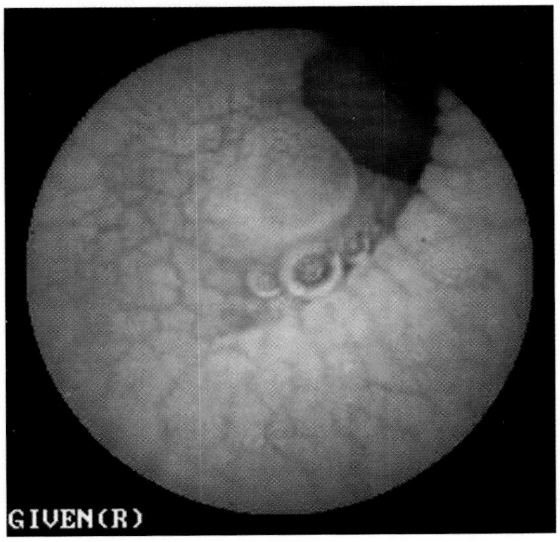

Polyposis Syndromes

Patients with **Peutz-Jeghers syndrome (PJS)** have a high prevalence of small intestinal polyps. In the past, many of them have undergone laparotomy for obstruction caused by large polyps. Video capsule endoscopy has been shown to be efficient in detecting small intestinal polyps too (■ Fig. 1.2-4) (Schulmann et al. 2005; Soares et al. 2004; Caspari et al. 2004). This has led to the suggestion of VCE as a first-line test for surveillance in PJS (Schulmann and Schmiegel 2004) (Chap. 7.3)

In **familial adenomatous polyposis (FAP)**, duodenal adenomas are frequently encountered. They may progress to duodenal cancer, which is the most frequent cause of death in patients with FAP, who have undergone colectomy. VCE can detect additional jejunal or ileal polyps in 76% of patients with duodenal adenomas (Schulmann et al. 2005). Especially in patients with stage III and IV duodenal adenomas, jejunal and ileal polyps could be recognized (Burke et al. 2005). However, in the absence of duodenal adenomas, polyps in the jejunum or ileum were found only in single cases (Mata et al. 2005; Schulmann et al. 2005). The clinical relevance of these findings has yet to be demonstrated.

Data on patients with **hereditary nonpolyposis colonic cancer (HNPCC)** and **juvenile polyposis syndrome (JPS)** are too sparse for recommendations, although in single cases VCE might be valuable.

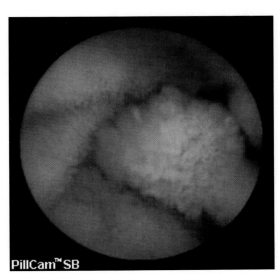

GIVEN(R)

■ **Fig. 1.2-3.** Long-standing celiac disease with polypoid lesion in the jejunum in a patient with new complaints

PillCam™SB

■ **Fig. 1.2-4.** One of multiple jejunal and ileal polyps in a patient with Peutz-Jeghers syndrome

Monitoring of Treatment

In special situations, VCE has been helpful in guiding therapy such as in **intestinal transplantation** (de Franchis et al. 2003; Chap. 9) and **acute gastrointestinal graft-versus-host reaction** after stem cell transplantation (Yakoub-Agha et al. 2004; Shapira et al. 2005; Chap. 6.7). The search for intestinal lesions caused by **radiation** therapy (◘ Fig. 1.2-5), however, is jeopardized by the risk of capsule retention (Lee et al. 2004).

Although small intestinal lesions caused by **nonsteroidal anti-inflammatory drugs (NSAIDs)** are detected frequently by VCE (Graham et al. 2005; Goldstein et al. 2005; Maiden et al. 2005; Chap. 6.6), the clinical relevance has not been studied as these lesions were asymptomatic and a potential complication such as obscure bleeding would be an indication by itself.

A consensus suggested VCE may have a unique role in assessing mucosal healing after medical therapy of **Crohn's disease** and for early postoperative recurrence to guide therapy (Kornbluth et al. 2005), although studies are pending.

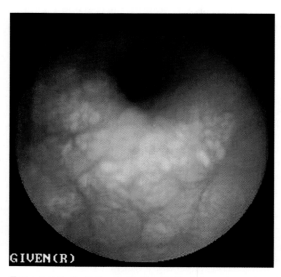

◘ **Fig. 1.2-5.** Radiation enteritis with ileal stenosis causing delayed passage of the capsule

Suspected Stenosis

Suspected intestinal stenoses are in general a contraindication for VCE, because a stenosis may lead to impaction of the capsule, probably requiring surgery. However, in patients with symptomatic stenosis, capsule endoscopy may provide a diagnosis leading to adequate endoscopic or surgical therapy (◘ Fig. 1.2-7). Preliminary data showed a diagnostic yield of 32% in patients with suspected stenosis but a retention rate of 16% (Cheifetz et al. 2004). Thus, VCE in patients with suspected stenosis can be justified if the patient is willing and fit to undergo surgery.

Tumor

The clinical presentation of small intestinal tumors is mainly bleeding (Schwartz and Barkin 2004), which is an indication for VCE by itself. However, in single cases the suspicion of a tumor may arise from abnormal radiological findings or the presence of hepatic metastases, especially in neuroendocrine tumors (Keuchel et al. 2004; Chap. 7.2).

In 25% of patients with gastric lymphoma, lesions in the small intestine were seen at VCE, partially confirmed by biopsy to be manifestations of lymphoma (Flieger et al. 2005). Gastric lymphoma may cause retention of the capsule endoscope due to impaired motility (◘ Fig. 1.2-6). The clinical impact of detecting additional intestinal lesions in these patients has to be documented in future.

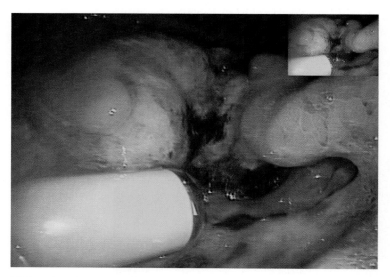

◘ **Fig. 1.2-6.** Gastric NK cell lymphoma. Capsule was temporarily retained at the ulcerated lymphoma. After endoscopic placement into the small intestine, uneventful passage occurred

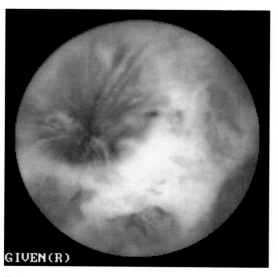

◘ **Fig. 1.2-7.** Symptomatic stenosis. Based on the VCE finding, surgery was performed, showing an ulcerated jejunal segment, most likely of ischemic origin

◧ **Table 1.2-1.** Established and potential fields of application for VCE

- Obscure, occult, or overt gastrointestinal bleeding with negative results on upper and lower gastrointestinal endoscopy
- Unexplained iron deficiency anemia
- Suspicion of small intestinal Crohn's disease after negative conventional diagnostic tests
- Staging and surveillance of patients with polyposis syndromes
- Refractory sprue or the recurrence of symptoms in patients previously treated for sprue
- Suspected tumor of the small bowel
- Selected cases of malabsorption after inconclusive prior studies
- Differentiation of indeterminate colitis
- Diagnosis of suspected symptomatic intestinal stenosis prior to surgery
- Monitoring and guidance of therapy in
  - Acute gastrointestinal graft-versus-host disease
  - Complications of NSAID medication
  - Intestinal transplantation
  - Early aggressive therapy of Crohn's disease
  - Assessing early postsurgical recurrence of Crohn's disease

Future Fields of Application of VCE in the Small Intestine

Future research might focus on diagnosis of intestinal manifestation in systemic diseases such as acquired or hereditary immunodeficiency syndromes, vasculitis, collagenosis, amyloidosis, hypobetalipoproteinemia, hereditary hemorrhagic teleangiectasias; studies on motility disorders; certain cases of malabsorption, monitoring of aggressive therapy of early Crohn's disease with biologicals or surveillance of patients with malignant melanoma for intestinal metastasis.

Application of VCE in Organs Other Than the Small Intestine

Esophageal VCE has been approved by the Food and Drug Administration (FDA) for diagnosis, screening and surveillance of esophageal diseases. Details are presented in Chap. 13. Capsules for the colon are undergoing clinical testing and capsules for the stomach have been designed.

References

Bar-Meir S, Eliakim R, Nadler M et al (2004) Second capsule endoscopy for patients with severe iron deficiency anemia. Gastrointest Endosc 60:711–713

Burke CA, Santisi J, Church J, Levinthal G (2005) The utility of capsule endoscopy small bowel surveillance in patients with polyposis. Am J Gastroenterol 100:1498–1502

Caspari R, von Falkenhausen M, Krautmacher C et al (2004) Comparison of capsule endoscopy and magnetic resonance imaging for the detection of polyps of the small intestine in patients with familial adenomatous polyposis or with Peutz-Jeghers' syndrome. Endoscopy 36:1054–1059

Cellier C, Green PH, Collin P, Murray J (2005) ICCE consensus for celiac disease. Endoscopy 37:1055–1059

Cheifetz AS, Sachar DB, Lewis BS (2004) Small bowel obstruction – indication or contraindication for capsule endoscopy. Gastrointest Endosc 59:AB102

Culliford A, Daly J, Diamond B et al (2005) The value of wireless capsule endoscopy in patients with complicated celiac disease. Gastrointest Endosc 62:55–61

Delvaux M, Fassler I, Gay G (2004) Clinical usefulness of the endoscopic video capsule as the initial intestinal investigation in patients with obscure digestive bleeding: validation of a diagnostic strategy based on the patient outcome after 12 months. Endoscopy 36:1067–1073

de Franchis R, Rondonotti E, Abbiati C et al (2003) Capsule enteroscopy in small bowel transplantation. Dig Liver Dis 35:728–731

Flieger D, Keller R, May A, Ell C, Fischbach W (2005) Capsule endoscopy in gastrointestinal lymphomas. Endoscopy 37:1174–1180

Graham DY, Opekun AR, Willingham FF, Qureshi WA (2005) Visible small-intestinal mucosal injury in chronic NSAID users. Clin Gastroenterol Hepatol 3:55–59

Goldstein JL, Eisen GM, Lewis B et al (2005) Video capsule endoscopy to prospectively assess small bowel injury with celecoxib, naproxen plus omeprazole, and placebo. Clin Gastroenterol Hepatol 3:133–141

Jones BH, Fleischer DE, Sharma VK (2005) Yield of repeat wireless video capsule endoscopy in patients with obscure gastrointestinal bleeding. Am J Gastroenterol 100:1058–1064

Keuchel M, Thaler C, Caselitz J, Hagenmüller F (2004) Diagnosis of small bowel tumors with video capsule endoscopy: report of 16 cases. Gastroenterology 126 [Suppl 2]: A347

Kornbluth A, Colombel JF, Leighton JA, Loftus E (2005) ICCE consensus for inflammatory bowel disease. Endoscopy 37:1051–1054

Krauss N, Cellier C, Collin P et al (2005) Evaluation of capsule endoscopy in celiac disease patients with ongoing symptoms on a gluten-free diet – a prospective, blinded European multicenter trial. Gastroenterology 128 [Suppl 2]:A-81

Kitiyakara T, Selby W (2005) Non-small-bowel lesions detected by capsule endoscopy in patients with obscure GI bleeding. Gastrointest Endosc 62:234–238

Lee DW, Poon AO, Chan AC (2004) Diagnosis of small bowel radiation enteritis by capsule endoscopy. Hong Kong Med J 10:419–421

Maiden L, Thjodleifsson B, Theodors A et al (2005) A quantitative analysis of NSAID-induced small bowel pathology by capsule enteroscopy. Gastroenterology 128:1172–1178

Mata A, Bordas JM, Feu F et al (2004) Wireless capsule endoscopy in patients with obscure gastrointestinal bleeding: a comparative study with push enteroscopy. Aliment Pharmacol Ther 20:189–194

Mata A, Llach J, Castells A et al (2005) A prospective trial comparing wireless capsule endoscopy and barium contrast series for small-bowel surveillance in hereditary GI polyposis syndromes. Gastrointest Endosc 61:721–725

Mow WS, Lo SK, Targan SR et al (2004) Initial experience with wireless capsule enteroscopy in the diagnosis and management of inflammatory bowel disease. Clin Gastroenterol Hepatol 2:31–40

Pennazio M, Santucci R, Rondonotti E et al (2004) Outcome of patients with obscure gastrointestinal bleeding after capsule endoscopy: report of 100 consecutive cases. Gastroenterology 126:643–653

Petroniene R, Dubcenco E, Baker JP (2005) Given capsule endoscopy in celiac disease: evaluation of diagnostic accuracy and interobserver agreement. Am J Gastroenterol 100:685–694

Rey JF, Gay G, Kruse A, Lambert R (2004) European Society of Gastrointestinal Endoscopy guideline for video capsule endoscopy. Endoscopy 36:656–658

Rösch T, Ell C (2004) Position paper on capsule endoscopy for the diagnosis of small bowel disorder. Z Gastroenterol 42:247–259

Schulmann K, Hollerbach S, Kraus K et al (2005) Feasibility and diagnostic utility of video capsule endoscopy for the detection of small bowel polyps in patients with hereditary polyposis syndromes. Am J Gastroenterol 100:27–37

Schulmann K, Schmiegel W (2004) Capsule endoscopy for small bowel surveillance in hereditary intestinal polyposis and non-polyposis syndromes. Gastrointest Endosc Clin N Am 14:149–158

Schwartz GD, Barkin JS (2004) Small bowel tumors detected by M2A capsule endoscopy. Am J Gastroenterol 99 [Suppl]:abstract 532

Selby W (2004) Can clinical features predict the likelihood of finding abnormalities when using capsule endoscopy in patients with GI bleeding of obscure origin? Gastrointest Endosc 59:782–787

Shapira MY, Adler SN, Jacob H (2005) New insights into the pathophysiology of gastrointestinal graft-versus-host disease using capsule endoscopy. Haematologica 90:1003–1004

Soares J, Lopes L, Vilas BG, Pinho C (2004) Wireless capsule endoscopy for evaluation of phenotypic expression of small-bowel polyps in patients with Peutz-Jeghers syndrome and in symptomatic first-degree relatives. Endoscopy 36:1060–1066

Triester SL, Leighton JA, Leontiadis GI et al (2005) A meta-analysis of the yield of capsule endoscopy compared to other diagnostic modalities in patients with obscure gastrointestinal bleeding. Am J Gastroenterol 100:2407–2418

Triester SL Leighton JA Leontiadis GI et al (2006) A meta-analysis of the yield of capsule endoscopy (CE) compared to other diagnostic modalities in patients with non-stricturing small bowel Crohn's disease. Am J Gastroenterol (in press)

Voderholzer W, Beinhoelzl J, Rogalla P et al (2005) Small bowel involvement in Crohn's disease. A prospective comparison of wireless capsule endoscopy and CT enteroclysis. Gut 54: 385–387

Yakoub-Agha I, Maunoury V, Wacrenier S (2004) Impact of small bowel exploration using video-capsule endoscopy in the management of acute gastrointestinal graft-versus-host disease. Transplantation 78:1697–1701

1.3   Procedure and Evaluation

1.3.1   Procedure

R. De Franchis

Technology

When the video capsule (◘ Fig. 1.3.1-1) is activated, it emits a strobe light from six light-emitting diodes (LEDs) at the rate of two flashes per second. Meanwhile, the image that reaches the CMOS chip camera (complementary metal oxide semiconductor with 256×256 pixels) through the optical dome window and lens is delivered by an application-specific integrated circuit (ASIC) to a radio transmitter (433 MHz), which transmits the images to an antenna array. The capsule itself does not store any data and is disposable. It is powered by two silver oxide batteries. The manufacturer has assigned the new name PillCam SB to the formerly called M2A/M2A plus video capsule endoscope.

> **Technical specifications of the PillCam SB video capsule (Given Imaging):**
>
> - Height 11 mm, width 27 mm, weight 3.7 g
> - Field of view 140°, magnification 1:8, resolution 0.1 mm
> - Nominal capsule operating time: 8 h
> - Total number of images: approximately 50,000–60,000

Informed Consent

The patient is informed about the preparations, conduct, contraindications, and risks associated with the procedure (Barkin and O'Loughlin 2004). A printed information sheet should be provided in addition to verbal counseling.

> **Contraindications to VCE:**
>
> - Strictures in the gastrointestinal tract
> - Pregnancy
> - Electromedical implants
> - Dysphagia
> - Planned magnetic resonance imaging
> - No therapeutic implications

Special situations such as swallowing disorders, pediatric patients, emergency procedures, patients with implanted pacemakers, or obesity are dealt with in Chap. 1.4.

Strictures in the gastrointestinal tract are the most important contraindication, but they are also the most difficult lesions to diagnose in preliminary tests. The principal risk factors are Crohn's disease, adhesions, prior extensive abdominal surgery, and prior abdominopelvic irradiation (Chap. 10). In these patients, consideration might be given to performing the Patency Capsule test (Chap. 1.5) before VCE.

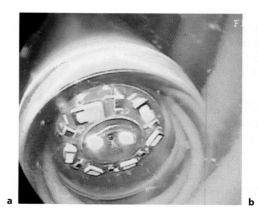
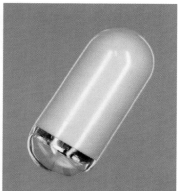
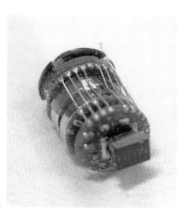

◘ **Fig. 1.3.1-1a–c.** Video capsule. **a** Endoscopic view of the video capsule in the small bowel, showing the optical window, the lens with holder, and six LEDs (white light-emitting diodes). **b** Side view of the capsule. **c** Contents of the video capsule: chip camera (*above*), batteries (*center*), and transmitter with antenna (*below*)

a   b   c

Capsule Endoscopy Procedure

Possible indications for VCE are discussed in Chap. 1.2.

The procedure for a VCE examination of the small intestine is outlined in ▣ Table 1.3.1-1 and illustrated in ▣ Figs. 1.3.1-2–1.3.1-13.

▣ **Table 1.3.1-1.** The capsule endoscopy procedure

Day before the examination	– Secure informed consent, review the indication, charge batteries for the data recorder – Evening: patient drinks 2 l of PEG solution at one time (optional)
Day of the examination	– Patient fasts after midnight – Early morning: 1 l of PEG solution (optional) – Enter the patient data into the PC and initialize the recorder – Affix the leads, and strap on the belt with recorder and battery pack – Administer a prokinetic agent (optional) – Administer simethicone (optional) – Patient swallows the capsule with a glass of water – One hour later, check the capsule position (optional; reached the small bowel?) – Patient may leave the office or hospital – Drinking is allowed 2 h after capsule ingestion (no carbonated beverages) – Eating and tablets are allowed 4 h after capsule ingestion – Examination is completed 8–9 h after capsule ingestion – Patient returns the data recorder and other equipment to the facility (may be done the next day)
Next day	– Download the data from the recorder to the PC – Review and interpret the examination – Save the VCE data on a CD and/or external hard disk

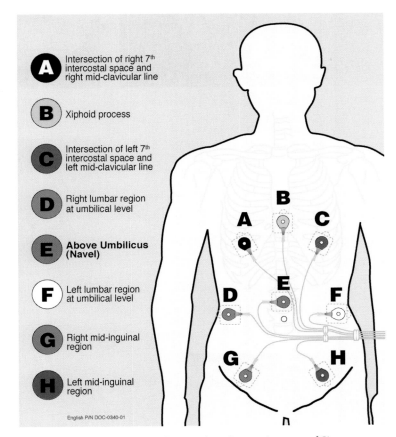

A Intersection of right 7th intercostal space and right mid-clavicular line

B Xiphoid process

C Intersection of left 7th intercostal space and left mid-clavicular line

D Right lumbar region at umbilical level

E **Above Umbilicus (Navel)**

F Left lumbar region at umbilical level

G Right mid-inguinal region

H Left mid-inguinal region

English P/N DOC-0340-01

▣ **Fig. 1.3.1-2.** Lead placement for capsule endoscopy (courtesy of Given Imaging)

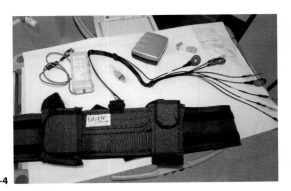

a

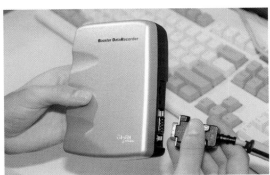

b

▣ **Fig. 1.3.1-3a, b.** Patient data are entered into the Rapid software template (**a**) and downloaded to the recorder (**b**) (▣ Figs. 1.3.1-3–1.3.1-13 by Wolfgang Lehmann)

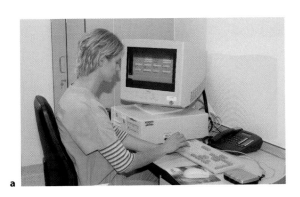

1.3.1-4

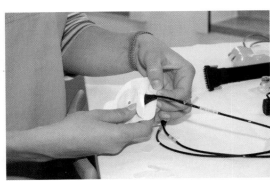

1.3.1-5

▣ **Fig. 1.3.1-4.** Equipment for VCE: belt (*front*), battery pack for recorder (*left*), packaged capsule and lead wires (*center*), data recorder (*top*)

▣ **Fig. 1.3.1-5.** The leads are slipped into adhesive pouches

1

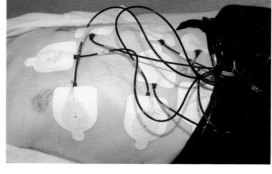

1.3.1-6

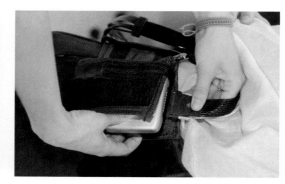

1.3.1-7

■ **Fig. 1.3.1-6.** The leads are affixed to the patient

■ **Fig. 1.3.1-7.** The lead cable is plugged into the data recorder

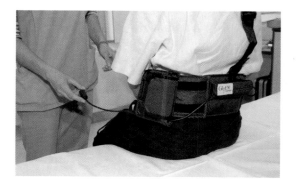

■ **Fig. 1.3.1-8.** A second cable connects the recorder to the battery pack

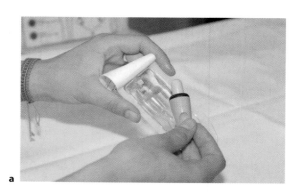

a

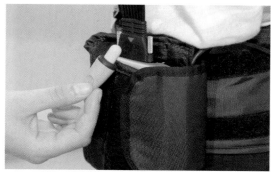

b

■ **Fig. 1.3.1-9a, b.** The capsule is activated by removal from the package **(a)**. The blinking light on the recorder indicates that the system is functioning **(b)**

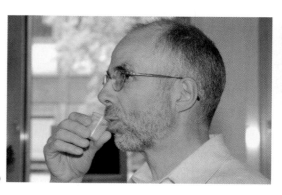

1.3.1-10

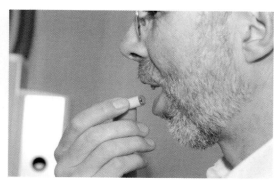

1.3.1-11

■ **Fig. 1.3.1-10.** A prokinetic agent is administered (optional)

■ **Fig. 1.3.1-11.** The patient swallows the capsule

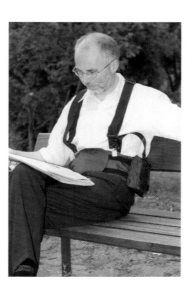

Fig. 1.3.1-12. The patient is free to leave the office or hospital during the examination

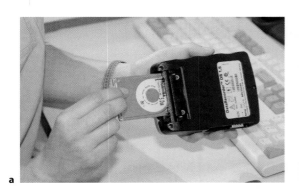

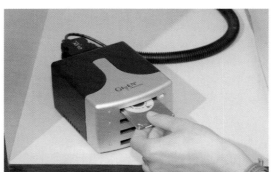

Fig. 1.3.1-13a, b. After the examination is completed, the image data are downloaded from the recorder to the PC. As an option, the data may be recorded onto a removable hard disk **(a)** that is plugged into a quad-port USB for downloading **(b,** booster)

a   b

Transit Time

The transit time of the capsule through the bowel is highly variable, and therefore normal values cannot be established. Approximate values are shown in ◻ Table 1.3.1-2.

The capsule reaches the colon during the image acquisition period in approximately 80% of cases (Rösch and Ell 2004). It is excreted while still transmitting in only 1% of cases. Excretion of the capsule after 5–14 days is defined (somewhat arbitrarily) as »delayed,« and an »impacted« capsule is one that has not been passed after 14 days.

Domperidone 20 mg (Keuchel et al. 2003), erythromycin 200 mg (Fireman et al. 2003), and metoclopramide 10 mg (Selby 2005) significantly shorten the gastric transit time to approximately 30 min. The observed effects of prokinetic agents on small bowel transit have been inconsistent. Tegaserod 6 mg may shorten small intestinal transit (Schmelkin 2004). At present, there is no consensus on indications for the use of prokinetic agents (▶ below).

◻ **Table 1.3.1-2.** Average transit times of the video capsule (without a prokinetic agent)

Location	Average transit time (mean±SD, n=93)	Range
Esophagus	Several seconds	No image to >8 h
Stomach	45 min±52 min	1 min to >8 h
Small bowel	3 h 37 min±90 min	48 min to >8 h
For comparison: total operating time of the PillCam SB	7 h 44 min	5 h 54 min to 9 h 13 min

1

Impediments

Since the bowel cannot be cleansed by irrigation and suction during VCE as it can during flexible endoscopy, adequate preparation is necessary to ensure satisfactory viewing conditions. According to the manufacturer, it is sufficient for the patient to fast overnight before swallowing the capsule. However, many centers routinely precede capsule endoscopy with bowel preparation, usually consisting of polyethylene glycol (PEG) solution. Analogous to the preparation for colonoscopy, we have the patient ingest 2 liters of the solution on the eve of the examination and another liter on the morning of the examination. There is increasing evidence to support the value of bowel preparation prior to VCE (Niv and Niv 2004; Viazis et al. 2004; Dai et al. 2005).

An expert consensus (de Franchis et al. 2005) stated that bowel preparation and prokinetics may reduce acceptance of the procedure. However, as VCE is not a screening method, but costly and time consuming, it should be performed under optimal conditions. Based on current evidence, it was concluded that bowel preparation probably improves the quality of small intestinal cleanliness. Prokinetics possibly shorten gastric and small intestinal transit time, possibly improving completeness of the examination. Possibly, postural tricks shorten gastric transit. Yet, current data are limited and inconsistent, especially concerning kind, amount, and timing of bowel preparation. A large randomized study on these issues is on the way.

A reduction of gas bubbles in the small bowel has been described after the administration of simethicone (Albert et al. 2004).

Possible impediments to VCE:

- Air bubbles
- Food residues
- Inspissated bile in the terminal ileum
- Oral medication, especially extended-release drugs and iron tablets
- Orally administered contrast medium, especially barium
- Blood (acute bleeding, biopsy just before VCE)

Carbonated beverages and upper gastrointestinal biopsy should be avoided just prior to VCE, as they might interfere with the study. Barium-containing contrast medium and iron tablets should not be ingested for about 3 days before the examination (◘ Fig. 1.3.1-14).

Essential medications should be changed to liquid, sublingual, rectal, or parenteral dosage forms whenever possible.

Space Requirements

The space requirements for VCE are modest: a place for the computer, a couch for the patient, and a storage area for the equipment. The patient is free to leave the office or hospital while the gastrointestinal images are being recorded.

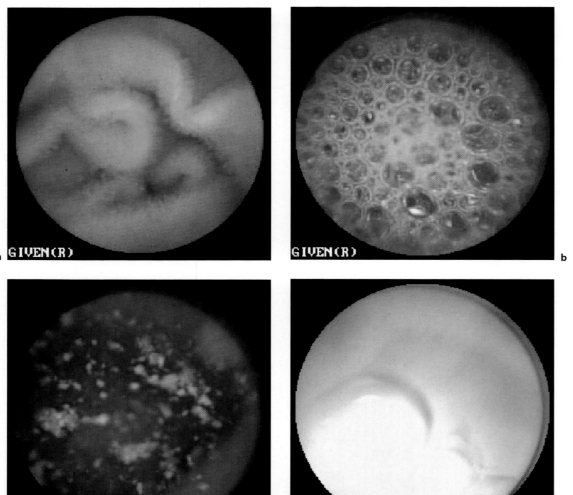

◘ **Fig. 1.3.1-14a–d.** Good examination conditions (**a**). Interpretation is hampered due to air bubbles (**b**); micropellets, tablets, and food residues (**c**); barium-containing contrast medium (**d**)

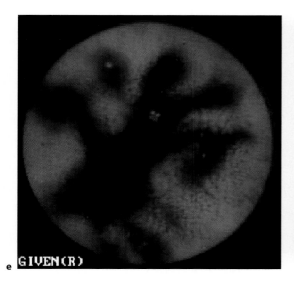
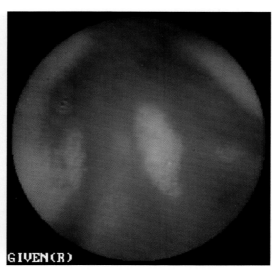

◨ **Fig. 1.3.1-14e,f.** Oral iron medication (**e**); bleeding biopsy site from a prior duodenoscopy (**f**)

Internet

www.givenimaging.com: Pill Cam is manufactured and marketed by Given Imaging Ltd., Yoqneam, Israel

www.capsuleendoscopy.org: European Capsule Endoscopy Group

References

Albert J, Göbel C, Leßke J et al (2004) Simethicone for small bowel preparation for capsule endoscopy: a systematic, single-blinded, controlled study. Gastrointest Endosc 59:487–491

Barkin JS, O'Loughlin C (2004) Capsule endoscopy contraindications: complications and how to avoid their occurrence. Gastrointest Endosc Clin N Am 14:61–65

Dai N, Gubler C, Hengstler P, Meyenberger C, Bauerfeind P (2005) Improved capsule endoscopy after bowel preparation. Gastrointest Endosc 61:28–31

de Franchis R, Avgerinos A, Barkin J et al (2005) ICCE consensus for preps and prokinetics. Endoscopy 37:1040–1045

Fireman Z, Mahajna E, Fish L et al (2003) Effect of erythromycin on gastric and small bowel (SB) transit time of video-capsule endoscopy (VCE). Gastrointest Endosc 57:AB163

Keuchel M, Voderholzer WA, Schenk G et al (2003) Domperidone shortens gastric transit time of video capsule endoscope. Endoscopy 35:A185

Niv Y, Niv G (2004) Capsule endoscopy: role of bowel preparation in successful visualization. Scand J Gastroenterol 39:1005–1009

Rösch T, Ell C (2004) Position paper on capsule endoscopy for the diagnosis of small bowel disorders. Z Gastroenterol 42:247–259

Schmelkin IJ (2004) Tegaserod decreases small bowel transit times in patients undergoing capsule endoscopy. Gastrointest Endosc 59:AB176

Selby W (2005) Complete small-bowel transit in patients undergoing capsule endoscopy: determining factors and improvement with metoclopramide. Gastrointest Endosc 61:80–85

Viazis N, Sgouros S, Papaxoinis K et al (2004) Bowel preparation increases the diagnostic yield of capsule endoscopy: a prospective, randomized, controlled study. Gastrointest Endosc 60:534–538

1

1.3.2 Evaluation of Capsule Endoscopic Images

B.S. Lewis

The Task of Reading

Though capsule endoscopy has grabbed the attention of physician and lay person alike, most overlook the importance and intensity of examining the wirelessly obtained images. Typical examinations obtain images over 8 h. Since images are obtained at a rate of 2 images/s, a total of 57,600 images are produced. The computer workstation allows images to be viewed singly or as a video stream (■ Fig. 1.3.2-1). Though obtained at 2 images/s, images may be reviewed up to 40 images/s. Since an abnormality may be present on only one image, most physicians familiar with the system feel that lesions could easily be missed at the faster rates (Ben-Soussan et al. 2004). A single image is only on the monitor for less than 2/100th of a second when viewing at 40 images/s. A consensus conference of users in 2002 agreed that 15 frames/s is the fastest acceptable rate of review. At this rate, 57,600 images can be seen in 64 min. This takes only into account running the images as a video without stopping to examine individual images.

We reported the viewing times of 20 exams performed using the Given system. We averaged 56 min to review only the small bowel images with a range of 34–94 min (Lewis and Swain 2002). Ell et al. also reported taking an average of 50 min in examining the small bowel data of 32 patients (Ell et al. 2002). The range was from 30 to 120 min. Costamagna et al. (2002) reported taking 2 h to review each study. It was unclear in this study if the images reviewed included the gastric and colonic portions. Average small bowel passage is 4 h and thus without viewing the gastric and colonic portions of the exam, a physician must review a minimum of 28,800 images. The time it takes to review the capsule study is extremely important, as it is a limiting factor to capsule endoscopy's acceptance by gastroenterologists. In an editorial, Fleischer (2002) stated that »the time required to read the studies (60-90 minutes) does not make economic or practice sense.« In an effort to shorten the review time, software has been developed to allow the reader to view up to four images simultaneously. This quad view image places four images, two full seconds of image collection, on one screen. This shortens the reading time by as much as 50%. In addition to the length of time the review takes, physicians are also concerned about reading the studies properly and not missing lesions. By placing four images on one screen each image changes at a slower pace to decrease the likelihood of missing abnormalities (■ Fig. 1.3.2-3). In addition, to aid physicians in this regard, software has been added to the system to identify red pixels as suspected bleeding areas. Fleischer also expressed concern that »without concentration on the part of the physician, a lesion could be missed.« So, in the end, despite great technologic advances, it comes down to the physician and the act of observation.

Vigilance

Lessons learned from anesthesiology (Petty et al. 2002) and airline pilots during long flights (Lavine et al. 2002) show that vigilance is especially necessary when the task is long and monotonous. The stress encountered by an individual being vigilant leads to fatigue and restlessness and this stress is determined by several factors. These factors include the type of event or cue that is being scanned for. Auditory cues are less stressful than visual events. The length of period of observation is also important. Periods greater than 50 min increase the stress to the observer no matter the cue or the event rate (Galinsky et al. 1993). Indeed,

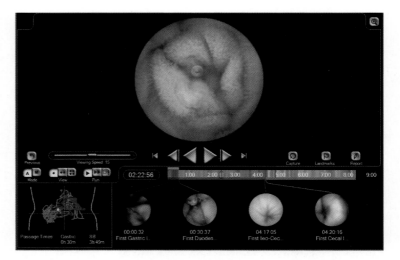

■ **Fig. 1.3.2-1.** RAPID III monitor showing endoscopic image (*top*), tool bar (*middle*), time bar in different colors, representing mean colors of the images in the corresponding segment and thumbnails of landmarks (*bottom*), localization left lower corner

the event rate is generally not related to creating stress. Thus if the thing being watched or listened for occurs frequently or rarely, the same vigilance is required. There are environmental factors as well. The background noise (Becker et al. 1995), the air temperature (Palinkas 2001), the nutrition of the individual (Lieberman et al. 2002), caffeine consumption (Lane and Phillips-Bute 1998), and the person's physical activity during the time of observation have all been found to be important factors in an individual's vigilance. Based on these factors, several suggestions have been made to improve vigilance during reading of a VCE examination (Lewis 2004).

> **Improvement of vigilance at VCE evaluation:**
> - Darkened but not black room
> - Comfortable seating and clothing
> - Carbohydrates (and caffeine?) prior to evaluation
> - Auditory distraction, e.g. music
> - Sessions limited to 1 h
> - Interruption of session in case of fidgetiness or restlessness

The Stress of Reading

It should also be remembered that the stress of reading a study is dependent on the indication for the study. Capsule exams performed for abdominal pain, malabsorption, or suspected Crohn's disease are generally less stressful to read than studies performed for obscure gastrointestinal bleeding. This is because the lesions or visual cues being looked for in the former group are generally larger and less easily missed when compared to a small vascular lesion that may be present on only a single image, when studying patients with bleeding. Most experienced physicians believe that the hardest study to read is the normal study. This requires the confidence of the reader that no lesion has been missed. With these issues in mind, physicians are reminded that prior to reading a capsule study they should be familiar with the patient's medical history not only including the indication for the study but also familiar with any surgical history. Prior knowledge of a surgical small bowel anastomosis (Chap. 9) can simplify the study's analysis.

Interpretation

In addition to vigilance, physicians must have experience in interpreting endoscopic images. Only one part of capsule endoscopy is the vigilant reader, who is able to identify an area that is different or abnormal from other areas examined. An equally important part of the exam is the proper identification of these abnormalities. The reader must be able to diagnose based on the images. This will allow the dismissal of normal variants and nonpathologic lesions and the identification of specific pathologies requiring specific therapies. The images obtained at capsule endoscopy are slightly different from traditional endoscopy since there is no air distention of the bowel wall and the capsule is at times located within millimeters of the mucosa. This is so-called »physiologic endoscopy«. The bowel is not altered by the process of the examination. There is no sedation used and thus there are no hemodynamic effects. There is no trauma caused by the capsule. There is no air insufflation to effect the microvasculature. Thus all findings are real and their location has not been altered by the exam. Expertise must be obtained to allow review of the images not only in an efficient manner but providing precise diagnosis.

The Steps to Efficient Reading

There are very specific steps that can be taken to ease the process of reading a capsule exam. A pattern of practice must be developed by the physician. This author will describe the pattern used by himself when viewing an exam. Initially, the very last image is examined to assure that the colon has been entered. The presence of stool will confirm this finding. After returning to the very first image, the next task is to activate blood detection software if the exam was performed in the setting of obscure gastrointestinal bleeding. To scan the entire study including the stomach, the first image is falsely identified as the first duodenal image on a thumbnail edit. This turns on the Suspected Blood Indicator (SBI) software (■ Fig. 1.3.2-4). Any positive findings can be quickly examined and thumbnails created. However, due to low sensitivity, the SBI software cannot replace careful personal examination of all images of the small intestine (D'Halluin et al. 2005). Once completed, the first image thumbnail is deleted. The third task is to identify the three specific locations needed to determine both the gastric and small bowel emptying times. Using a single view image, but increasing the image rate to 25 frames/s, the images are played forward in an automatic mode. The esophagogastric junction is quickly seen and the first gastric image is duly noted on a thumbnail edit. Using the time bar, the images are quickly advanced forwards and backwards until the first image of the duodenum is identified. This too is noted on a thumbnail edit.

It should be remembered that the capsule can move backwards and forwards through the pylorus several times prior to its final passage and further advancement into the small bowel.

Again the time bar is used to identify the ileocecal valve. This is the landmark that proves to be quite difficult for many physicians. The presence of formed stool is a definite indicator of the colon. It can take some time for the beginning reader to reliably identify this landmark and then note it on a thumbnail edit.

Once the landmarks have been thumbnailed, the images are viewed. The gastric portion of the exam should be examined but can be viewed at a rapid rate. In the small bowel starting at the first image of the duodenum, this author uses the multiviewer function to scan two images at a total rate of 20 frames/s or 10 frames/s of the individual images (■ Fig. 1.3.2-2). A mouse with jogwheel is always at the ready. If reading is performed on a laptop computer, a mouse is attached, since this greatly eases the reading process. When an area moves by too quickly or if a possible abnormality is seen, movement of the jogwheel will stop the progress of the images and allow review of the passed images. The capsule moves extremely quickly in the proximal small bowel as compared to the distal sections. In the duodenum, the frame-to-finding ratio is quite high and thus the duodenum often requires using the jogwheel to examine each individual image. The frame-to-finding ratio in the ileum is quite low and the use of the jogwheel diminishes distally. When an abnormality is identified, a thumbnail is created. This author routinely creates thumbnails for every 30 min of images viewed. This allows the reader to stop and know where the reading stopped and also prevents having to start over should the reader lose his or her place.

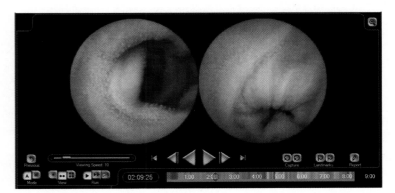

■ **Fig. 1.3.2-2.** Double image view

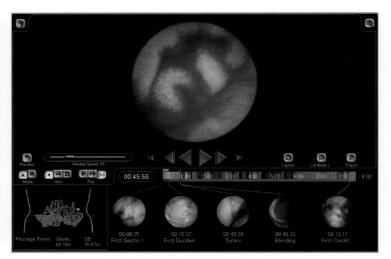

□ **Fig. 1.3.2-3.** Quadruple image mode, combining four different consecutive images

□ **Fig. 1.3.2-4.** Activation of the SBI turns the *arrows* of the tool bar into *red*. Little *red lines* at the appropriate places of the time bar indicate blood

Use of Localization Software

In addition to interpreting individual images, localization data must also be learned. The advantage to localization data is that it allows a physician to know if an identified abnormality is within reach of a push enteroscope (□ Fig. 1.3.2-5). The information can also guide subsequent surgery. Generally, the localization drawing identifies the duodenum and ligament of Treitz well. The physician derives location of an abnormality within the jejunum or ileum from a compilation of data. This includes the quadrant location provided by the localization drawing with an accuracy of about 6 cm (Fischer et al. 2004), the time of passage from the pylorus to the lesion, the amount of bowel visually passed by the capsule in route to the lesion, and the amount of bowel traversed from the lesion to the ileocecal valve. This information is difficult to quantify but qualitative judgments by an experienced physician can be quite accurate in providing a location and thus a differentiation between those patients treated with push enteroscopy and those requiring double-balloon enteroscopy or surgical intervention.

Generally, lesions found within 30 min of passage from the pylorus and those located in the left abdomen (□ Fig. 1.3.2-5a) are generally within reach of a 2.5-m long push enteroscope.

This statement is based on a typical small bowel passage time of 4 h and a normal progression of the capsule within the proximal small bowel. Occasionally, a capsule can stay a prolonged time in the duodenal bulb, altering the above generalizations. Double-balloon enteroscopy can be used to reach lesions further inside the small bowel (Chap. 2.2).

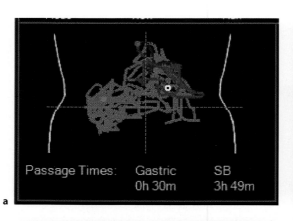

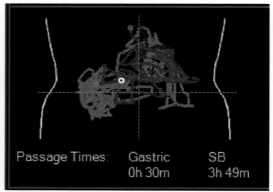

□ **Fig. 1.3.2-5a–d.** Localization software. Progression of the capsule from jejunum (**a**), mid-small intestine (**b**), ileum (**c**) to colon (**d**)

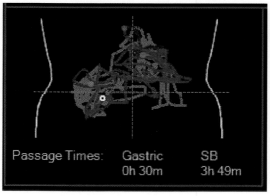

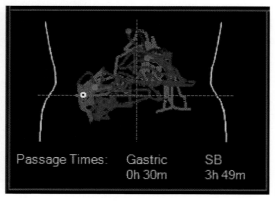

Difficult Images

There are specific problems when interpreting some capsule images. These include single image abnormalities, proper identification of submucosal processes, and differentiating dark blood from dark bile. Unlike traditional endoscopy, a single image abnormality cannot be viewed from different angles but rather must be identified by a single 0.5-s image. This is dependent on the experience and confidence of the reader. Equally troubling for the beginner, a submucosal lesion can be mistaken for the bulge created by another loop of bowel overlying the loop being inspected. There are visual cues that allow for this differentiation. The presence of bridging folds speaks for a submucosal process (◘ Fig. 1.3.2-7f). Capsule images can also clearly show the stretching of the mucosa as well as mucosal edema. Conversely, overlying loops (◘ Fig. 1.3.2-6) can be suspected when the indentation moves with peri-

stalsis indicating its softness. Lymphangiectatic cysts typically have a more soft appearance, yellow color shining through the mucosa above the entire mass, visible vessels on the surface, yellow color, and sometimes whitish villi on their surface differentiating them from other solid submucosal tumors (◘ Fig. 1.3.2-8).

Attests to submucosal lesions:

- Stretched or lobulated mucosa (◘ Fig. 1.3.2-7d)
- Bridging folds (◘ Fig. 1.3.2-7f)
- Central umbilication (◘ Fig. 1.3.2-7b)
- Surface ulcerations (◘ Fig. 1.3.2-7c)
- Villous alterations on surface (◘ Fig. 1.3.2-7a)

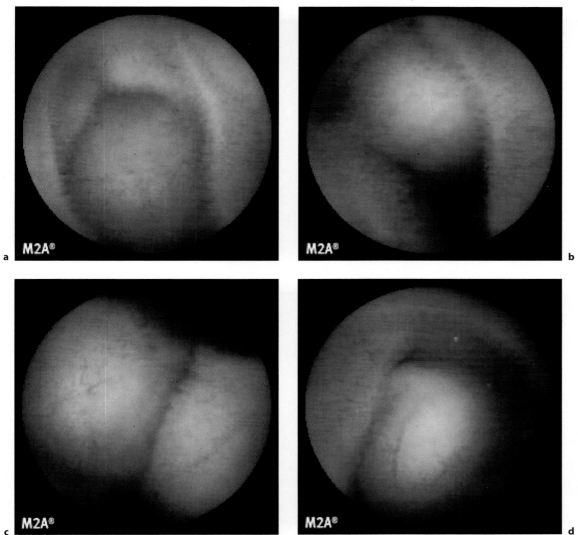

◘ **Fig. 1.3.2-6a–d.** Bulges from adjacent loops with normal mucosa and normal villi

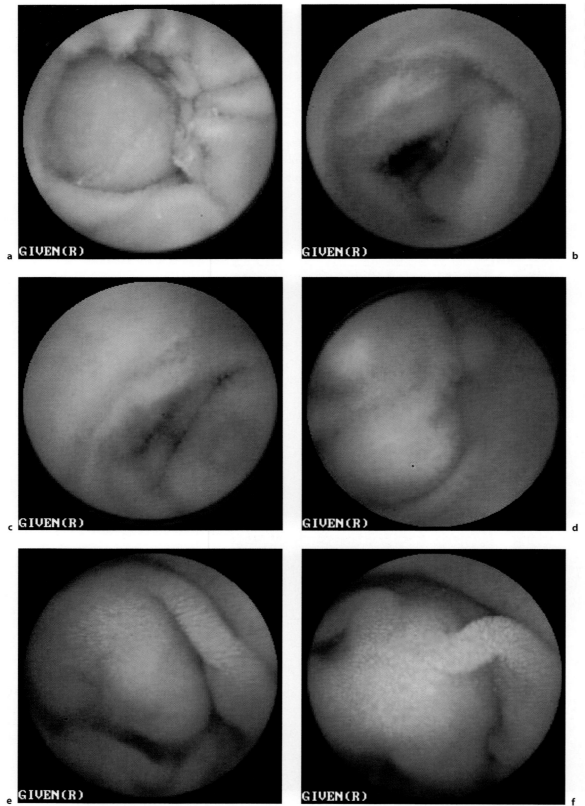

■ **Fig. 1.3.2-7.** **a** Altered villi on surface. **b** Central umbilication. **c** Surface ulceration. **d** Lobulated and stretched mucosa. **e** Thickened fold. **f** Bridging folds come up to but not across the bulge

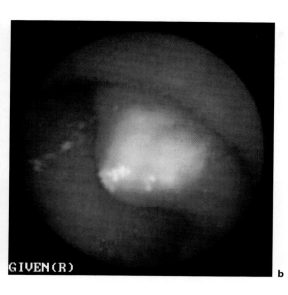

Fig. 1.3.2-8. a Carcinoid (courtesy of André Van Gossum, M.D.). **b** Cystic lymphangiectasia

Dark bile is another situation that can be difficult for the beginning reader, who can mistake bile for dark blood. This is avoided by examining the mucosa beyond the stained area to see if coffee ground (■ Fig. 1.3.2-9a, b) or bloody material (■ Fig. 1.3.2-9c, d) is seen. Its absence indicates likely bile proximally. Air bubbles create light reflection and can give the false impression of absent villi (■ Fig. 1.3.2-10), while floating debris may resemble ulceration (■ Fig. 1.3.2-11). White lines on the edges of folds are a normal finding (■ Fig. 1.3.2-12). Mucosa touching the optical dome of the capsule endoscope can resemble a red spot (■ Fig. 1.3.2-13). Red lesions are easily diagnosed as angiectasias, if they are sharply demarcated and of bright red color (■ Fig. 1.3.2-14a). Other red spots can be diffuse, multiple, shallow, or petechia-like

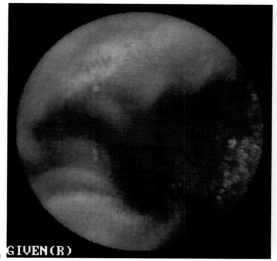

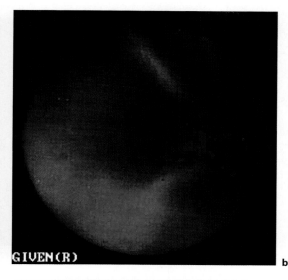

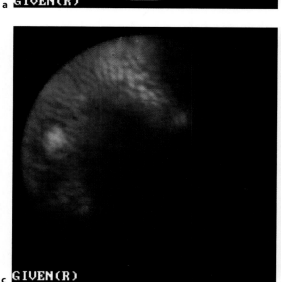

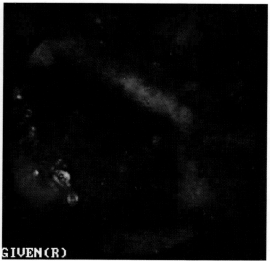

Fig. 1.3.2-9a–d. a, b Dark bile. **c** Dark blood. **d** Coffee grounds

(■ Figs. 1.3.2-14b–d). In these cases, additional findings at VCE such as ulcers, masses, and fibrosis may be necessary along with knowledge of clinical history to make a presumptive diagnosis. Definitive diagnosis may warrant histological confirmation. White lesions are mainly related to villi. Hence, characterization of white lesions should consider the morphology of villi, as totally or partially absent in villous atrophy (■ Fig. 1.3.2-15c) or enlarged in lymphangiectasia (■ Fig. 1.3.2-15b). Duodenal adenomas are typically whitish and re-semble a villous structure, but no single villus can be differentiated (■ Fig. 1.3.2-15d).

❗ Capsule endoscopy is a new field of endoscopy, but it is endoscopy. Experience gained through standard endoscopy is invaluable to the identification and then interpretation of abnormalities. In addition, the following image atlas is aimed to aid in this interpretation.

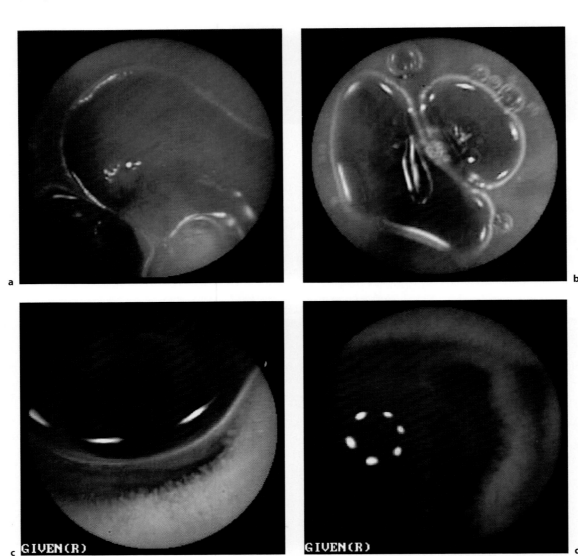

■ Fig. 1.3.2-10a–d. a, b Air bubbles create light reflection and can give false impression of absent villi. **c** Air bubble (*above*) and underwater view with magnification effect. **d** Reflection of the LEDs of the video capsule at the surface of an air bubble

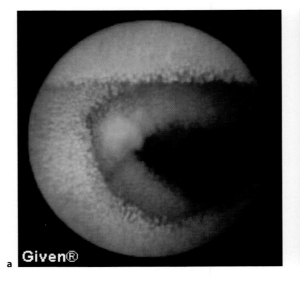
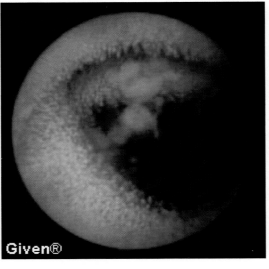

■ Fig. 1.3.2-11. a Ulcer? **b** Floating debris, normal mucosa

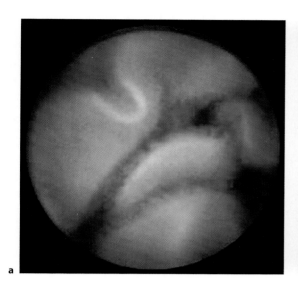

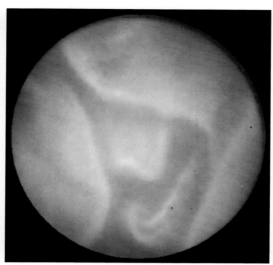

▣ **Fig. 1.3.2-12a, b.** White lines are a normal finding

a   b

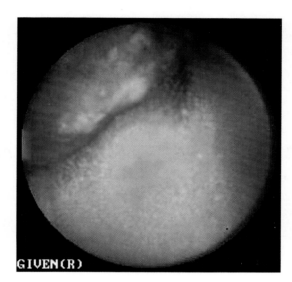

▣ **Fig. 1.3.2-13.** Mucosa touching the optical dome of the capsule endoscope resembles a red spot. The finding is in the left top corner—a tumor

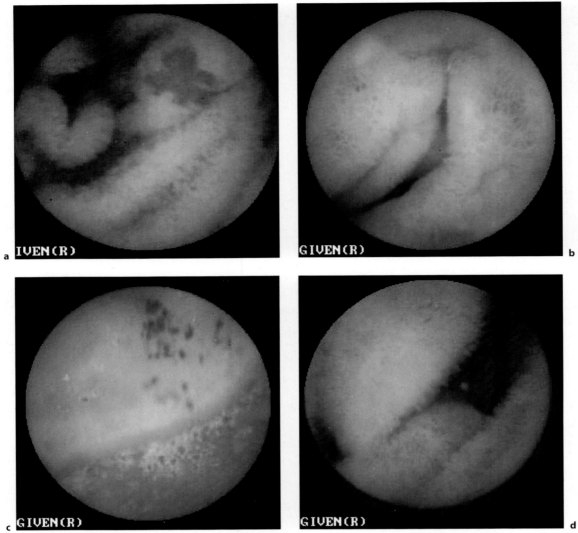

■ **Fig. 1.3.2-14a-d.** Red spots. **a** Sharply demarcated angiectasia with bright red color. **b** Shallow reddening with discrete mucosal fibrosis in radiation enteritis. **c** Infiltrating carcinoid with multiple petechial red spots. **d** Diffuse shallow reddening in NSAID enteropathy

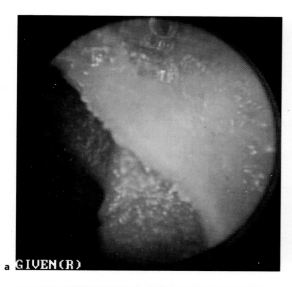

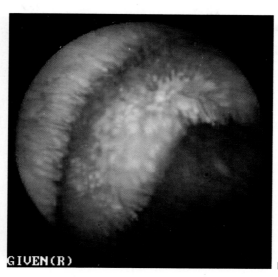

a GIVEN(R)

b GIVEN(R)

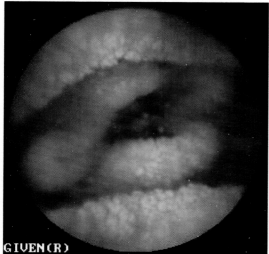

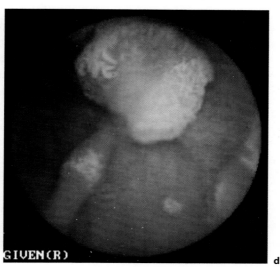

c GIVEN(R)

d GIVEN(R)

◘ **Fig. 1.3.2-15a–d.** White spots. **a** Dry mucosa with reflection artifacts. **b** White villi in genuine lymphangiectasia. **c** Villous atrophy with whitish remnants of villi. **d** Slightly elevated multifocal duodenal adenoma with gyriform appearance

References

Becker A, Warm J, Dember W, Hancock P (1995) Effects of jet engine noise and performance feedback on perceived workload in a monitoring task. Int J Aviat Psychol 5:49–62

Ben-Soussan E, Lecleire S, Ramirez S (2004) Is there a way to improve reading performance of wireless capsule by the Multi-view® System using maximal speed. Gastrointest Endosc 59:AB174

Costamagna G, Shah S, Riccioni M et al (2002) A prospective trial comparing small bowel radiographs and video capsule endoscopy for suspected small bowel disease. Gastroenterology 123:999–1005

D'Halluin PN, Delvaux M, Lapalus MG et al (2005) Does the »Suspected Blood Indicator« improve the detection of bleeding lesions by capsule endoscopy? Gastrointest Endosc 61:243–249

Ell C, Remke S, May A et al (2002) The first prospective controlled trial comparing wireless capsule endoscopy with push enteroscopy in chronic gastrointestinal bleeding. Endoscopy 34:685–689

Fischer D, Schreiber R, Levi D, Eliakim R (2004) Capsule endoscopy: the localization system. Gastrointest Endosc Clin N Am 14:25–31

Fleischer D (2002) Capsule endoscopy: the voyage is fantastic – will it change what we do. Gastrointest Endosc 56:452–456

Galinsky T, Rosa R, Warm J, Dember W (1993) Psychophysical determinants in sustained attention. Hum Factors 35:603–614

Lane J, Phillips-Bute B (1998) Caffeine deprivation affects vigilance performance and mood. Physiol Behav 65:171–175

Lavine R, Sibert J, Gokturk M, Dickens B (2002) Eye-tracking measures and human performance in a vigilance task. Aviat Space Environ Med 73:367–372

Lewis B, Swain P (2002) Capsule endoscopy in the evaluation of patients with suspected small intestinal bleeding: results of a pilot study. Gastrointest Endosc 56:39–43

Lewis BS (2004) How to read wireless capsule endoscopic images: tips of the trade. Gastrointest Endosc Clin N Am 14:11–16

Lieberman H, Falco C, Slade S (2002) Carbohydrate administration during a day of sustained aerobic activity improves vigilance. Am J Clin Nutr 76:120–127

Palinkas L (2001) Mental and cognitive performance in the cold. Int J Circumpolar Health 60:430–439

Petty W, Kremer M, Biddle C (2002) A synthesis of the Australian Patient Safety Foundation Anesthesia Incident Monitoring Study, the American Society of Anesthesiologists Closed Claims Project, and the American Association of Nurse Anesthetists Closed Claims Study. AANA J 70:193–202

1

1.4   Special Situations

1.4.1 Swallowing and Motility Disorders, Pacemakers, and Obesity

M. Keuchel, M.H. Dirks, E.G. Seidman

Swallowing Disorders

Difficulties in swallowing the capsule are rarely encountered in adults (Keuchel et al. 2003). Nevertheless, any history of dysphagia or swallowing disorders should be elicited prior to capsule endoscopy (Barkin and O'Loughlin 2004). Psychogenic or neurological factors usually underlie a patient's inability or refusal to swallow the capsule. Esophageal strictures, diverticula, webs, or rings may be problematic. A history of previous surgery involving the ENT tract and esophagus should also be elicited.

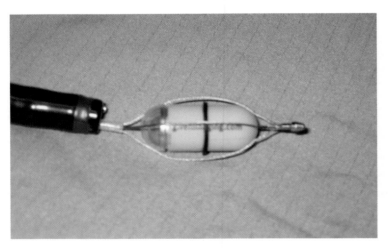

◻ **Fig. 1.4.1-1.** Technique to »front-load« a gastroscope in order to deliver the capsule endoscope directly into the duodenum in patients incapable of swallowing the device. Use of a basket with a variceal ligator placed around the waist of the capsule to secure its grip and prevent its sliding out (reprinted from Seidman et al. 2004 with permission from Elsevier)

In terms of pediatric candidates for capsule endoscopy, children under the age of 8 are rarely able to swallow medication tablets, let alone the larger PillCam SB capsule (measuring 26.4 mm in length and 11 mm in diameter). This problem may be encountered in older patients as well (Sant'Anna et al. 2005). In order to preclude the loss of a capsule (the battery is activated upon removal of the capsule from its package), we recommend that patients should be first instructed to practice by swallowing candies (Seidman et al. 2004). It is worthwhile to have young patients demonstrate that they are capable of swallowing a similar sized vitamin tablet or jelly bean prior to undergoing the test.

For individuals judged unable to swallow the capsule, or those with severe dysphagia or swallowing disorders, the study can be safely undertaken by introducing the capsule into the proximal duodenum endoscopically, under direct vision (Seidman et al. 2004). This can be accomplished by »front loading« the capsule on a gastroscope, holding it in place using a foreign body retrieval net, a polyp retriever snare or a basket (◻ Fig. 1.4.1-1). In our experience, the Roth net is more secure than using a snare. However, it may be difficult to open the net and release the capsule into the small space offered by the proximal duodenum in smaller children. When using a snare for such cases, it is advisable to place a variceal ligator band around the waist of the capsule, as shown in ◻ Fig. 1.4.1-1, in order to secure the capsule and prevent it from slipping off (Seidman et al. 2004). In all cases, it is advisable to employ endotracheal intubation in order to protect the patient's airway.

In adult patients, it has been suggested that the capsule be placed into the stomach endoscopically using an overtube (◻ Fig. 1.4.1-2), using a polypectomy snare, or a foreign body retrieval net (Carey et al. 2004; Tóth et al. 2004). Alternatively, others have reported simply placing the capsule into the overtube and pushing it forward into the stomach with the reinserted endoscope (Leung and Sung 2004; Skogestad and Tholfsen 2004). However, this entails the risk that the study fails if the capsule remains in the stomach for a prolonged period, resulting in an incomplete visualization of the small bowel.

The same techniques of transferring the capsule endoscopically from the stomach into the duodenum can be employed in patients with severe gastroparesis (Carey et al. 2004; Seidman et al. 2004). In our experience, capsules may be retained in the stomach for prolonged periods in diabetics and in patients receiving medications which delay gastric emptying, such as narcotics.

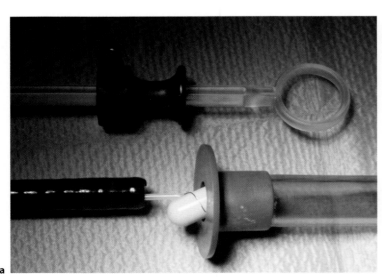

a

◻ **Fig. 1.4.1-2a, b.** Use of an overtube to insert the capsule into the stomach using a gastroscope. **a** Overtube (*right*) with inserted video capsule, held by a polypectomy snare inserted through a gastroscope (*left*) and handle of the snare

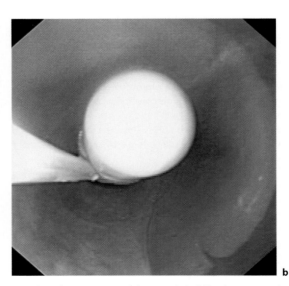

b

(*top*). **b** Endoscopic view of the capsule held by the snare at the distal end of the overtube, which is inserted into the esophagus

In a patient with a Zenker's diverticulum, endoscopic placement of the capsule has been described after insertion of the endoscope over a guide wire through the working channel. The capsule is held externally at the distal end by a polypectomy snare fixed on the outer surface of the endoscope (Aabakken et al. 2003).

More recently, a capsule delivery device (AdvanCE, US Endoscopy) has been developed (■ Figs. 1.4.1-3–1.4.1-5): a wire is inserted through the working channel of a standard gastroscope. Subsequently, the capsule holder is screwed onto the wire, and the capsule is pressed into the holder. The esophagus can then be intubated either blindly using this device pulled back to the scope, or under direct vision if the device is pushed 1–2 cm forward. Once the duodenum is reached, the capsule is released by pulling the device's handle.

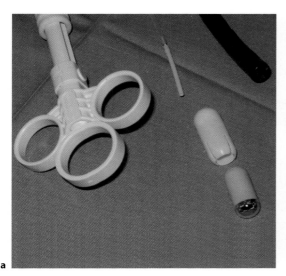

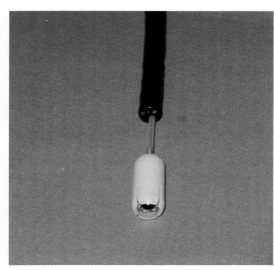

■ Fig. 1.4.1-3a–c. Specific capsule delivery device. **a** Device prior to assembling. **b** Mounted device with capsule secured. **c** The capsule has been released by pushing the inner wire forward using the handle

a

b

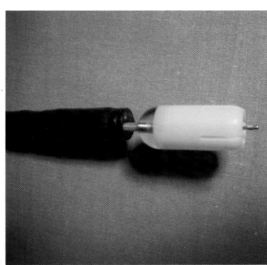

c

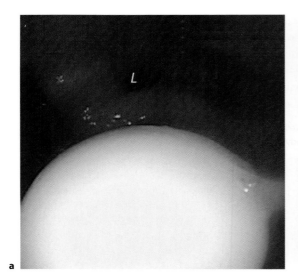

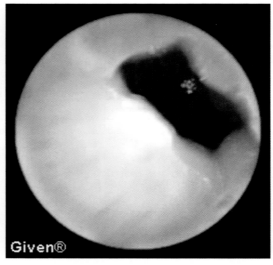

Fig. 1.4.1-4. a Capsule delivery device inserted endoscopically under direct visualization of hypopharynx and larynx (*L*) while the capsule endoscope is passing the upper esophageal sphincter (**b**)

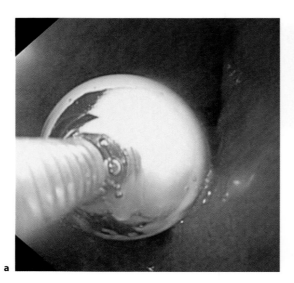

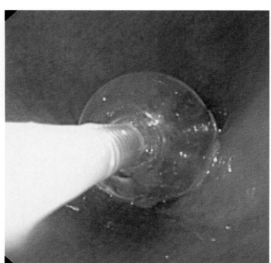

Fig. 1.4.1-5. a Capsule delivery device with capsule in the duodenum. **b** Empty cup of the delivery device after release of the capsule

Management of Gastric Motility Problems

One method of detecting delayed gastric passage is by performing a parallel, approximately 10-min-long recording with a second, separately initialized recorder with its own electrode leads and battery pack (Seitz et al. 2002). The clothed patient lies on a couch while wearing the recorder belt. The leads for the second recorder are placed loosely on the patient's clothing, approximating the standard sensor layout for capsule endoscopy (**Fig. 1.4.1-6**). After the data have been downloaded from the second recorder, one can quickly determine whether the capsule has reached the small intestine or is still in the stomach or even the esophagus.

If the capsule is still in the stomach after 1 h, a prokinetic agent can be given. We have obtained good results by infusing erythromycin. A dose of 3 mg/kg i.v. has been proposed, based on gastric emptying studies in healthy subjects (Boivin et al. 2003). An alternate approach we have employed in diabetics who might have gastroparesis is to keep the patient fasting and take a plain abdominal radiograph 2 h after the capsule was swallowed. If the capsule still remains in the gastric cavity, it can then be placed in the duodenum endoscopically, as described above. However, both of these approaches can result in considerable time delays. We feel that endoscopic insertion of the capsule into the duodenum is a more effective option in patients with known gastroparesis.

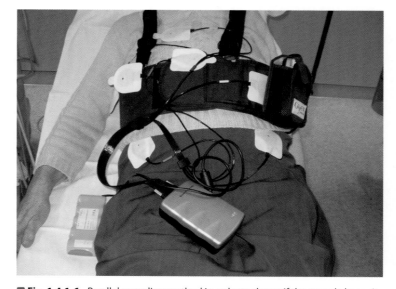

Fig. 1.4.1-6. Parallel recording method in order to detect if the capsule has exited the stomach. Patient with regular recording equipment and a second recording system placed loosely over the clothes

Various instruments can be used to grasp and transport the swallowed capsule across the pylorus (■ Figs. 1.4.1-7–1.4.1-8): a foreign body grasping forceps (Spera et al. 2004), a Roth net (Fleischer et al. 2003), a polypectomy snare (Hollerbach et al. 2003), or a Dormia basket.

A three-prong foreign body grasper does not hold the capsule securely enough. The use of such insertion instruments has not been associated with damage to the capsule, to date.

■ Fig. 1.4.1-7a–i. Instruments used to grasp a swallowed capsule in the stomach in order to deposit into the duodenum. **a** Capsule held securely with foreign body grasping forceps. **b** Roth net. **c** Capsule viewed through the Roth net. **d** Polypectomy snare with capsule proximal to the pylorus. **e** Snare viewed from the capsule

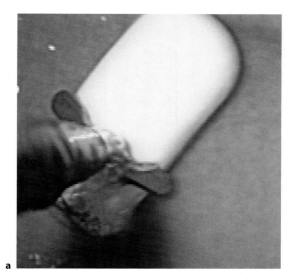

a

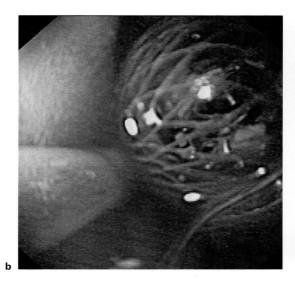

b

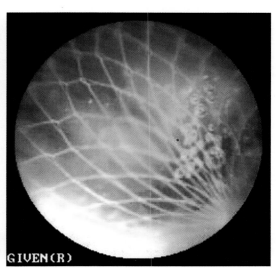

c

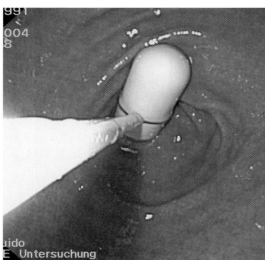

d

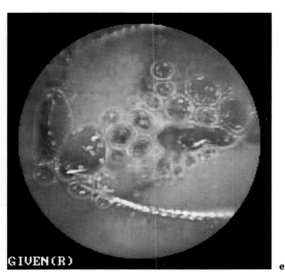

e

1

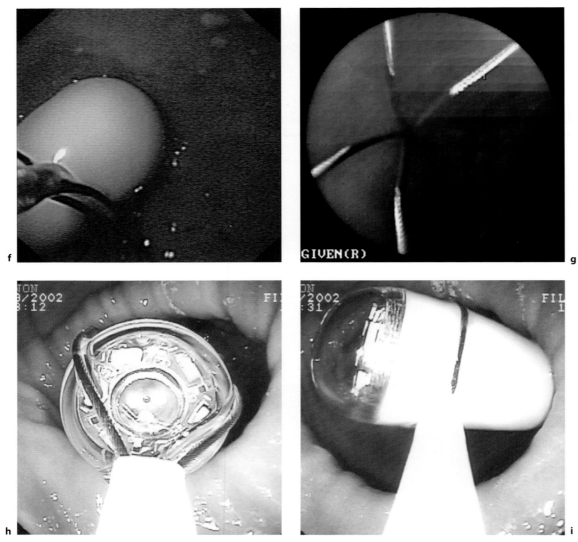

GIVEN(R)

f

g

h

i

□ **Fig. 1.4.1-7f–i. f** Capsule held in a Dormia basket. **g** Basket viewed from the capsule. **h** Capsule held lengthwise and crosswise (**i**) in a Dormia basket

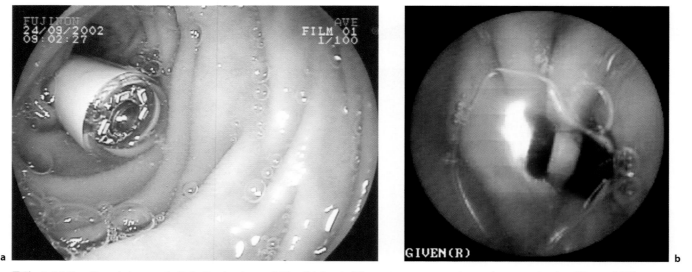

a

b

GIVEN(R)

□ **Fig. 1.4.1-8. a** Capsule transported into the duodenum. **b** The distal end of the gastroscope extends past the upper duodenal flexure (VCE)

Pacemakers

The presence of a cardiac pacemaker or other electromechanical implants such as defibrillators had been considered a contraindication to the procedure. On the other hand, initial observations in patients with a bipolar cardiac pacemaker have shown no evidence of danger or interference (Perez Piqueras et al. 2004). Capsule endoscopy in patients with a bipolar cardiac pacemaker has even been recently recommended as an outpatient procedure (Leighton et al. 2004). The patient should nevertheless be informed about the theoretical risk of interference. Direct hindrance with capsule endoscopy recording has been reported (Guyomar et al. 2004) from a pacemaker in VV0 mode implanted into the abdominal wall. In general, the risk is probably greater if the battery and signal emitting device is inserted in the abdominal area, rather than the usual thoracic (clavicular) area.

If a capsule study is performed during electrocardiographic monitoring at the bedside or during telemetry, interference with the recording of the images may occur. Testing the system by activating the capsule and observing whether the light on the recorder is blinking before swallowing the capsule should be performed in the unit where the patient is being monitored (ICU, etc), rather than in the endoscopy suite. In case of malfunction, the patient may be transferred to another location for the procedure.

Obesity

In patients with marked obesity, signals from the capsule's transmitter might not be powerful enough to reach the sensor fields placed on the abdomen. Alternatively, it has been suggested to place the sensor field in corresponding positions on the patient's back (◘ Fig. 1.4.1-9) in order to shorten the distance between capsule and sensors (Seitz and Soehendra 2003). In order to make the localization software work properly, the sensor electrodes are placed inversely on the back.

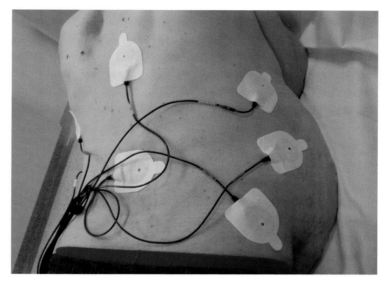

◘ **Fig. 1.4.1-9.** Obese patient (140 kg) with electrodes placed inversely on his back

Internet

www.usendoscopy.com: Manufacturer of AdvanCE capsule delivery device

References

Aabakken L, Blomhoff JP, Jermstad T, Lynge AB (2003) Capsule endoscopy in a patient with Zenker's diverticulum. Endoscopy 35:799

Barkin JS, O'Loughlin C (2004) Capsule endoscopy contraindications: complications and how to avoid their occurrence. Gastrointest Endosc Clin N Am 14: 61–65

Boivin MA, Carey MC, Levy H (2003) Erythromycin accelerates gastric emptying in a dose-response manner in healthy subjects. Pharmacotherapy 23:5–8

Carey EJ, Heigh RI, Fleischer DE (2004) Endoscopic capsule endoscope delivery for patients with dysphagia, anatomical abnormalities, or gastroparesis. Gastrointest Endosc 59:423–426

Fleischer DE, Heigh R, Nguyen CC et al (2003) Videocapsule impaction at the cricopharyngeus: first report of this complication and its successful resolution. Gastrointest Endosc 57:427–428

Guyomar Y, Vandeville L, Heuls S, Coviaux F, Graux P, Cornaert P, Filoche B (2004) Interference between pacemaker and video capsule endoscopy. Pacing Clin Electrophysiol 27:1329–1330

Hollerbach S, Kraus K, Willert J, Schulmann K, Schmiegel W (2003) Endoscopically assisted video capsule endoscopy of the small bowel in patients with functional gastric outlet obstruction. Endoscopy 35:226–229

Keuchel M, Thaler C, Csomós G et al (2003) Video capsule endoscopy: technical and medical failures. Endoscopy 35 [Suppl]:A6

Leighton JA, Sharma VK, Srivathsan K, Heigh RI, McWane TL, Post JK, Robinson SR, Bazzell JL, Fleischer DE (2004) Safety of capsule endoscopy in patients with pacemakers. Gastrointest Endosc 59:567–569

Leung WK, Sung JJ (2004) Endoscopically assisted video capsule endoscopy. Endoscopy 36:562–563

Sant'Anna AMGA, Dubois J, Miron MJ, Seidman EG (2005) Wireless capsule endoscopy for obscure small bowel disorders: final results of the first pediatric controlled trial. Clin Gastroenterol Hepatol 3:264–270

Perez Piqueras J, Payeras E, Selva E, Mendez M, Jimenez A, Purrinos J, Cabrera A (2004) Protocol for pacemaker patient study (abstract). 3rd International Conference on Capsule Endoscopy, Miami, FL, USA, 29 February–3 March 2004

Seidman EG, Sant'Anna AMGA, Dirks MH (2004) Potential applications of wireless capsule endoscopy in the pediatric age group. Gastrointest Endosc Clin N Am 14:207–218

Seitz U, Bohnacker S, Soehendra N (2002) A simple method to determine the location of the capsule and thus whether prokinetic drugs are needed during video capsule endoscopy. Endoscopy 34:1027

Seitz U, Soehendra N (2003) Solving the problem of video recording gaps in capsule endoscopy of overweight patients. Endoscopy 35:714

Skogestad E, Tholfsen JK (2004) Capsule endoscopy: in difficult cases the capsule can be ingested through an overtube. Endoscopy 36:1038

Spera G, Spada C, Riccioni ME, Perri V, Costamagna G (2004) Video capsule endoscopy in a patient with a Billroth II gastrectomy and obscure bleeding. Endoscopy 36:931

Toth E, Fork FT, Almqvist P, Thorlacius H (2004) Endoscopy-assisted capsule endoscopy in patients with swallowing disorders. Endoscopy 36:746–747

1.4.2 Video Capsule Endoscopy in the Emergency Room

D.R. Cave, R. Sachdev

Special Considerations in Acute Bleeding

Video capsule endoscopy has been used extensively and effectively for the detection of the source of obscure gastrointestinal bleeding (Pennazio et al. 2004). The possible role of capsule endoscopy in acute gastrointestinal bleeding has received scant attention. We hypothesize that it may have a role in helping facilitate detection of the origin of non-hematemesis gastrointestinal bleeding. Obviously the symptom of hematemesis implies a source of bleeding within range of the conventional gastroscope, usually in the esophagus, stomach, or duodenum. However, when this population is excluded and patients with melena and hematochezia are assessed, the diagnostic yield is much smaller when using esophagogastroduodenoscopy (EGD) and colonoscopy (COL). This in part is due to the poor predictive value of both melena and hematochezia as to the precise source of bleeding. Melena can be present in those patients with epistaxis to a right colonic bleed (Lee and Cave 2003). This lack of precision often results in the need to perform both EGD and COL. Since most gastrointestinal bleeding stops spontaneously, many of these procedures are performed after bleeding has ceased, further reducing the reliability of the observations as to where bleeding originated. We therefore performed a randomized pilot study to examine the possible benefit of capsule endoscopy in this context (Sachdev et al. 2004).

> Contraindications to VCE as first-line diagnostic test in acute bleeding:
>
> — Dysphagia
> — Gastroparesis
> — Known Zenker's or other large necked diverticula in the stomach or duodenum
> — Uncooperative patient
> — Pregnancy
> — Implanted pacemakers and defibrillators

VCE as First-Line Test in Acute Non-Hematemesis Bleeding

A study was designed to determine if early vs late use of the capsule might help in the evaluation of patients in whom the origin of gastrointestinal bleeding was unclear. The PillCam SB (Given Imaging, Yoqneam, Israel) capsule was allowed to traverse the intestines for 8 h. The data were downloaded and read as soon as possible for the early capsules. Results were then provided to the team taking care of the patient to facilitate work-up. Results from patients who ingested the capsule before discharge and after the conventional work-up was completed were provided to the patient's physician as they became available (■ Fig. 1.4.2-1).

A total of 138 patients entering the emergency room with gastrointestinal bleeding were screened over a 6-month period and 24 were eligible, having non-hematemesis acute gastrointestinal bleeding, and were able to sign a consent form. The early group ingested their capsule an average of 1.2 h after entry into the emergency room (■ Fig. 1.4.2-2). The late group ingested their capsule a mean of 63 h after admission. Of the 16 (75%) patients in the early capsule endoscopy group, 12 had

Study Design

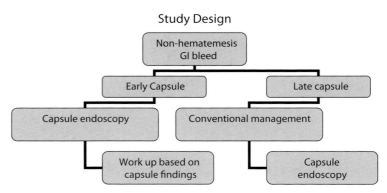

■ **Fig. 1.4.2-1.** Study design

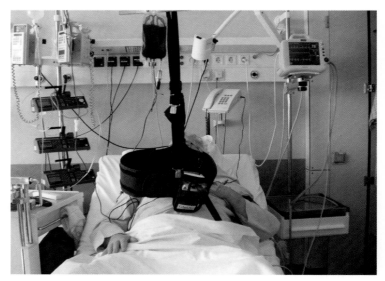

■ **Fig. 1.4.2-2.** VCE under emergency conditions in acute bleeding

a presumptive source of bleeding detected by capsule endoscopy (10), EGD (1), and COL (1) vs 3 of 8 (38%) patients (EGD, 3) in the capsule endoscopy late group (*p*=0.099) within 24 h of enrollment. The median time to presumptive diagnosis by any diagnostic device was 19 h in the early capsule endoscopy group vs 35 h in the capsule endoscopy late group (*p*=0.06). Overall, active bleeding was detected by capsule endoscopy in 13 of 24 (54%) patients, 2 of 17 (11%) by EGD, and 0 of 13 (0%) by COL. Capsule endoscopy provided no useful information in 4 of 24 (17%) patients because of inability to swallow the capsule (1) or because of gastric retention (3). Examples of findings from this study are presented below (■ Figs. 1.4.2-3–1.4.2-6). The anatomic site from which the bleeding originated, as determined by the video capsule, is summarized in ■ Table 1.4.2-1.

We have demonstrated that capsule endoscopy is feasible in the emergency room setting. Our entry criteria for the study were clearly defined and we failed to screen only 11 of 138 patients over a 6-month period and there were no complications.

This pilot study does suggest that the use of capsule endoscopy, in this selected but common scenario, can accelerate the time to diagnosis compared to conventional endoscopic intervention. There was no shortening of time spent in hospital. However, this study was too small and not designed to examine this issue, which would require a much larger study. Similarly, we did not examine cost effectiveness.

Comparative data on the exact population we studied is not available since it is usually included in a more general population of gastrointestinal bleeding. The number of patients studied was small, and the diagnostic yield by capsule endoscopy was numerically smaller than that reported by Pennazio et al. (2004) who noted that in their patients with obscure bleeding, if active bleeding was occurring, the diagnostic yield was 92%.

Table 1.4.2-1. Anatomic origin of source of bleeding

	Late capsule	Early capsule
Retained capsule	1	3
Stomach	2	4
Small bowel	2	4
Colon	1	1
Unknown	2	4

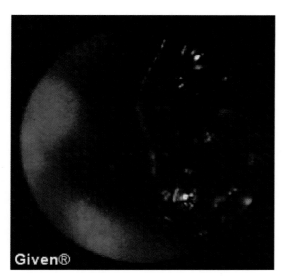

Fig. 1.4.2-3. Patient A. Late capsule. Melena in the ileum. Conventional work-up was negative. Colonoscopy was refused. Precise origin of bleeding not seen

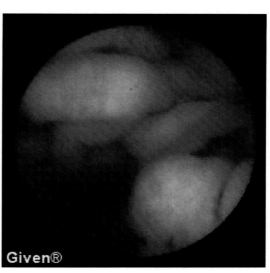

Fig. 1.4.2-4. Patient B. Early capsule. Active bleeding in the duodenum

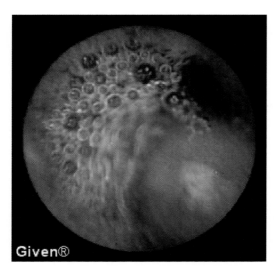

Fig. 1.4.2-5. Patient C. Late capsule. Ulcer in the distal ileum associated with use of nonsteroidal anti-inflammatory drugs. This was the probable source of bleeding. Colonoscopy showed diverticulosis

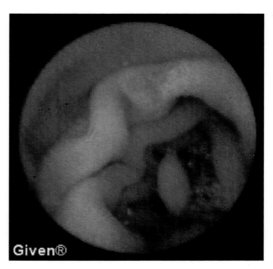

Fig. 1.4.2-6. Patient D. Early capsule. Angiectasia in the small intestine. Upper endoscopy demonstrated portal hypertensive gastropathy

1

Special Aspects of VCE in Acutely Ill Patients

Three patients retained the capsule in the stomach. This is not surprising as these patients were acutely ill and probably subject to increased vagal tone that impaired gastric emptying. This problem could possibly be reduced by the use of prokinetics in future studies to accelerate gastric emptying. Erythromycin or tegaserod may be useful since we had a much higher gastric retention rate than previously reported. Some acceleration of the capsule should not be very important, as in this context we are looking for bleeding more than fine detail.

No interference was seen in our study suggesting that monitoring equipment does not interfere with the capsule telemetry and recording. It is unlikely that the capsule will interfere with other diagnostic tests since it only lasts for 8 h. Magnetic resonance imaging would have to be withheld until excretion of the capsule. However, an experiment we conducted demonstrated that placing the capsule inside the magnetic field of a scanner exerted very little force on the capsule, certainly nothing that would injure a patient.

We have not seen an increase in aspiration risk and would not anticipate this problem since all patients studied were hemodynamically stable and fully conscious.

VCE in Severe Acute Bleeding After Negative EGD and COL

VCE is widely used in the context of obscure gastrointestinal bleeding. This implies its use in a non-emergent manner after conventional technology has failed. This may be the antithesis of its eventual role in the detection of hard to locate severe small intestinal bleeding, which is often intermittent. We would advocate its use as soon as possible and appropriate after conventional endoscopy has failed to demonstrate a bleeding site. This approach has been validated by the recent report by Pennazio et al. (2004) who demonstrated a 92% yield in the presence of active bleeding. Furthermore, in the context of recurrent bleeding, we suggest using the capsule as soon as there is evidence for renewed bleeding and avoiding further conventional endoscopy, which yields very little, thus allowing time for bleeding to cease.

Future Concepts

The concept of real-time interrogation of the capsule will be available in 2006. This would mean plugging in a handheld computer to the capsule recording device to check at any time where the video capsule was in the alimentary canal and whether or not there was blood or melena present in the lumen. Such a device would have important implications for the reduction of capsule procedure time and reading, particularly in a patient with acute bleeding. As real-time reading devices become available, the use of the capsule will become even more useful, since once active bleeding is detected, therapy can be initiated without waiting the 8 h of capsule transit time plus downloading and reading time.

The improved yield of VCE in the acute setting suggests that we should be much more aggressive in its application than is currently the case.

References

Lee H, Cave D (2003) Melena and its anatomic sources. Gastrointest Endosc 57: AB169

Pennazio M, Santucci R, Rondonotti E, Abbiati C, Beccari G, Rossini FP, de Franchis R (2004) Outcome of patients with obscure gastrointestinal bleeding after capsule endoscopy: report of 100 consecutive cases. Gastroenterology 126:643–653

Sachdev R, Hibberd P, Perlmutter M, Cave D (2004) Capsule endoscopy in the emergency room for acute non-hematemesis gastrointestinal bleeding. Am J Gastroenterol 99:S295

1.5   Patency Capsule

G. Costamagna, M.E. Riccioni, M. Keuchel

Principle

The Patency Capsule (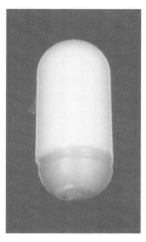 Fig. 1.5-1) is designed to remain intact in the gastrointestinal (GI) tract for about 40–100 h. A new device with two plugs, dissolving after about 30 h (AGILE Patency Capsule) has been developed. Following this period of time, if still inside the body it disintegrates spontaneously. Surface erosions caused by the gastric and intestinal fluids form a hole in the plug over the designated time period (Fig. 1.5-4). Fluids penetrate through this hole to reach the body of the capsule and dissolve the lactose-barium mixture, leaving behind the parylene C coating and the metal tag (Fig. 1.5-5).

Retention of the test capsule can be detected radiographically (Fig. 1.5-2) or with an external detector (Fig. 1.5-3) that responds to a small induction coil inside the capsule (Fig. 1.5-5).

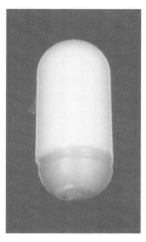

Fig. 1.5-1. Commercially available Patency Capsule

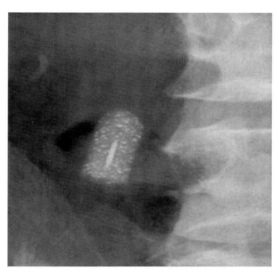

Fig. 1.5-2. Radiograph shows an intact Patency Capsule with internal coil and flecks of barium in the lactose filler

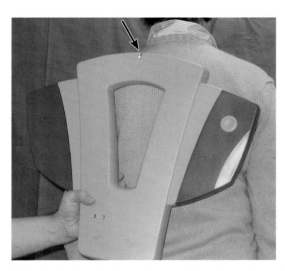

Fig. 1.5-3. The blue light at the top of the detector (*arrow*) indicates the presence of the coil. It cannot be determined, however, whether the coil is still inside an intact capsule or has been released from a disintegrated capsule

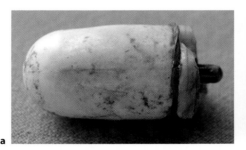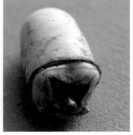

Fig. 1.5-4a, b. Beginning disintegration of the Patency Capsule (prototype). As the maximal diameter is conserved, passing of such a capsule still indicates intestinal patency

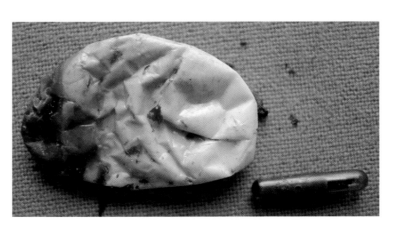

Fig. 1.5-5. Disintegrated Patency Capsule, leaving coating and tag

1

Procedure

After obtaining informed consent, including risk of retention with need for surgery, the patients swallow the Patency Capsule with a glass of water. Although recommended by the manufacturer, there is no need to fast prior to ingestion. Hereafter, the patient has to look carefully for the capsule with every bowel movement.

If the capsule is not excreted the next day, the presence of the tag can be proven with a detector. This detector recognizes the intracorporeal tag via induction. However, it can neither discriminate whether the Patency Capsule is still intact or already dissolved nor whether the tag or capsule are lodged in the small bowel or have passed into the colon.

Therefore, X-ray films of the abdomen are preferable if the Patency Capsule was not excreted. Repeated X-rays on subsequent days document whether the capsule is lodged, moves into the colon, or dissolves (◘ Fig. 1.5-7).

If only the collapsed shell of the capsule (◘ Fig. 1.5-5) is excreted instead of the intact Patency Capsule, a significant stenosis has to be assumed. In this case, VCE is contraindicated unless surgery is scheduled. VCE is also contraindicated if the X-ray documents disintegration of the Patency Capsule by showing the tag without surrounding capsule (◘ Fig. 1.5-7b).

❶ Note: The only evidence of intestinal patency with this test is the excretion of the intact Patency Capsule (◘ Fig. 1.5-9).

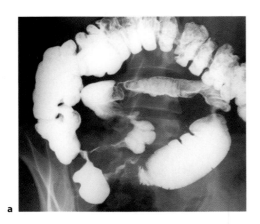 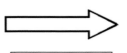 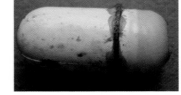 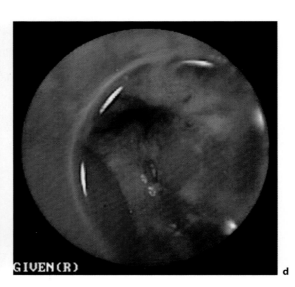

◘ **Fig. 1.5-6a–e.** Crohn's disease patient with radiological tight ileal strictures (**a**). The intact Patency Capsule was excreted intact 27 h after ingestion, without adverse events (**b**). Patient underwent VCE that showed ileal ulcerations and stenosis. The PillCam passed uneventfully (**c–e**)

27 hours later

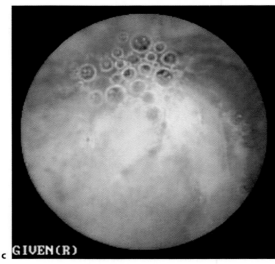

GIVEN(R)
c

GIVEN(R)
d

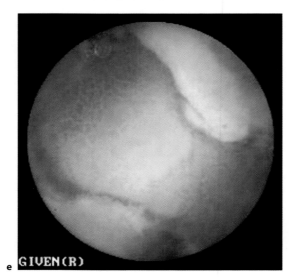

GIVEN(R)
e

Indication

The Patency Capsule may offer information on functional intestinal patency and may be used as a test before VCE in patients with:

- Established diagnosis of Crohn's disease
- Suspicion of intestinal stenosis based on clinical, radiologic, or sonographic findings
- Prior abdominopelvic radiation
- Prior small bowel resection
- Prior major abdominal surgery with a possibility of adhesions

Clinical Application

The Patency Capsule has received CE (European Conformity) certification. First studies have assessed the clinical value of this device. Some patients have complained of transient abdominal pain. One patient with Crohn's disease and a long small intestinal stricture had to undergo surgery for small intestinal obstruction before the Patency Capsule was able to dissolve (Boivin et al. 2004; ◻ Fig. 10-20). Another patient developed temporary obstruction (Gay et al. 2005; ◻ Fig. 10-21); 39 patients who passed an intact Patency Capsule underwent VCE despite a known or presumed stenosis (◻ Fig. 1.5-6). In all cases the imaging capsule was passed without incident (Boivin et al. 2005; Delvaux et al. 2005; Spada et al. 2005).

Cave		
In a long stenosis, the Patency Capsule may cause obstruction requiring surgery.		

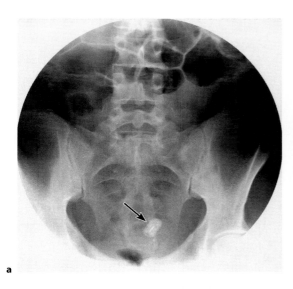

a

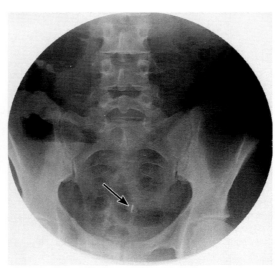

b

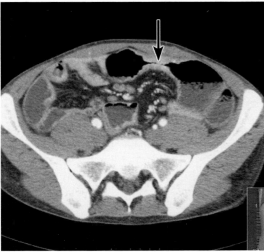

c

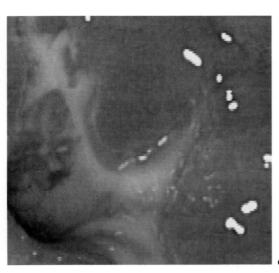

d

◻ **Fig. 1.5-7a–d.** Crohn's disease with stricture. **a** Intact Patency Capsule (*arrow*) at 24 h. **b** At 50 h only the tag (*arrow*) is visible, and therefore VCE is contraindicated. **c** CT shows circumscribed thickening with stenosis (*arrow*), dilatation, and small lymph nodes (sonography Fig. 2.4-1a). **d** Enteroscopy demonstrates an impassable ulcerated jejunal stenosis

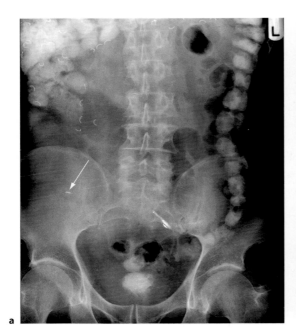

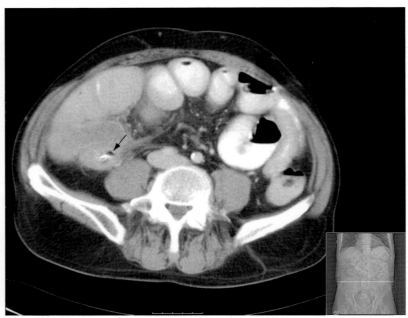

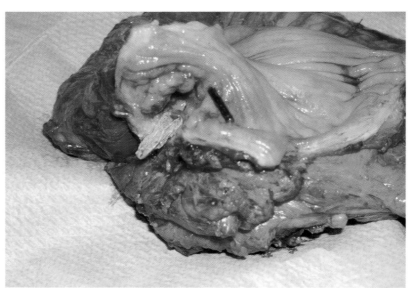

■ **Fig. 1.5-8a–c.** Patient with obscure bleeding after resection of colonic carcinoma. Because of postprandial abdominal discomfort, the Patency Capsule was given prior to a scheduled VCE. **a** Abdominal X-ray shows clips after surgery, and the coil of the dissolved Patency Capsule. **b** CT depicts the coil in a narrow ileal lumen (courtesy of Ernst Malzfeldt, M.D.). **c** Surgery reveals metastatic small bowel adenocarcinoma with stenosis and remnants of the Patency Capsule (courtesy of Christopher Pohland, M.D.)

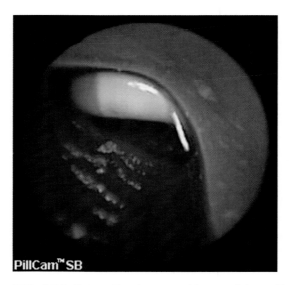

■ **Fig. 1.5-9.** Patency Capsule seen on video capsule image. The patient had reported the excretion of the Patency Capsule. Both capsules finally passed uneventfully

References

Boivin ML, Lochs H, Voderholzer WA (2005) Does passage of a patency capsule indicate small-bowel patency? A prospective clinical trial. Endoscopy 37:808–815

Delvaux M, Ben Soussan E, Laurent V et al (2005) Clinical evaluation of the use of the M2A patency capsule system before a capsule endoscopy procedure, in patients with known or suspected intestinal stenosis. Endoscopy 37:801–807

Gay G, Delvaux M, Laurent V et al (2005) Temporary intestinal occlusion induced by a »patency capsule« in a patient with Crohn's disease. Endoscopy 37:174–177

Spada C, Spera G, Riccioni M et al (2005) A novel diagnostic tool for detecting functional patency of the small bowel: the Given patency capsule. Endoscopy 37:793–800

1.6   Terminology

M. Delvaux, L.Y. Korman, M. Keuchel

Introduction

A standard terminology is essential for the reproducible, internationally uniform, and electronic data processing (EDP)-compatible reporting of endoscopic findings. A standard terminology has been developed for VCE (Korman 2004), following the model of the Minimal Standard Terminology (MST) created by a collaboration between the European, American, and Japanese Endoscopy Societies under the sponsorship of the *Organisation Mondiale d'Endoscopie Digestive* (OMED) for the fields of esophagogastroduodenoscopy, endoscopic retrograde cholangiopancreatography, and colonoscopy (Maratka 1992; Delvaux et al. 2000; Delvaux et al. 2002). The Capsule Endoscopy Structured Terminology (CEST) has been developed following the rules established for MST and adapted to the specific needs for the reporting of findings and diagnoses in capsule endoscopy findings. The CEST has been validated in a retrospective trial (Delvaux et al. 2005) and published for an open access use in softwares and scientific applications (Korman et al. 2005). The CEST supports the structured reporting of all data necessary for an examination, including pathological findings. This chapter provides an overview and examples of the use of the CEST for reporting a VCE examination.

Structured Documentation of an Examination

The VCE examination report follows the general MST structure for endoscopic reporting to provide the necessary documentation of the procedure.

> **Documentation of a VCE examination:**
>
> — Patient data
> — Procedural data (date, examiner)
> — Reason (indication) for the examination
> — Limitations (viewing conditions, completeness of the examination)
> — Complications
> — Description of findings
> — Localization
> — Diagnosis
> — Recommendations

Findings

The »Findings« section is based on a hierarchy of descriptive levels that starts with categories of findings called »Headings« (see below). Below the headings are terms, followed by attributes and attribute values.

> **The following headings are used for the structured description of findings in the small bowel:**
>
> — Normal
> — Lumen
> — Contents
> — Mucosa
> — Flat lesions
> — Protruding lesions
> — Excavated lesions

For example, fresh blood in the bowel lumen due to active bleeding is described as follows: contents (heading) – blood (term) – kind of blood (attribute) – red (attribute value). In some cases a finding is an aggregate of different observations described under multiple headings. For example: stenosing tumor: tumor (protruding lesion) and stenosis (lumen) or diverticulitis: diverticulum (excavated lesion) and ulcer (excavated lesion) and erythema (mucosa).

Localization

— By **time:** proximal, middle, or distal third of the small bowel. The time between the initial images of the duodenum and of the cecum is divided into three equal segments. Any delay of the capsule in the duodenum or terminal ileum and any variations in transit speed are ignored.
— By **organ** (esophagus, stomach, duodenum, small bowel, terminal ileum, colon) or by anatomical landmarks (Z line, pylorus, papilla, ileocecal valve).
— By using **localization software** that shows an abdominal-wall projection of the capsule location (■ Fig. 1.6-1).

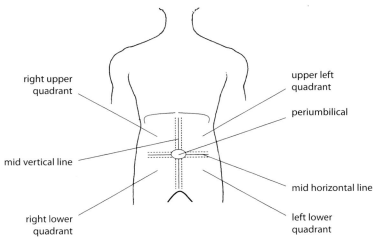

■ **Fig. 1.6-1.** Capsule localization based on four quadrants, the periumbilical area, a vertical line through the umbilicus (above/below), and a horizontal line through the umbilicus (right/left)

Normal

Lumen

Stenosis	Type	– Extrinsic compression – Intraluminal (intrinsic) benign – Intraluminal (intrinsic) malignant
	Traversed	Yes/no
Dilated	Longitudinal extent	Short segment/ long segment/ whole organ
	Wall contractions	Present/absent
Evidence of previous surgery	Type Suture material	Specify Yes/no

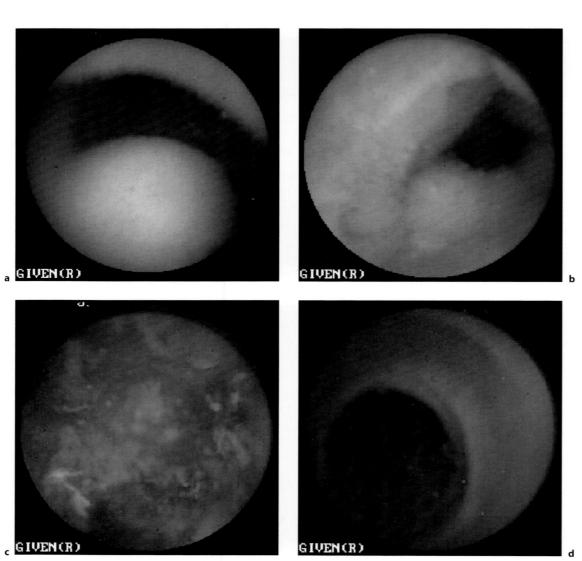

Fig. 1.6-2a–d. Stenosis/dilatation: **a** extrinsic stenosis, **b** intrinsic benign stenosis, **c** intrinsic malignant stenosis, **d** dilatation

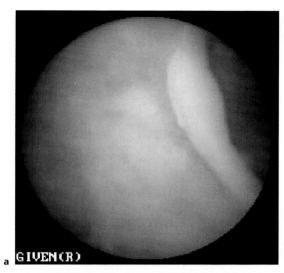

GIVEN(R)

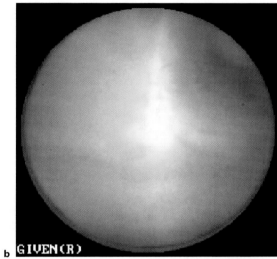

GIVEN(R)

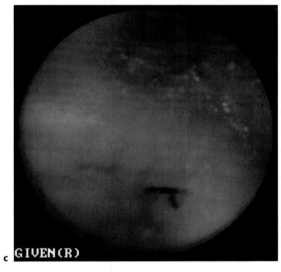

GIVEN(R)

Fig. 1.6-3a–c. Signs of previous surgery: **a** anastomosis, **b** scar, **c** suture material

Contents

Blood	Type	Red/clot/hematin
Bile		
Parasites	Type	Specify
Foreign body	Type	Specify
Food	Type	Specify
Feces		

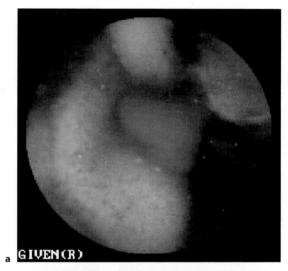

GIVEN(R)

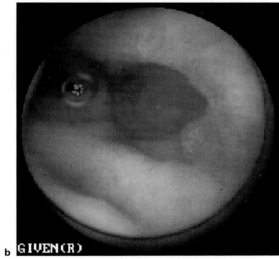

GIVEN(R)

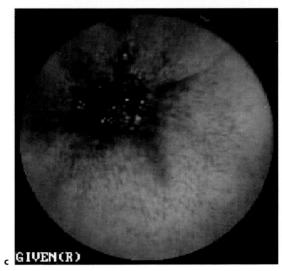

GIVEN(R)

Fig. 1.6-4a–c. Description of contents: **a** red blood, **b** clot, **c** hematin

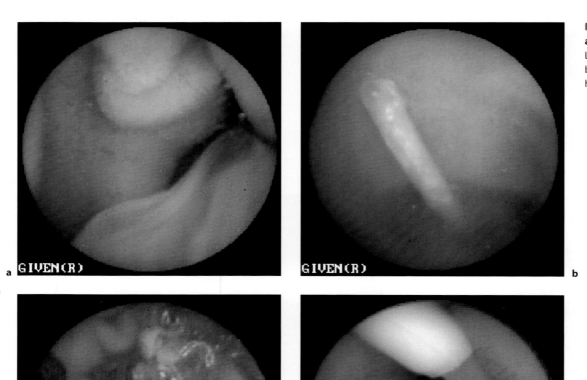

Fig. 1.6-5a–d. Description of contents: **a** bile, **b** parasite (courtesy of Wilfred Landry, M.D.), **c** food (plant parts), **d** foreign body (tube; courtesy of Wilfried Voderholzer, M.D.)

Mucosa

Erythematous	Distribution pattern	Localized/patchy/diffuse
	Longitudinal extent	Short segment/long segment/whole organ
Pale	Distribution pattern	Localized/patchy/diffuse
	Longitudinal extent	Short segment/long segment/whole organ
Edematous (congested)	Distribution pattern	Localized/patchy/diffuse
	Longitudinal extent	Short segment/long segment/whole organ
Granular	Distribution pattern	Localized/patchy/diffuse
	Longitudinal extent	Short segment/long segment/whole organ

Nodular	Distribution pattern	Localized/patchy/diffuse
	Longitudinal extent	Short segment/long segment/whole organ
Atrophic	Distribution pattern	Localized/patchy/diffuse
	Longitudinal extent	Short segment/long segment/whole organ
Abnormal villi	Shape	Convoluted/swollen/blunted/absent
	Color	Whitish/yellow
	Distribution pattern	Localized/patchy/diffuse
	Longitudinal extent	Short segment/long segment/whole organ

▼

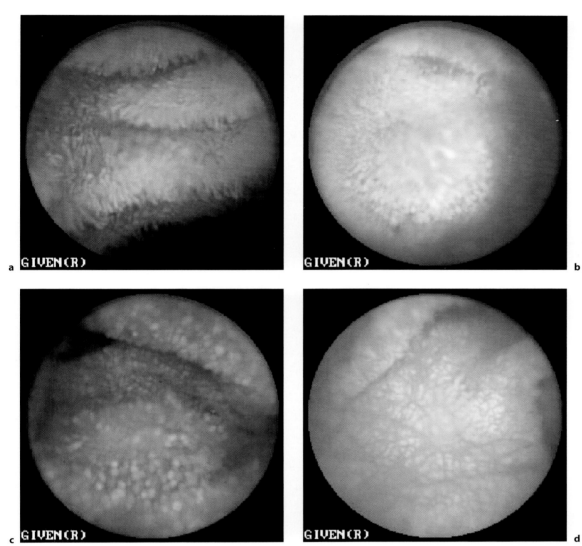

■ **Fig. 1.6-6a–d.** Abnormal villi: **a** convoluted, **b** blunted, **c** swollen, **d** absent villi

1

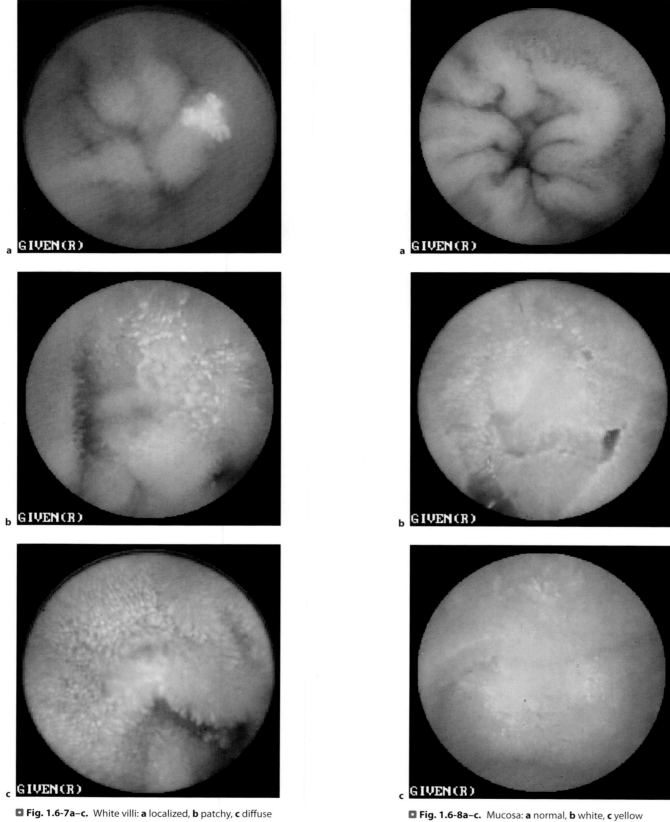

■ **Fig. 1.6-7a–c.** White villi: **a** localized, **b** patchy, **c** diffuse

■ **Fig. 1.6-8a–c.** Mucosa: **a** normal, **b** white, **c** yellow

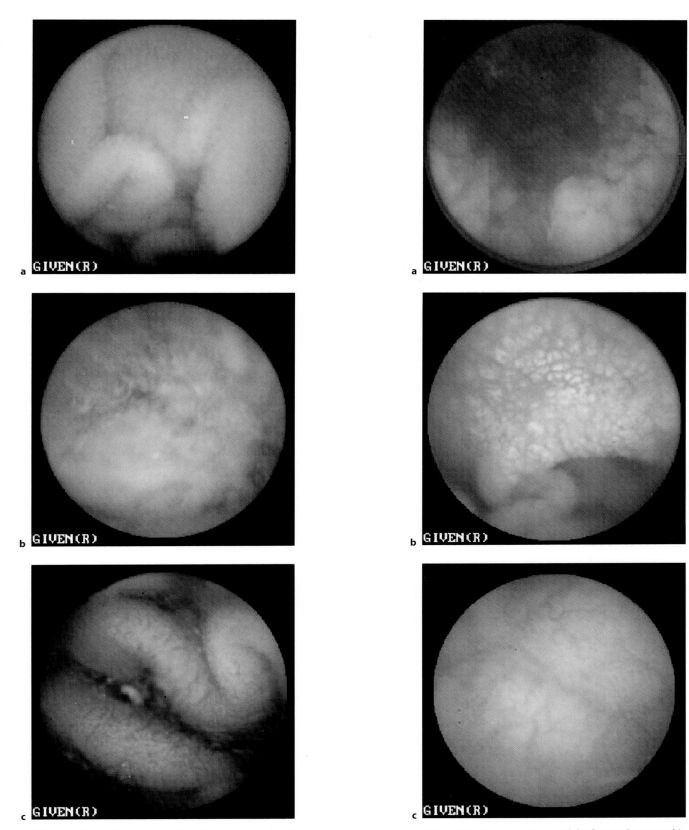

□ **Fig. 1.6-9a–c.** Mucosa: **a** pale, **b** erythematous, **c** edematous

□ **Fig. 1.6-10a–c.** Mucosa: **a** nodular, **b** granular, **c** atrophic

Flat Lesions

Spot		
	Number	Single/multiple
	Type	Red/white/black
	Bleeding	Yes/no
	Distribution pattern	Localized/patchy/diffuse
	Longitudinal extent	Short segment/ long segment/ whole organ

Plaque		
	Number	Single/multiple
	Type	Red/white/black
	Distribution pattern	Localized/patchy/diffuse
	Longitudinal extent	Short segment/ long segment/ whole organ

▼

Angiectasia		
	Number	Single/multiple
	Size	Small/medium/large
	Arborization	Yes/no
	Bleeding	Yes/no
	Stigmata of bleeding	Yes/no
	Bleeding potential	Yes/possible/no
	Distribution pattern	Localized/patchy/diffuse
	Longitudinal extent	Short segment/ long segment/ whole organ

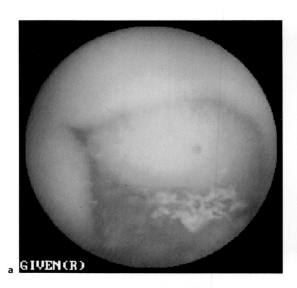

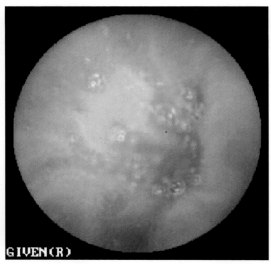

a GIVEN(R)   b GIVEN(R)

◨ Fig. 1.6-11a–d. Angiectasias:
a small, **b** medium, **c** large with arborization, **d** large in colon

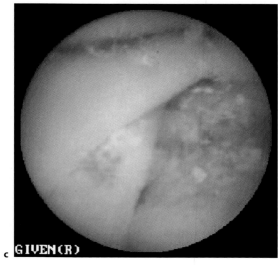

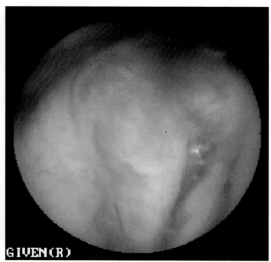

c GIVEN(R)   d GIVEN(R)

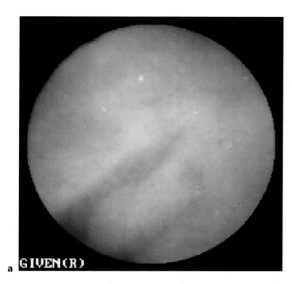

GIVEN(R)

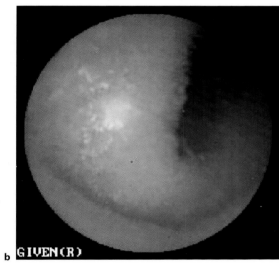

GIVEN(R)

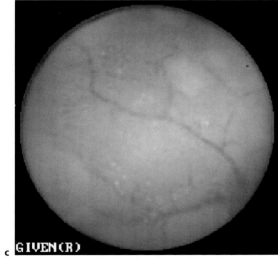

GIVEN(R)

Fig. 1.6-12a–c. Spots: **a** red spot, **b** yellow spot, **c** white spot

Protruding Lesions

Nodules	Number	Single/few/multiple
	Bleeding	Yes/no
	Stigmata of bleeding	Yes/no
	Distribution pattern	Localized/patchy/diffuse
	Longitudinal extent	Short segment/ long segment/ whole organ
Polyps	Number	Single/few/multiple
	Size	Small/medium/large
	Pedicle	Sessile/pedunculated/ unknown
	Bleeding	Yes/no
Mass/tumor	Size	Small (<5 mm)/ medium (5–20 mm)/ large (>20 mm)
	Type	Submucosal/fungating/ ulcerated/frond-like/ villous
	Bleeding	Yes/no
	Stigmata of bleeding	Yes/no
Venous structure	Type	Venous lake/bleb/varix
	Number	Single/few/multiple
	Bleeding	Yes/no
	Stigmata of bleeding	Yes/no
	Bleeding potential	Yes/possible/no
	Distribution pattern	Localized/patchy/diffuse
	Longitudinal extent	Short segment/ long segment/ whole organ

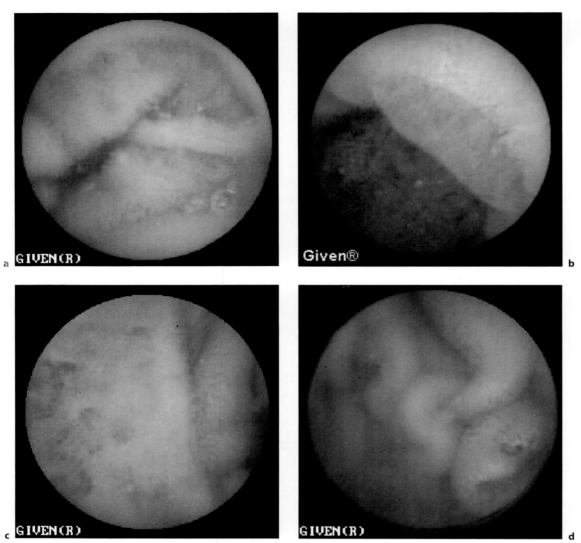

Fig. 1.6-13a–d. Veins: **a** venous lake, **b** bleb, **c** varix, **d** bleeding potential present (eroded surface)

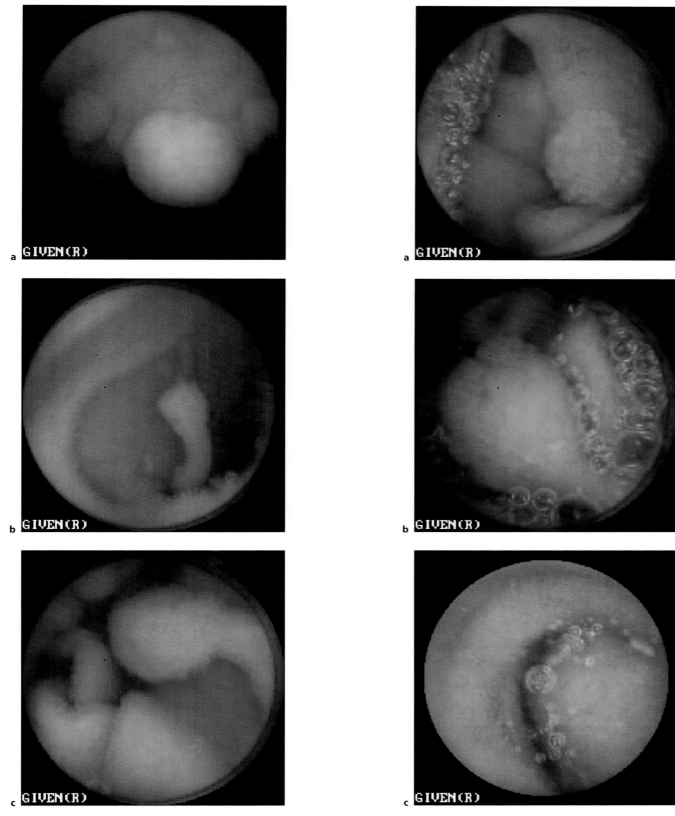

Fig. 1.6-14a–c. Polyps: **a** sessile, **b** pedunculated, c questionable

Fig. 1.6-15a–c. Polyps: **a** small, **b** medium, **c** large

1

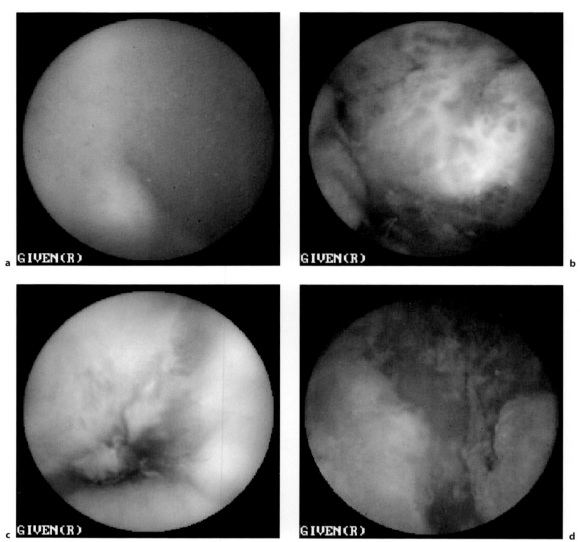

▫ **Fig. 1.6-16a–d.** Tumors: **a** submucosal, small, **b** ulcerated, large, **c** infiltrative, **d** villous

Excavated Lesions

Aphtha	Number	Single/few/multiple
	Distribution pattern	Localized/patchy/diffuse
	Longitudinal extent	Short segment/ long segment/ whole organ

Erosion	Number	Single/few/multiple
	Bleeding	Yes/no
	Stigmata of bleeding	Yes/no
	Distribution pattern	Localized/patchy/diffuse
	Longitudinal extent	Short segment/ long segment/ whole organ

Ulcer	Number	Single/few/multiple
	Bleeding	Yes/no
	Stigmata of bleeding	Yes/no
	Distribution pattern	Localized/patchy/diffuse
	Longitudinal extent	Short segment/ long segment/ whole organ

Scar		

Diverticulum		Single/multiple

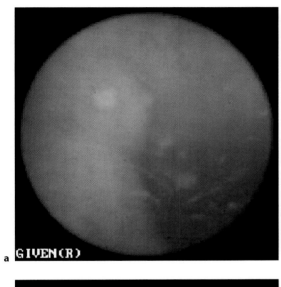
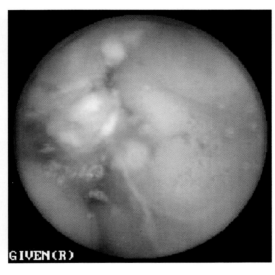
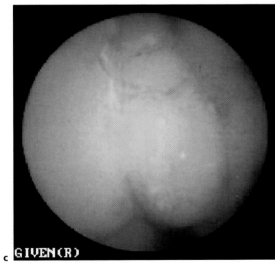
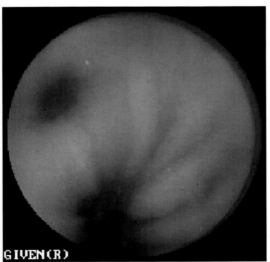

a GIVEN(R)

b GIVEN(R)

c GIVEN(R)

d GIVEN(R)

Fig. 1.6-17a–d. Excavated lesions:
a aphtha, **b** erosion, **c** ulcer, **d** diverticulum

Diagnoses

The diagnosis represents the opinion of the examiner based on clinical history and findings. The examiner should try to distinguish the diagnosis from the findings. For example, small bowel erosions can be found in both nonsteroidal anti-inflammatory drug (NSAID)-induced enteropathy and Crohn's disease. The examiner should select the diagnoses from the following list that represents the range of common and rare small bowel diagnoses. The list of diagnoses, as proposed by the CEST, is divided into two lists of terms, the *main diagnoses* and *other diagnoses* being classified according to their frequency in clinical practice.

Main diagnoses:

- Normal
- Angiectasia
- Erosion
- Ulcer
- Crohn's disease
- Celiac disease
- NSAID enteritis
- Tumor
    - Benign
    - Malignant
- Bleeding of unknown origin

Other diagnoses:

- Diverticulum
- Tropical sprue
- Parasites
- Dieulafoy's lesion
- Hemobilia
- Phlebectasia
- Varices
- Intestinal lymphangiectasia
- Ischemic enteritis
- Vasculitis
- Radiation enteritis
- Post-transplant lymphoproliferative disorder
- Graft-versus-host disease
- Enteropathy
    - Erosive
    - Erythematous
    - Congestive
    - Hemorrhagic
- Brunner's gland hyperplasia
- Lipoma
- Xanthelasma
- Neuroendocrine tumor
- Melanoma
- GIST (gastrointestinal stromal tumor)
- Kaposi's sarcoma
- Lymphoma
- Polyp
- Juvenile polyposis
- Familial adenomatous polyposis
- Peutz-Jeghers syndrome

Internet

www.omed.org/mst: source for downloading the Minimal Standard Terminology (MST)

References

Delvaux M, Crespi M, Armengol-Miro JR et al (2000) Minimal standard terminology for digestive endoscopy: results of prospective testing and validation in the GASTER project. Endoscopy 32:345–355

Delvaux M, Crespi M, Korman LY, Fujino MA (2002) Minimal standard terminology for digestive endoscopy. Terms and attributes, Version 2.0. Normed Verlag, Bad Homburg, Englewood NJ

Delvaux M, Friedman S, Keuchel M et al (2005) Structured terminology for capsule endoscopy: results of retrospective testing and validation in 766 small-bowel investigations. Endoscopy 37:945–950

Korman LY (2004) Standard terminology for capsule endoscopy. Gastrointest Endosc Clin N Am 14:33–41

Korman LY, Delvaux M, Gay G et al (2005) Capsule endoscopy structured terminology (CEST): proposal of a standardized and structured terminology for reporting capsule endoscopy procedures. Endoscopy 37:951–959

Maratka Z (1992) The OMED data base: standard for nomenclature. Endoscopy 24 [Suppl 2]:455–456

Complementary Procedures

2

2.1 Duodenoscopy, Ileocolonoscopy, Push Enteroscopy

F. Hagenmüller, M. Keuchel

Duodenoscopy

Before the entire small bowel is imaged by video capsule endoscopy, a careful esophagogastroduodenoscopy (EGD) should be performed. In several studies, missed sources of bleeding within the reach of a gastroscope were detected in a significant percentage, e.g., in 42% of patients referred for push enteroscopy (Hayat et al. 2000).

In many cases also the portion of the duodenum beyond the papilla can be visualized by EGD (■ Fig. 2.1-1). For special investigations, intravital staining can be used during endoscopy to bring out fine details in the mucosa (■ Fig. 2.1-3) (Kiesslich et al. 2003). Zoom endos-copy allows detailed visualization of villi (■ Fig. 2.1-7a) (Cammarota et al. 2005). Endoscopic ultrasound can also be performed to investigate protruding or infiltrating lesions (■ Fig. 2.1-4a). A side-viewing duodenoscope allows a superior view of the papillary region (■ Fig. 7.2-28).

Duodenal biopsies are important in patients with suspected celiac sprue and other diseases such as Whipple's disease, genuine lymphangiectasia, or suspected giardiasis after negative stool tests.

If necessary, therapeutic procedures can be added to the examination. These include control of bleeding by injection of saline, epinephrine, or fibrin glue as well as coagulation procedures or placement of hemoclips (■ Fig. 2.1-2). Snare polypectomy of pedunculated polyps can be carried out during duodenoscopy. Mucosectomy of flat adenomas may require prior injection of saline or hyaluronic acid. Special endoscopes with a second working channel are advantageous for special therapeutic procedures, allowing the application of a forceps together with a snare for mucosectomy (■ Fig. 2.1-4b–d) or more powerful suction during bleeding.

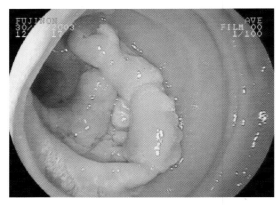

■ Fig. 2.1-1. Duodenoscopy: carcinoma of the distal duodenum

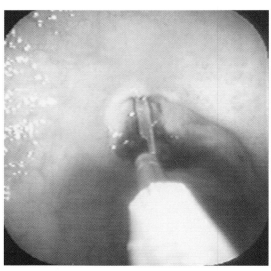

■ Fig. 2.1-2. Duodenal ulcer with vascular stump and clot, treated by clipping

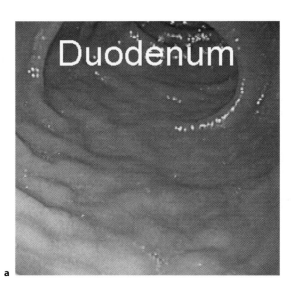

a

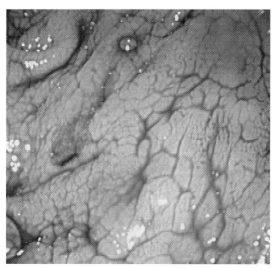

b

■ Fig. 2.1-3a, b. Villous atrophy. **a** Native endoscopic view. **b** Chromoendoscopy with methylene blue

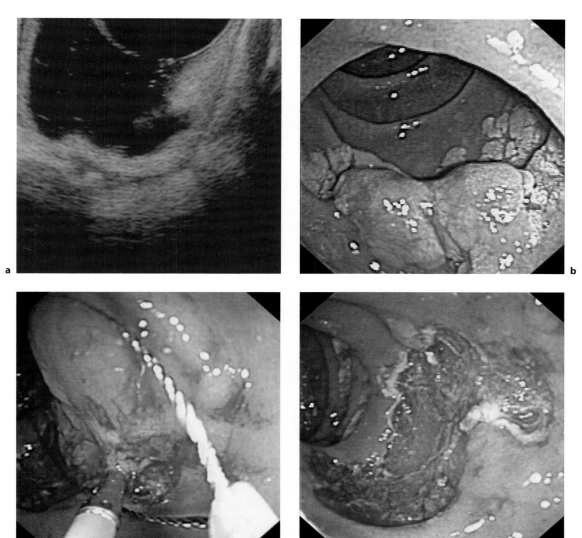

◧ Fig. 2.1-4a–d. Large broad-based duo-denal adenomas. **a** Endoscopic ultrasound image. **b** Endoscopic image. **c** Mucosecto-my using double-channel therapeutic endoscope. **d** Result after mucosectomy

Ileocolonoscopy

Colonoscopy is the method of choice for diagnosis and increasingly for therapy of lower gastrointestinal (GI) diseases (Cappel and Friedel 2002a, b). In patients with GI bleeding, colonoscopy can provide diagnosis of the underlying disease in most cases with normal EGD. Diagnoses include diverticular disease, colonic polyps and cancer, angiectasias especially of the cecum, inflammatory bowel disease (IBD), or infection.

Ileocolonoscopy is still the mainstay for the diagnosis of IBD (Hommes and van Deventer 2004). Approximately 5–30 cm of the terminal ileum can be visualized after intubation of the ileocecal valve during colonoscopy (◘ Fig. 2.1-5a). Endoscopic evaluation and optional biopsy of the terminal ileum are of particular importance in the diagnosis of Crohn's disease (◘ Fig. 2.1-5c) and lymphoma (◘ Fig. 2.1-5b). Microbiologic investigation of biopsies from ulcers in the terminal ileum, ileocecal valve, or colon may give the diagnostic clue in infections that are hardly diagnosed from stool specimens as in tuberculosis or cytomegalovirus infection.

Bowel strictures due to scarring can be treated by balloon dilatation (◘ Fig. 2.1-5d).

> ❶ EGD or ileocolonoscopy prior to video capsule endoscopy may cause mucosal defects due to biopsy, endoscope passage, or coagulation which should not be confused with preexisting lesions.

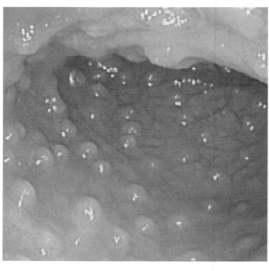
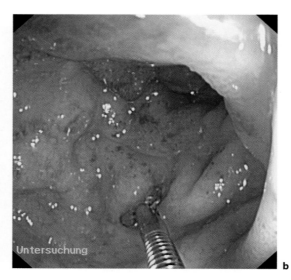
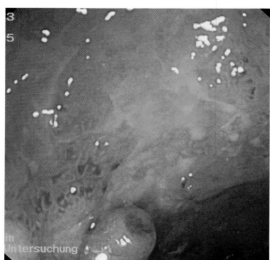
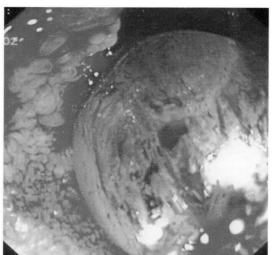

◘ **Fig. 2.1-5a–d.** Ileoscopy. **a** Lymph follicle hyperplasia in a child. **b** Biopsy of a lymphoma. **c** Non-stricturing Crohn's disease. **d** Balloon dilatation of a Crohn's stricture

Push Enteroscopy

The proximal part of the small bowel can be visualized with an extended length endoscope introduced perorally. A pediatric colonoscope or special enteroscope can be used for this purpose. These instruments have all the functions of an ordinary gastroscope such as steering, irrigation, air insufflation, suction, and a standard working channel with a length of up to 250 cm. Special accessories such as biopsy forceps, snares, injection needles, and argon plasma coagulation probes enable the examiner to perform any kind of diagnostic and therapeutic procedure (◘ Figs. 2.1-6–2.1-8) (Landi et al. 1998; Rossini and Gay 1998; Swain 1999).

No more than about 50% of the small bowel is accessible to push enteroscopy. In practice, the attainable depth of insertion is often considerably less. In one report, intubation 61 cm past the pylorus could be increased to 72 cm by using an overtube to prevent looping of the enteroscope within the stomach (Benz et al. 2001). A similar gain was described with a variable stiffness enteroscope (Harewood et al. 2003). The limited insertion depth accounts for the poorer diagnostic yield of push enteroscopy compared with VCE. However, a high incidence of bleeding lesions in the jejunum as in chronic renal failure (Lepere et al. 2005) may justify primary application of push enteroscopy after inconclusive EGD.

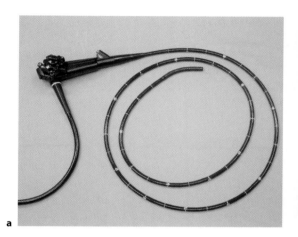
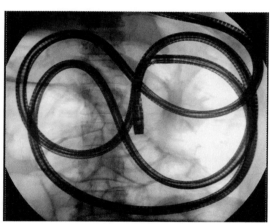

a   b

◘ **Fig. 2.1-6.** **a** SIF Q140 enteroscope. **b** Position checked by fluoroscopy

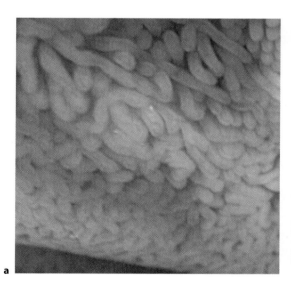
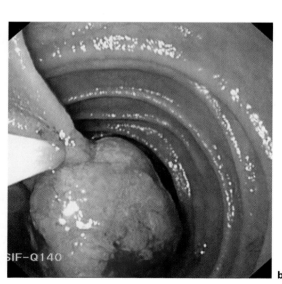

a   b

◘ **Fig. 2.1-7.** **a** Zoom enteroscopy. **b** Polypectomy

2

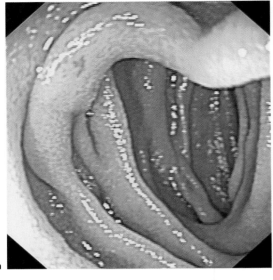

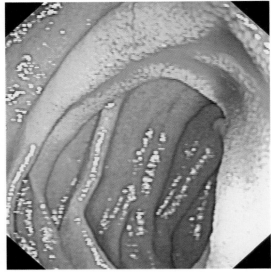

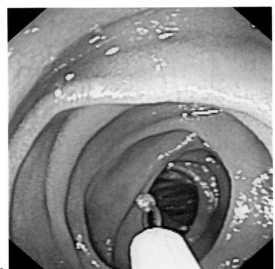

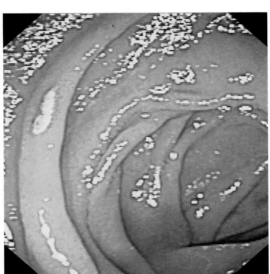

Fig. 2.1-8a–d. Push enteroscopy. Small vascular ectasia of the jejunum (**a**) bleeds actively only in response to air insufflation and instrument passage (**b**). **c** Tip of a polypectomy snare for electrocoagulation. **d** Scar after coagulation of the vascular ectasia, hemostasis

References

Benz C, Jakobs R, Riemann JF (2001) Do we need the overtube for push enteroscopy? Endoscopy 33:658–661

Cammarota G, Cianci R, Gasbarrini G (2005) High-resolution magnifying video endoscopy in primary intestinal lymphangiectasia: a new role for endoscopy? Endoscopy 37:607

Cappell MS, Friedel D (2002a) The role of sigmoidoscopy and colonoscopy in the diagnosis and management of lower gastrointestinal disorders: endoscopic findings, therapy, and complications. Med Clin North Am 86:1253–1288

Cappell MS, Friedel D (2002b) The role of sigmoidoscopy and colonoscopy in the diagnosis and management of lower gastrointestinal disorders: technique, indications, and contraindications. Med Clin North Am 86:1217–1252

Harewood GC, Gostout CJ, Farrell MA, Knipschield MA (2003) Prospective controlled assessment of variable stiffness enteroscopy. Gastrointest Endosc 58:267–271

Hayat M, Axon AT, O'Mahony S (2000) Diagnostic yield and effect on clinical outcomes of push enteroscopy in suspected small-bowel bleeding. Endoscopy 32:369–372

Hommes DW, van Deventer SJ (2004) Endoscopy in inflammatory bowel diseases. Gastroenterology 126:1561–1573

Kiesslich R, Mergener K, Naumann C et al (2003) Value of chromoendoscopy and magnification endoscopy in the evaluation of duodenal abnormalities: a prospective, randomized comparison. Endoscopy 35:559–563

Landi B, Tkoub M, Gaudric M et al (1998) Diagnostic yield of push-type enteroscopy in relation to indication. Gut 42:421–425

Lepere C, Cuillerier E, Van Gossum A et al (2005) Predictive factors of positive findings in patients explored by push enteroscopy for unexplained GI bleeding. Gastrointest Endosc 61:709–714

Rossini FP, Gay G (1998) Atlas of enteroscopy. Springer, Milan

Sharma BC, Bhasin DK, Makharia G et al (2000) Diagnostic value of push-type enteroscopy: a report from India. Am J Gastroenterol 95:137–140

Swain CP (1999) The role of enteroscopy in clinical practice. Gastrointest Endosc Clin N Am 9:135–144

2.2   Double-Balloon Endoscopy

H. Yamamoto, C. Ell, H. Kita, A. May

The method of double-balloon endoscopy introduced by Yamamoto (Yamamoto et al. 2001) permits the noninvasive endoscopic evaluation of the small bowel while also providing therapeutic access (May et al. 2003; Yamamoto et al. 2003; Ell et al. 2005; Di Caro et al. 2005; May et al. 2005a). A specifically designed video endoscope (outer diameter 8.5 mm for the regular type, Fujinon EN450 P5, and 9.4 mm for the therapeutic type, Fujinon EN450 T5, working length 200 cm) with an attachable balloon at its tip and a soft overtube (length 145 cm) with another balloon at the distal end are used together (◘ Fig. 2.2-1a). In order to make insertion procedures safe as well as effective, latex soft balloons are used for both the endoscope and the overtube, and a specifically designed pump has also been developed, which can inflate and deflate the balloons with one touch while accurately monitoring the balloon pressure (◘ Fig. 2.2-1b). First the overtube is inflated in the duodenum to fix its position, and the endoscope is advanced deeper into the bowel through the stationary outer tube. Next the balloon at the distal end of the endoscope is inflated to fix the position of the scope, and the overtube balloon is deflated and advanced. If the endoscope and overtube are now withdrawn with both balloons inflated, the small bowel will invaginate over the outertube, shortening and pleating like an accordion. The endoscope can then be deflated and advanced even farther distally. This process is repeated, aided by intermittent fluoroscopy, until all relevant portions of the small bowel have been examined (◘ Fig. 2.2-2a, b). This technique can be used from the anal side as well (◘ Fig. 2.2-3a, b) (Miyata et al. 2004). A combination of oral and anal approaches can be used for a patient to examine the entire small bowel if necessary. Total enteroscopy can be confirmed by reaching an ink mark from the opposite approach that was placed during the initial examination. The success rate of total enteroscopy using the double-balloon endoscopy is reported to be over 80% by combination of both approaches (Yamamoto et al. 2004). A model using porcine organs for training purposes has been developed (May et al. 2005b).

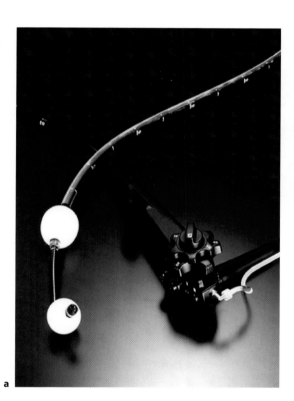

a

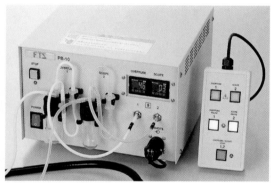

b

◘ Fig. 2.2-1a, b. Double-balloon endoscope (Fujinon EN-450P5/20): working length 200 cm, outer diameter of endoscope 8.5 mm, working channel 2.2 mm (**a**), with air pump for inflating both balloons (**b**) (reprinted from Yamamoto 2005 with permission from the American Gastroenterological Association)

2

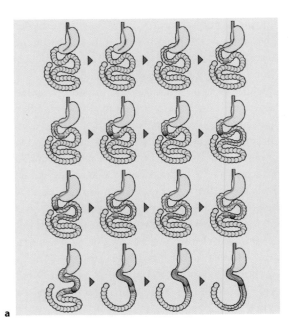

a

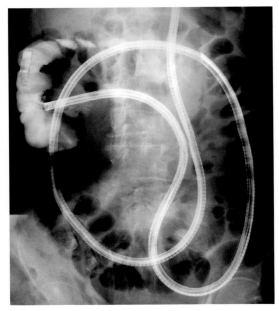

b

Fig. 2.2-2a, b. Illustrations demonstrate the sequential maneuvers of the instruments in the oral insertion of the double-balloon endoscopy (**a**) (reprinted from Yamamoto 2005 with permission from the American Gastroenterological Association). X-ray image of enteroscope inserted from the mouth to the ascending colon (**b**) (reprinted from Yamamoto et al. 2003 with permission from the American Gastroenterological Association)

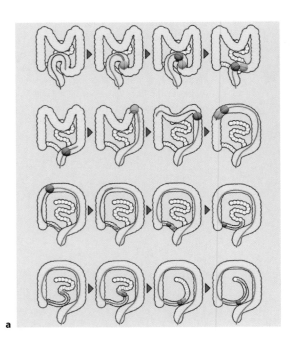

a

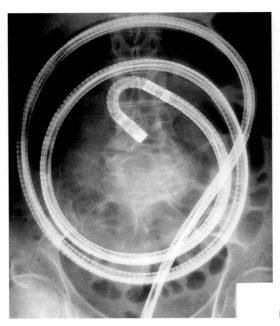

b

Fig. 2.2-3a, b. Illustrations demonstrate the sequential maneuvers of the instruments in the anal insertion of the double-balloon endoscopy (**a**) (reprinted from Yamamoto 2005 with permission from the American Gastroenterological Association). X-ray image of enteroscope with anal approach (**b**) (reprinted from Yamamoto et al. 2003 with permission from the American Gastroenterological Association)

Double-balloon endoscopy also enables endoscopic observation of a blind loop or afferent loop (Kuno et al. 2004), and is also even applicable for the evaluation of strictures of the small bowel (Sunada et al. 2004). Moreover, to and fro observation of an affected area with controlled movement of the endoscope with an accessory channel enables interventions, including biopsies, hemostasis (◻ Figs. 2.2-4a–c to 2.2-5a, b) (Nishimura et al. 2004), balloon dilatation (◻ Fig. 2.2-6a–d), stent placement, polypectomy (◻ Fig. 2.2-7a, b) (Kita et al. 2005), and endoscopic mucosal resection (◻ Fig. 2.2-8a, b). Thus, the double-balloon endoscopy has distinct advantages that can complement the limitation of capsule endoscopy.

Double-balloon endoscopy may well eliminate the need for intraoperative enteroscopy in many patients.

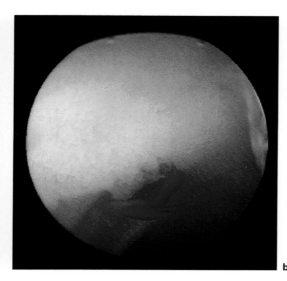
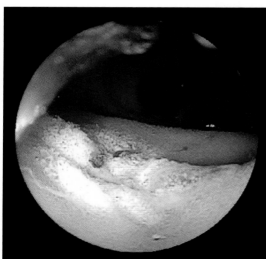

a

b

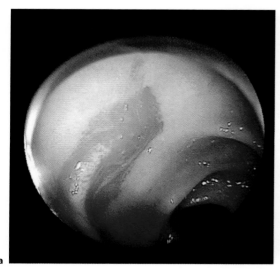

c

◻ Fig. 2.2-4a–c. Endoscopic hemostasis using electrosurgical coagulation for bleeding from jejunal angiodysplasia. Endoscopic image of bleeding angiodysplasia (**a**). Observation of the same angiodysplasia in water (**b**). Endoscopic image of the region after hemostasis (**c**) (reprinted from Yamamoto et al. 2004 with permission from the American Gastroenterological Association)

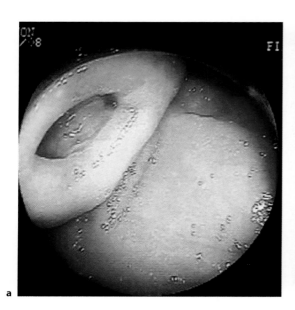
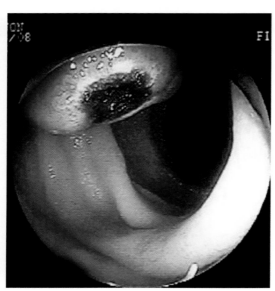

a

b

◻ Fig. 2.2-5a, b. Endoscopic hemostasis using electrosurgical coagulation for bleeding from jejunal gastrointestinal stromal tumor. Tumor with central ulceration (**a**). Endoscopic image of the region after hemostasis (**b**) (reprinted from Nishimura et al. 2004)

2

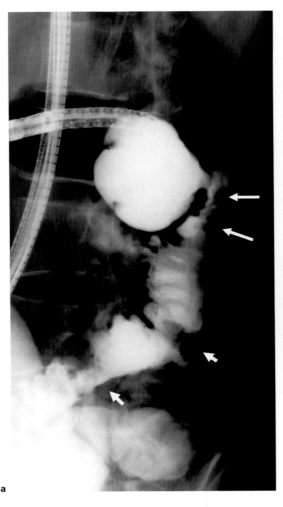

a

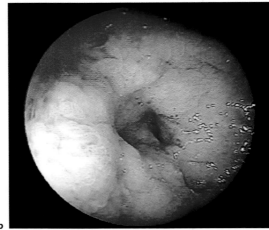

b

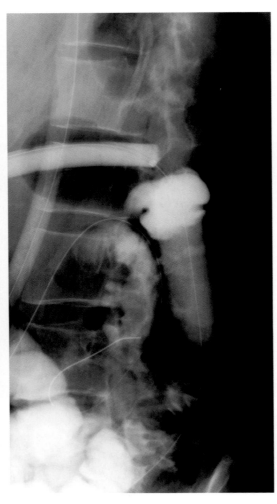

c

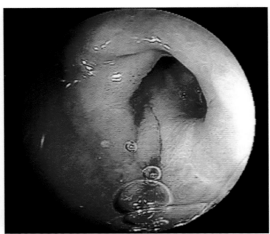

d

◘ Fig. 2.2-6a–d. Fluoroscopic image of the water-soluble contrast study of the small bowel while inflating the balloon on the tip of the endoscope showing one major stricture segment (*arrows*) and multiple smaller strictures (*arrowheads*) (**a**). Endoscopic view of the tight fibrotic stricture in the small bowel before dilation (**b**). Insertion of the balloon catheter into the major stricture through the overtube with the assistance of a guidewire (**c**). Endoscopic view after dilatation (**d**) (reprinted from Sunada et al. 2004 with permission from Blackwell Publishing Asia)

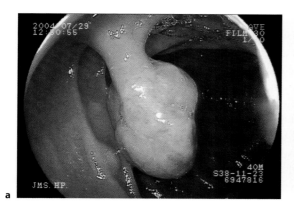

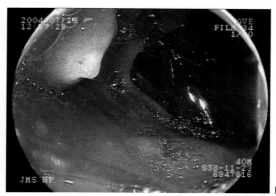

Fig. 2.2-7a, b. Endoscopic view of Peutz-Jeghers polyp in the jejunum (**a**). Endoscopic view showing the polypectomy site (**b**)

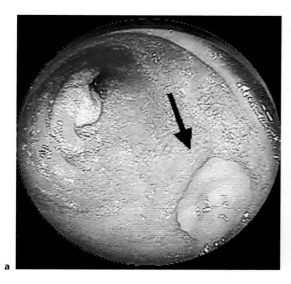

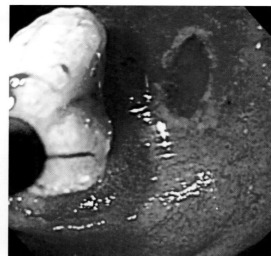

Fig. 2.2-8a, b. Endoscopic view of the tumor (*arrow*) near closed end of the duodenal afferent loop (**a**). Endoscopic view showing endoscopic mucosal resection site and tumor in the forceps (**b**) (reprinted from Kuno et al. 2004 with permission from the American Society for Gastrointestinal Endoscopy)

References

Di Caro S, May A, Heine DG et al (2005) The European experience with double balloon enteroscopy: indications, methodology, safety and clinical impact. Gastrointest Endosc 62:545–550

Ell C, May A, Nachbar L, Cellier C, Landi B, di Caro S, Gasbarrini A (2005) Push-and-pull enteroscopy in the small bowel using the double-balloon technique: results of a prospective European multicenter study. Endoscopy 37:613–616

Kita H, Yamamoto H, Nakamura T et al (2005) Bleeding polyp in the mid small intestine identified by capsule endoscopy and treated by double-balloon endoscopy. Gastrointest Endosc 61:628–629

Kuno A, Yamamoto H, Kita H et al (2004) Application of double-balloon enteroscopy through Roux-en-Y anastomosis for the endoscopic mucosal resection of an early carcinoma in the duodenal afferent limb. Gastrointest Endosc 60:1032–1034

May A, Nachbar L, Wardak A et al (2003) Double-balloon enteroscopy: preliminary experience in patients with obscure gastrointestinal bleeding or chronic abdominal pain. Endoscopy 35:985–991

May A, Nachbar L, Ell C (2005a) Double-balloon enteroscopy (push-and-pull enteroscopy) of the small bowel: feasibility and diagnostic and therapeutic yield in patients with suspected small bowel disease. Gastrointest Endosc 62:62–70

May A, Nachbar L, Schneider M et al (2005b) Push-and-pull enteroscopy using the double-balloon technique: method of assessing depth of insertion and training of the enteroscopy technique using the Erlangen Endo-Trainer. Endoscopy 37:66–70

Miyata T, Yamamoto H, Kita H et al (2004) A case of inflammatory fibroid polyp causing small bowel intussusception in which retrograde double-balloon enteroscopy was useful for the preoperative diagnosis. Endoscopy 36:344–347

Nishimura M, Yamamoto H, Kita H et al (2004) Gastrointestinal stromal tumor in the jejunum: diagnosis and control of bleeding with electrocoagulation by using double-balloon enteroscopy. J Gastroenterol 39:1001–1004

Ohmiya N, Taguchi A, Shirai K et al (2005) Endoscopic resection of Peutz-Jeghers polyps throughout the small intestine at double-balloon enteroscopy without laparotomy. Gastrointest Endosc 61:140–147

Sunada K, Yamamoto H, Kita H et al (2004) Case report: successful treatment with balloon dilatation in combination with double-balloon enteroscopy of a stricture in the small bowel of a patient with Crohn's disease. Digestive Endoscopy 16:237–240

Yamamoto H (2005) Double balloon endoscopy. Clin Gastroenterol Hepatol 3 [Suppl 1]: S27-S29

Yamamoto H, Kita H, Sunada K et al (2004) Clinical outcomes of double-balloon endoscopy for the diagnosis and treatment of small-intestinal diseases. Clin Gastroenterol Hepatol 2:1010–1016

Yamamoto H, Sekine Y, Sato Y et al (2001) Total enteroscopy with a nonsurgical steerable double-balloon method. Gastrointest Endosc 53:216–220

Yamamoto H, Sugano K (2003) A new method of enteroscopy – the double-balloon method. Can J Gastroenterol 17:273–274

Yamamoto H, Yano T, Kita H et al (2003) New system of double-balloon enteroscopy for diagnosis and treatment of small intestinal disorders. Gastroenterology 125:1556; author reply 1556–1557

Yoshida N, Wakabayashi N, Nomura K et al (2004) Ileal mucosa-associated lymphoid tissue lymphoma showing several ulcer scars detected using double-balloon endoscopy. Endoscopy 36:1022–1024

Internet

www.fujinon.de/produkte: double-balloon enteroscope: Fujinon Europe
tv.fujinon.jp/products/endoscope/shouchou/index.html: Fujinon Japan

2.3   Intraoperative Endoscopy

D. Hartmann, H.J. Schulz, J.F. Riemann

Intraoperative enteroscopy is generally carried out as the ultimate diagnostic procedure for complete evaluation and treatment of the small bowel. Due to the potential for associated morbidity and mortality, the use of this procedure is recommended only after less invasive procedures have failed to yield a diagnosis. Exploratory laparotomy without intraoperative enteroscopy is not recommended because it subjects the patient to all the risks of surgery without the benefit of a complete endoscopic examination to detect subtle mucosal lesions that can be missed by palpation and transillumination alone.

Technique

Laparotomy has been coupled with the passage of an endoscope orally, transnasally (using a sonde endoscope), per rectum, or through enter-

otomies performed on the small bowel (□ Fig. 2.3-1). The standard procedure consists of a laparotomy followed by one or two small enterotomy incisions through which the endoscope (standard colonoscope, preferably pediatric, push enteroscope, sonde enteroscope (D'Agostino et al. 1997), or even a standard gastroscope) is introduced. A laparoscopically assisted total enteroscopy has also been described (Ingrosso et al. 1999). The advantages of intraoperative enteroscopy through an enterotomy include elimination of intestinal dead space (i.e., esophagus, stomach, and duodenum or colon and rectum) that presumably was already extensively examined before intraoperative enteroscopy and decreased trauma to the bowel.

After enterotomy the endoscope is advanced through the small bowel with the assistance of the surgeon, who pleats the small bowel over the endoscope. Examination is performed while the endoscope is being advanced because surgical manipulation can create artifacts that can be mistaken for potential bleeding lesions.

Treatment may be performed endoscopically, or the affected small bowel segments may be identified endoscopically and then treated surgically, usually in the form of a segmental resection (Douard et al. 2000; Rodriguez-Bigas et al. 1995).

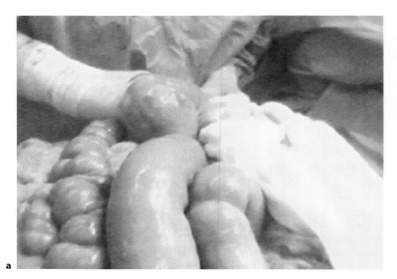
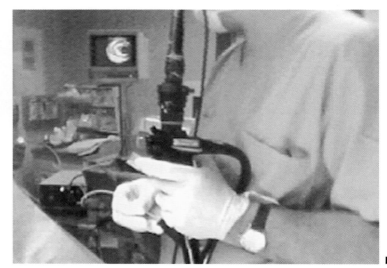

a   b

□ **Fig. 2.3-1a, b.** Intraoperative enteroscopy. **a** Intraoperative view of the exposed small bowel. **b** Endoscopist with a mobile endoscopy unit in the operating room

Complications

Complications include mucosal laceration, intramural hematomas, mesenteric hemorrhage, perforation, prolonged ileus, Ogilvie's syndrome, intestinal ischemia, intestinal obstruction, wound infection, and postoperative pulmonary infection. Mortality related to the procedure or to postoperative complications has been up to 11% (Lewis et al. 1991; Desa et al. 1991).

Diagnostic Yield

When performed for obscure gastrointestinal bleeding, the ability of intraoperative enteroscopy to identify potential bleeding lesions (◘ Figs. 2.3-2–2.3-4) has been impressive, ranging from 70 to 100% (◘ Table 2.3-1).

◘ **Table 2.3-1.** Intraoperative enteroscopy in obscure gastrointestinal bleeding

Author	Patients (n)	Diagnostic yield
Bowden et al. 1980	18	89%
Lau et al. 1987	15	80%
Flickinger et al. 1989	14	93%
Lewis et al. 1991	23	87%
Desa et al. 1991	12	83%
Ress et al. 1992	44	70%
Szold et al. 1992	30	93%
Lopez et al. 1996	16	88%
Dourad et al. 2000	20	80%
Kendrick et al. 2001	70	74%
Jakobs et al. 2006	81	84%

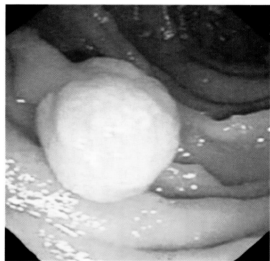

◘ **Fig. 2.3-2.** Intraoperative endoscopy: large Peutz-Jeghers polyp in the distal jejunum

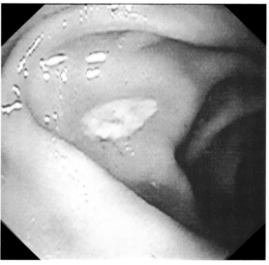

◘ **Fig. 2.3-3.** Intraoperative view of a small ulcer in the proximal jejunum due to chronic nonsteroidal anti-inflammatory drug intake

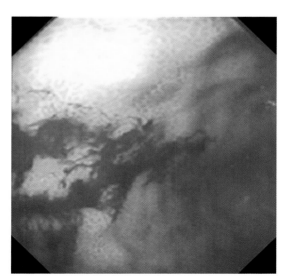

◘ **Fig. 2.3-4.** Intraoperative view of a bleeding angiectasia

Video Capsule Endoscopy and Intraoperative Enteroscopy

To calculate the sensitivity and specificity of video capsule endoscopy, we performed a prospective, blinded study to compare the diagnostic yield of capsule endoscopy with intraoperative enteroscopy as the gold standard in patients (*n*=47) with obscure digestive bleeding and negative standard endoscopic work-up (Hartmann et al. 2005). Within

7 days after video capsule endoscopy, intraoperative enteroscopy was performed during open laparotomy (◘ Fig. 2.3-5). Compared with intraoperative enteroscopy, the sensitivity, specificity, positive and negative predictive value of capsule endoscopy were 95, 75, 95, and 86%, respectively. Based on these data we suggest that patients with obscure gastrointestinal bleeding and with negative bidirectional endoscopy are candidates for use of video capsule endoscopy in clinical practice.

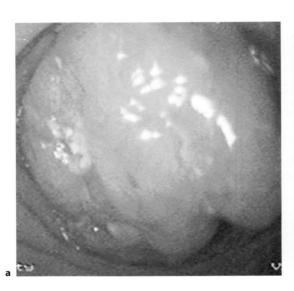

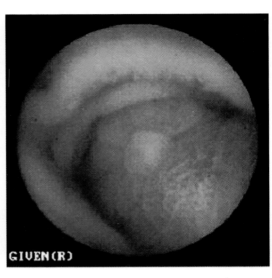

◘ Fig. 2.3-5a–c. Large hyperplastic polyp of the jejunum in a patient with obscure gastrointestinal bleeding: **a** intraoperative view, **b** video capsule endoscopy, **c** segmental resection of the jejunum

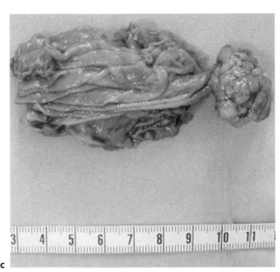

References

Bowden TA Jr, Hooks VH 3rd, Mansberger AR Jr (1980) Intraoperative gastrointestinal endoscopy. Ann Surg 191:680–687

D'Agostino JA, Petros JG, Semegran AB et al (1997) Complete intraoperative Sonde enteroscopy in the evaluation of recurrent partial small-bowel obstruction. Gastrointest Endosc 46:577–578

Desa LA, Ohri SK, Hutton KA et al (1991) Role of intraoperative enteroscopy in obscure gastrointestinal bleeding of small bowel origin. Br J Surg 78:192–195

Douard R, Wind P, Panis Y et al (2000) Intraoperative enteroscopy for diagnosis and management of unexplained gastrointestinal bleeding. Am J Surg 180:181–184

Flickinger EG, Stanforth AC, Sinar DR et al (1989) Intraoperative video panendoscopy for diagnosing sites o f chronic intestinal bleeding. Am J Surg 157:137–144

Hartmann D, Schmitt H, Bolz G et al (2005) A prospective two-center study comparing wireless capsule endoscopy with intraoperative enteroscopy in patients with obscure gastrointestinal bleeding. Gastrointest Endosc 61:826–832

Ingrosso M, Prete F, Pisani A et al (1999) Laparoscopically assisted total enteroscopy: a new approach to small intestinal diseases. Gastrointest Endosc 49:651–653

Jakobs R, Hartmann D, Benz C et al (2006) Diagnosis of obscure gastrointestinal bleeding by intra-operative enteroscopy in 81 consecutive patients. World J Gastroenterol 12:313–316

Kendrick ML, Buttar NS, Anderson MA et al (2001) Contribution of intraoperative enteroscopy in the management of obscure gastrointestinal bleeding. J Gastrointest Surg 5:162–167

Lau WY, Fan ST, Wong SH et al (1987) Preoperative and intraoperative localisation of gastrointestinal bleeding of obscure origin. Gut 28:869–877

Lewis BS, Wenger JS, Waye JD (1991) Small bowel enteroscopy and intraoperative enteroscopy for obscure gastrointestinal bleeding. Am J Gastroenterol 86:171–174

Lopez MJ, Cooley JS, Petros JG, Sullivan JG, Cave DR (1996) Complete intraoperative small-bowel endoscopy in the evaluation of occult gastrointestinal bleeding using the sonde enteroscope. Arch Surg 131:272–277

Ress AM, Benacci JC, Sarr MG (1992) Efficacy of intraoperative enteroscopy in diagnosis and prevention of recurrent, occult gastrointestinal bleeding. Am J Surg 163:94–98

Rodriguez-Bigas MA, Penetrante RB, Herrera L et al (1995) Intraoperative small bowel enteroscopy in familial adenomatous and familial juvenile polyposis. Gastrointest Endosc 42:560–564

Szold A, Katz LB, Lewis BS (1992) Surgical approach to occult gastrointestinal bleeding. Am J Surg 163:90–92

2.4 Non-endoscopic Imaging Studies

E.-J. Malzfeldt, A.K. Hara, O.-H. Wegener

Ultrasound

Ultrasound is a noninvasive modality for examining the small bowel. Sites of wall thickening, stenoses (◼ Fig. 2.4-1a), and abscesses can be demonstrated, depending on their location. As a real-time study, ultrasound can be used to evaluate intestinal peristalsis, and color Doppler can be added to define the vascularity of the bowel wall (◼ Fig. 2.4-1b).

Because sonographic signs are often nonspecific, the role of ultrasound is basically limited to preliminary examinations and follow-ups. Patient-related factors such as obesity and tympanites can greatly limit the accuracy of the ultrasound study, whose quality also depends critically on the experience of the examiner.

Radiographic Methods

Plain Abdominal Radiograph

The plain abdominal radiograph is a simple but nonspecific tool in the diagnosis of certain abdominal diseases. Image analysis is based largely on the distribution of fluids, calcifications, and especially gases. Attention is given to fluid levels, the shape and width of the bowel loops, and the presence of gas in the bowel wall, blood vessels, bile ducts, and abdominal cavity. Perforations and bowel obstructions can usually be confidently identified (◼ Fig. 2.4-2), but generally their cause cannot be determined from abdominal radiographs alone.

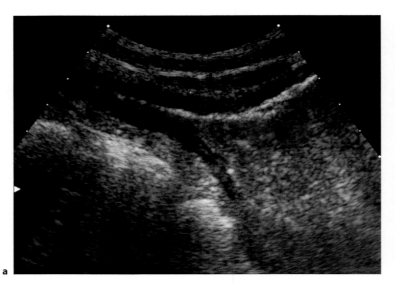

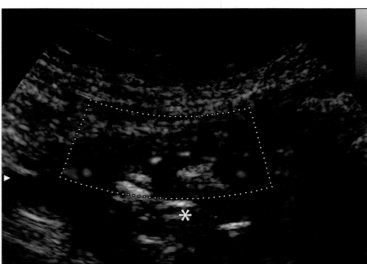

◼ **Fig. 2.4-1a, b.** Crohn's disease: thickened loop of small bowel with marked prestenotic dilatation (**a**) and thickened loop of small bowel with increased perfusion at power Doppler; adjacent conglomerate mass* (**b**)

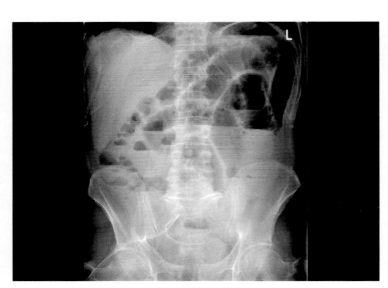

◼ **Fig. 2.4-2.** Plain abdominal radiograph: small bowel obstruction and free intraperitoneal air

Upper Gastrointestinal Series

The upper gastrointestinal series after oral contrast administration provides information on the dynamics and disturbances of intestinal transit. A detailed evaluation requires a small bowel follow through (SBFT), which includes an alternating series of survey views and spot views aided by palpation. Mucosal lesions, diverticula, fistulae, and stenoses can be detected and localized with this technique. Drawbacks are the unpredictable transit time and the frequent difficulty of evaluating coils of intestine within the pelvis.

Enteroclysis

Enteroclysis is a small bowel enema using barium and methylcellulose administered by duodenal intubation (Sellink method). The mucosa can be clearly evaluated within the uniformly distended and opacified bowel lumen. The indications for this study have declined with the increasing refinement of cross-sectional imaging modalities, but it is still used in the diagnosis of stenoses (◻ Fig. 2.4-3) and the differential diagnosis of mucosal abnormalities (Antes 2003; Nolan and Traill 1997).

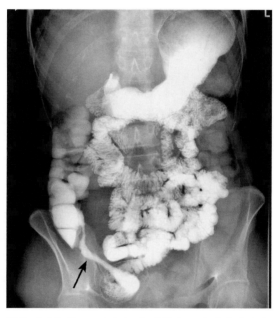

◻ **Fig. 2.4-3.** Enteroclysis by the Sellink method: Crohn's disease with a long stenotic segment of terminal ileum (*arrow*)

Cross-sectional Imaging Modalities

Computed Tomography (CT), CT Enterography/Enteroclysis (CTE)

CT is a cross-sectional imaging modality that is a rapid, noninvasive method of evaluating the small bowel (Maglinte et al. 2003). A CT examination delivers a radiation dose that is approximately equal to that in an enteroclysis study. While CT provides less soft tissue contrast than magnetic resonance imaging (MRI), it offers higher spatial resolution with a very short examination time and a high resistance to artifacts. The advantage compared to enteroclysis is the ability to provide non-superimposed views of all small bowel loops as well as any mesenteric and extraintestinal lesions that are present (◻ Fig. 2.4-4). As a rule, these capabilities offset the disadvantage of decreased mucosal surface details compared with enteroclysis.

The CTE technique usually requires distention of the small bowel lumen with 1200–1500 cc of a low-density, negative oral contrast such as water or a 0.1% weight/volume barium sulfate suspension. The intraluminal contrast can be administered either following nasojejunal intubation or orally. Intravenous contrast is also routinely administered to allow assessment of mucosal vascularity and bowel wall enhancement.

Magnetic Resonance (MR) Enterography/Enteroclysis (MRE)

MRE is another cross-sectional imaging modality being used to evaluate the small bowel, particularly in patients with Crohn's disease. Like CT, oral and intravenous contrast is used. Unlike CT, radiation is not used. MRE provides better soft tissue discrimination (◻ Fig. 2.4-5) but is more susceptible to extraneous disturbances and motion artifacts. Longer examination times, claustrophobia, and the presence of metallic implants also limit its use.

Today both CTE and MRE are evolving at a rapid pace, permitting the increasingly accurate diagnosis of inflammatory, vascular, and neoplastic diseases of the small bowel (Horton et al. 2004; Schmidt et al. 2003; Umschaden et al. 2000). It remains to be seen whether the results will justify the added cost and complexity of the examinations.

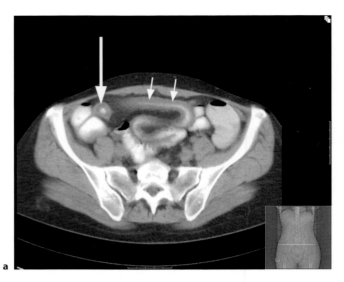

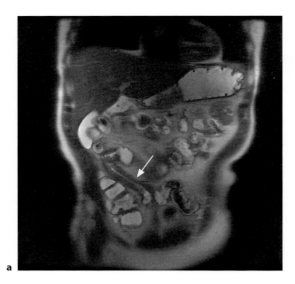

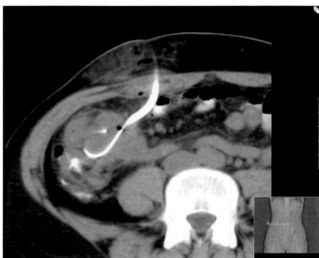

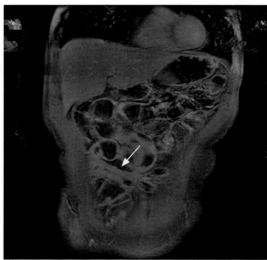

Fig. 2.4-4a, b. Abdominal CT scans in Crohn's disease. **a** Inflammatory wall thickening and stenosis of the neoterminal ileum after ileocecal resection (*thin arrows*), complicated by an adjacent loop abscess (*thick arrows*). **b** Appearance following CT-guided drain insertion

Fig. 2.4-5a, b. MR enterography (MRE) in a patient with Crohn's disease. **a** Coronal T2-weighted MRE demonstrates marked thickening of the terminal ileum. **b** Coronal gadolinium-enhanced MRE shows marked enhancement in the terminal ileum.

Angiography

Angiography provides detailed views of blood flow disturbances in the small bowel, especially at the level of the smaller vessels as in non-occlusive ischemia. Occlusive diseases of the large vessels can generally be diagnosed adequately and noninvasively by computed tomography.

In patients with gastrointestinal bleeding, angiography permits a targeted search for vascular lesions (e.g., vascular ectasias), making it possible to identify the bleeding source even between bleeding episodes (Fig. 2.4-6a) and guide an interventional procedure (Fig. 2.4-6b). Angiography can detect active bleeding in 39–67% of cases in selected patient groups, although this requires fairly profuse bleeding with a blood loss of at least 0.5–3.0 ml/min. This results in a high rate of false-negative findings (Pennoyer et al. 1997).

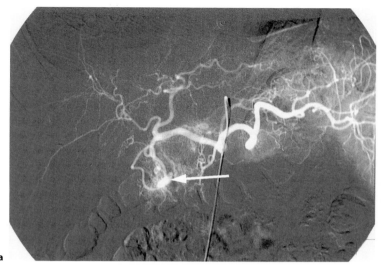
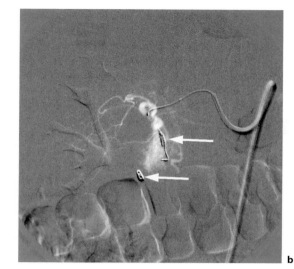

◼ Fig. 2.4-6a, b. Superselective digital subtraction angiography of the gastroduodenal artery: aneurysm (*arrow*) before (**a**) and after (**b**) the placement of metal coils (*arrows*) for embolization

Nuclear Medicine Studies

Because technetium pertechnate is secreted by gastric mucosa, radionuclide imaging can detect a Meckel's diverticulum if it contains ectopic gastric mucosa (Jewett et al. 1970; ◼ Fig. 4-6d). Since this ectopic tissue occurs in only 30–65% of all symptomatic adults, the findings are positive in only about 50% of cases. False-positive results may be caused by obstructions, inflammatory bowel disease, and arteriovenous malformations.

Gastrointestinal bleeding can be detected with Tc-Sn II-labeled erythrocytes at bleeding rates as low as 0.05–1 ml/min (◼ Fig. 2.4-7). Since the radiotracer is retained in the blood for up to 24 h, this method is ideally suited to the intermittent character of gastrointestinal bleeds and provides a sensitivity greater than 90%.

References

Antes G (2003) Konventionelle Dünn- und Dickdarmdiagnostik bei entzündlichen Darmerkrankungen. Radiologe 43:9–16

Horton KM, Fishman EK (2004) Multidetector-row computed tomography and 3-dimensional computed tomography imaging of small bowel neoplasms: current concept in diagnosis. J Comput Assist Tomogr 28:106–116

Jewett TC, Duszynski DO, Allen JE (1970) The visualization of Meckel's diverticulum with 99m Tc-pertechnetate. Surgery 68:567–570

Maglinte DD, Bender GN, Heitkamp DE, Lappas JC, Kelvin FM (2003) Multidetector-row helical CT enteroclysis. Radiol Clin North Am 41:249–262

Nolan DJ, Traill ZC (1997) The current role of the barium examination of the small intestine. Clin Radiol 52:809–820

Pennoyer W, Vignati P, Cohen J (1997) Mesenteric angiography for lower gastrointestinal hemorrhage: are there predictors for a positive study? Dis Colon Rectum 40:1014–1018

Schmidt S, Lepori D, Meuwly JY et al (2003) Prospective comparison of MR enteroclysis with multidetector spiral-CT enteroclysis: interobserver agreement and sensitivity by means of »sign-by-sign« correlation. Eur Radiol 13:1303–1311

Umschaden HW, Szolar D, Gasser J, Umschaden M, Haselbach H (2000) Small-bowel disease: comparison of MR enteroclysis images with conventional enteroclysis and surgical findings. Radiology 215:717–725

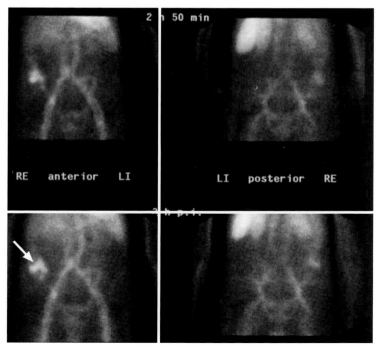

◼ Fig. 2.4-7. Radionuclide imaging with Tc-Sn II-labeled erythrocytes in a patient with occult gastrointestinal bleeding. The scans demonstrate a bleeding source in the terminal ileum with drainage into the cecum (*arrow*)

Normal Small Intestine

M. Keuchel, F. Hagenmüller, A. von Herbay

Macroscopic Anatomy

The small bowel is a tubular organ of 3–5 m in length, which starts at the pylorus and terminates at the ileocecal valve (von Herbay 1999). It is usually subdivided into the duodenum, jejunum, and ileum. The most proximal portion is the C-shaped duodenum, approximately 25 cm long, which is almost a fixed retroperitoneal structure. Four subdivisions of the duodenum are recognized: the first or superior portion (bulb, D1), the second or descending portion which includes the papilla of Vater (D2), the third or horizontal portion (D3), and the fourth or ascending portion (D4). At the duodenojejunal flexure (so-called ligament of Treitz), which is left of midline at the level of the second lumbar vertebra, the duodenum becomes continuous with the intra-abdominal small intestine. Just by convention, the jejunum comprises the upper two-fifths of the intraperitoneal small intestine, while the distal three-fifths are designated as ileum. The multiple intra-abdominal coils are mobile; they are attached to the mesentery (◘ Fig. 3-1).

The lumen of the small bowel is ringed by circular mucosal folds, the so-called valvulae conniventes (Kerckring's folds), which gradually decrease distally.

The arterial blood is supplied to the jejunum and ileum by anastomosing branches of the superior mesenteric artery. The duodenum additionally receives blood from the celiac trunk. Venous drainage is towards the portal venous system via the superior mesenteric veins and is parallel to the arteries. Lymphatic drainage starts in the villi with lymphatic capillaries which become confluent to form a central chylous vessel, passes through a submucous network into mesenteric lymphatic vessels and lymph nodes, finally entering via the thoracic duct into the venous circulation.

Microscopic Anatomy

The anatomical layers of the small bowel wall are, from the inside out: the mucosa, submucosa, muscularis propria, and serosa.

The mucosal surface is characterized by leaflike and fingerlike extensions, the villi. Intervening and beneath the villi are short tubular depressions, the crypts of Lieberkühn.

The epithelium is composed of specialized columnar cells, the enterocytes, mucus-producing goblet cells, secretory Paneth's cells, and diverse endocrine cells. A distinctive feature of the duodenum is the presence of mucoid Brunner's glands (Dobbins 1990).

While there are multiple disseminated lymphoid follicles along the duodenum, jejunum, and ileum, the terminal ileum contains aggregates of lymphoid follicles known as Peyer's plaques. They are covered by a specialized immunocompetent epithelium [microfold (M) cells]. Together they form the mucosa-associated lymphatic tissue (MALT).

Function

Two of the major functions of the small bowel are to break down and absorb nutrients, and to absorb water and electrolytes. The absorption of vitamin B_{12} occurs exclusively in the terminal ileum. Further functions are secretion, endocrine activity, motility, and immunological defense.

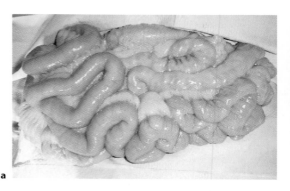

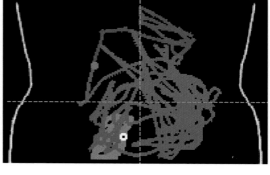

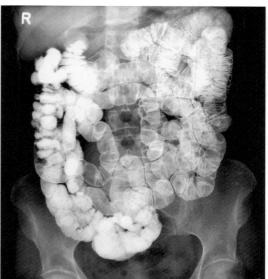

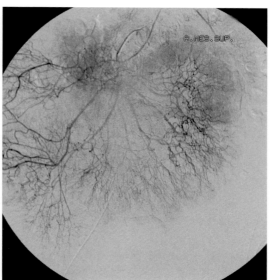

a

b

c

d

◘ **Fig. 3-1a–d.** Small bowel. **a** Intraoperative view (courtesy of Thomas Mansfeld, M.D.). **b** Localization software: passage of the video capsule through the small bowel (white ring: ileocecal valve; blue: stomach; green: small bowel; gray: cecum). **c** Contrast radiograph of the normal small bowel. **d** Selective digital subtraction angiography of the superior mesenteric artery demonstrating blood supply of the small bowel (courtesy of Doris Welger, M.D.)

Normal Video Capsule Endoscopy of the Small Intestine

The resolution of VCE provides a detailed view of the bowel mucosa including the villi.

Characteristics of the normal small bowel at VCE:

- Yellow-orange colored mucosa
- Circular folds
- Villi
- Small vessels, occasional larger veins
- Peristalsis: propulsive and occasional retropulsive contractions
- Bile, air bubbles, debris in secretions
- Lymph follicles in the terminal ileum

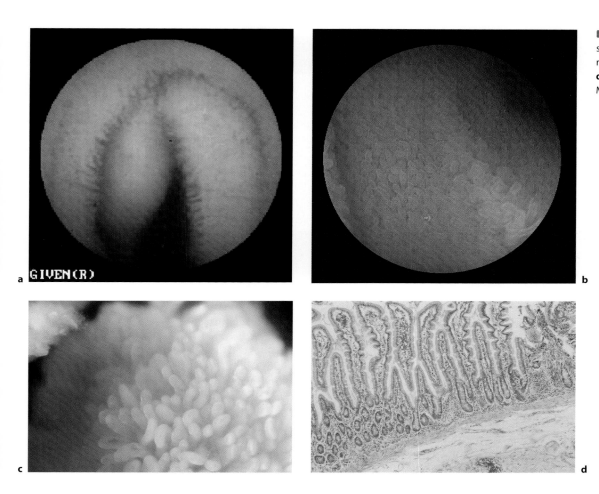

■ **Fig. 3-2a–d.** Villi in close-up, fluid-filled small bowel. **a** VCE. **b** Double ballon enteroscopy. **c** Reflected light microscopy. **d** Histology (H&E, courtesy of Jörg Caselitz, M.D.)

Villi

The villi in the fluid-filled small bowel can be very clearly seen and evaluated when viewed at a tangential angle (■ Fig. 3-2a, b). The high resolution of modern video endoscopy and VCE has substituted reflected light microscopy (■ Fig. 3-2c). The villi in the duodenal bulb (■ Fig. 3-9a) are broader and flatter than in the more distal small bowel. The villous architecture of the jejunum and ileum, on the other hand, can hardly be distinguished by endoscopic inspection (■ Fig. 3.3a, b).

3

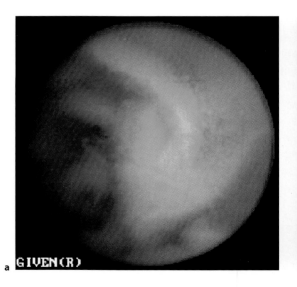

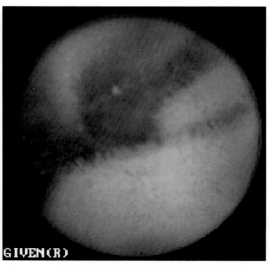

◨ **Fig. 3-3a, b.** The jejunum (**a**) and ileum (**b**) cannot be distinguished by endoscopy reliably just by the appearance of their villi

Vessels

Blood vessels are most clearly visualized when viewed directly from above. The vascular pattern in the ileum (◨ Fig. 3-4) is more distinct than in the other segments.

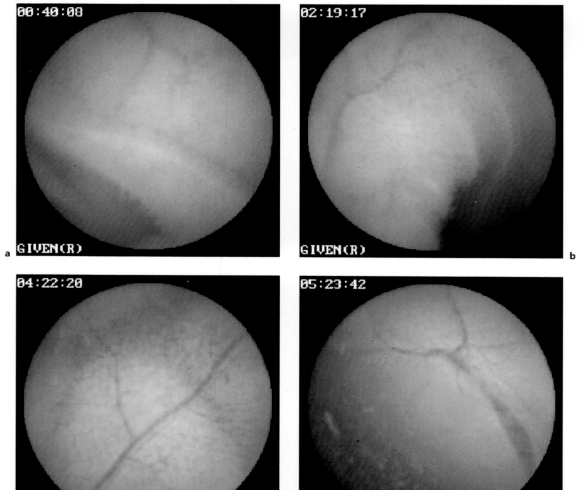

◨ **Fig. 3-4a–d.** The vascular markings tend to become more conspicuous as the capsule proceeds distally

Motility

The small bowel shows brisk peristaltic activity, recognized by the contraction and migration of the valvulae conniventes and small superimposed folds. The contractions show varying temporal patterns, with smaller bidirectional movements and intermittent forceful, propulsive contractions (◘ Fig. 3-5). This may temporarily arrest the movement of the capsule, propel it quickly forward, or occasionally cause it to move backward. In contrast to flexible endoscopy, bowel mobility can be observed during VCE with no effects from air insufflation (◘ Fig. 3-6) or sedatives. However, use of prokinetic drugs to shorten gastric passage of the capsule as well as bowel preparation before VCE may have a significant influence on small intestinal transit time. Transit times have been measured in patients (Chap. 1.3-1), whereas data on healthy subjects are sparse. Small intestinal transit in a small number of healthy volunteers was 143 min (Gat et al. 2001). So far there have been no relevant reports of experience in interpreting motility observations.

❶ The capsule may move past the same lesion several times due to bidirectional peristalsis, mimicking the presence of multiple lesions.

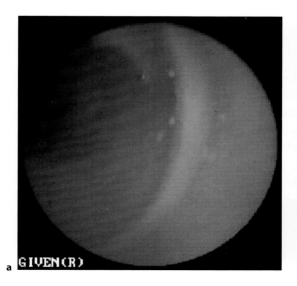
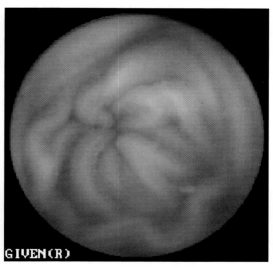

a   b

◘ **Fig. 3-5a, b.** Fluid-filled small bowel lumen (**a**), contracted lumen on the right side (**b**)

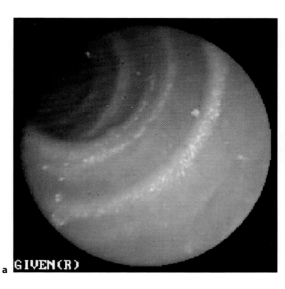
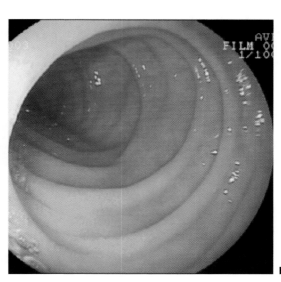

a   b

◘ **Fig. 3-6a, b.** Air-filled small bowel lumen with valvulae conniventes. VCE (**a**) and push enteroscopy (**b**). Compare with colonic motility (◘ Fig. 8.3-2)

Subdivision of the Small Intestine, Anatomical Landmarks

As there are no anatomical landmarks available, the subdivision of the small bowel in VCE interpretation is purely based on pragmatic considerations. The time that elapses between the reference points of the pylorus and the first cecal image is divided into three equal parts.

The jejunum and ileum are hardly distinguishable by their endoscopic features, but the duodenum and terminal ileum can be identified. Localization software is occasionally helpful in distinguishing the distal duodenum from the jejunum and the terminal ileum from the mid-ileum. These boundaries cannot be precisely defined, however.

Small bowel segments in VCE:

- Duodenum
- Proximal third of the small bowel
- Middle third of the small bowel
- Distal third of the small bowel
- Terminal ileum

Duodenum

While the capsule is still in the stomach, it is occasionally possible to get a transpyloric view into the duodenal bulb (☐ Fig. 3-7a). If the capsule is pointing in a favorable direction, the distal aspect of the pylorus may be visible from within the bulb as a circular ridge (☐ Fig. 3-7b). This should not be mistaken for abnormal folds or tumors, especially since this view may reappear after some time due to retrograde movement of the capsule. Brunner's glands may produce a nodular mucosal pattern (☐ Fig. 3-8). Folds are first seen past the apex of the bulb (☐ Fig. 3-9a), and circular folds first appear in the descending duodenum (☐ Fig. 3-9b). Bile is usually visible in the bowel lumen at this level.

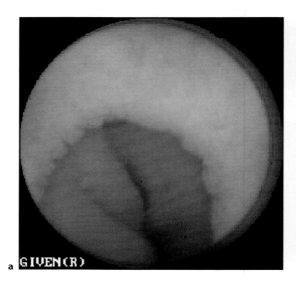

a   GIVEN(R)

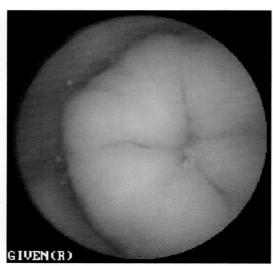

GIVEN(R)   b

☐ **Fig. 3-7.** **a** View through the pylorus into the duodenal bulb. **b** Retrograde view of the pylorus from within the duodenal bulb

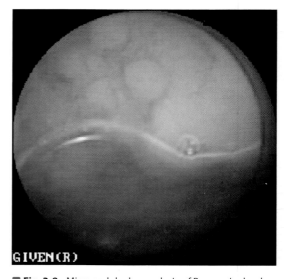

GIVEN(R)

☐ **Fig. 3-8.** Micronodular hyperplasia of Brunner's glands in the duodenal bulb

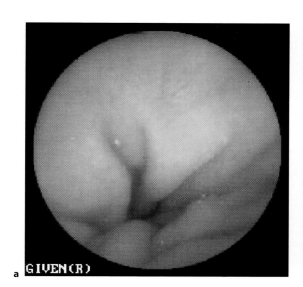

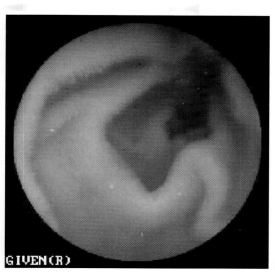

Fig. 3-9. a Duodenum, distal bulb.
b Duodenum, descending portion

Papilla of Vater

The papilla of Vater (■ Fig. 3-10) is rarely imaged by VCE.

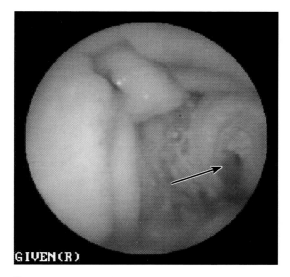

Fig. 3-10. Papilla of Vater with flow of bile from the pylorus (*arrow*)

3

Terminal Ileum

A characteristic feature of the terminal ileum is the presence of multiple small lymph follicles (□ Fig. 3-11). The vascular markings are more conspicuous than in the proximal small bowel. Sometimes vision is obscured due to inspissated bile, air bubbles, or feces.

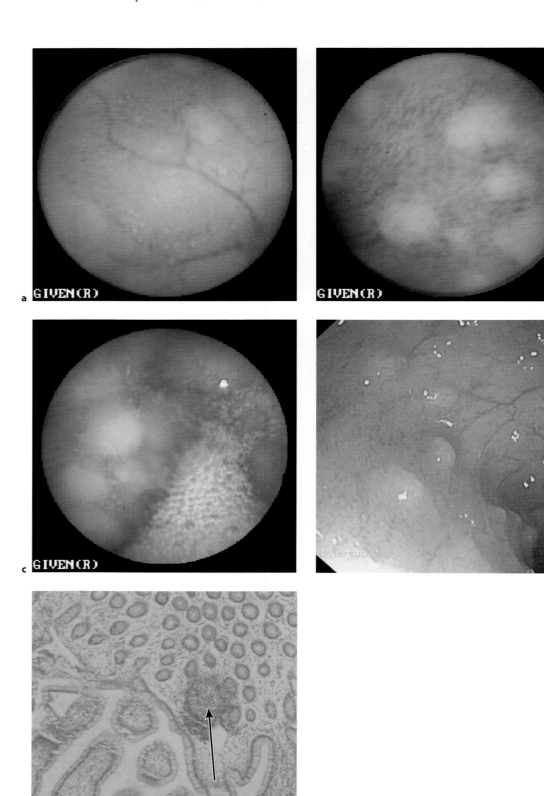

□ **Fig. 3-11a–e.** Terminal ileum with lymph follicles of varying prominence. **a–c** VCE. **d** Ileoscopy. **e** Histology; *arrow* indicates a lymph follicle (H&E, courtesy of Jörg Caselitz, M.D.)

Ileocecal Valve

The ileocecal valve (■ Figs. 3-12 and 3-13) is not consistently visualized. The capsule may move back and forth in the terminal ileum for some time. Passage of the capsule through the valve itself is usually very abrupt, yielding only an initial image of the colon.

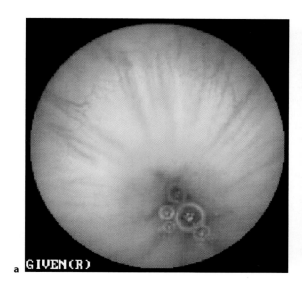

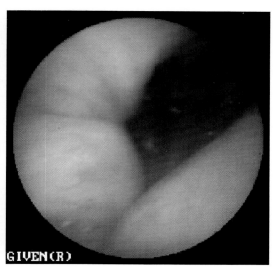

■ **Fig. 3-12. a** Closed ileocecal valve with longitudinal vessels. **b** Opened valve

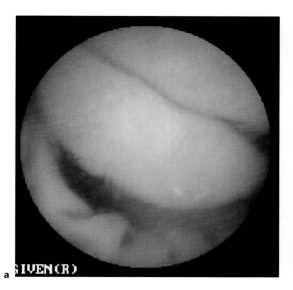

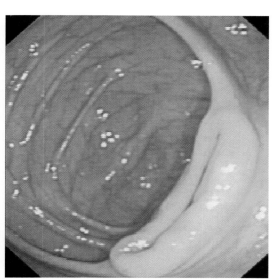

■ **Fig. 3-13. a** VCE, looking back from the cecum at the two lips of the ileocecal valve. **b** Colonoscopic view of the ileocecal valve

References

Dobbins WO III (1990) Diagnostic pathology of the intestinal mucosa. An atlas and review of biopsy interpretation. Springer, Berlin Heidelberg New York

Gat D, Fireman Z, Scapa E et al (2001) Transit times for the capsule endoscope-effect of colon prep on small bowel transit time of the capsule. Endoscopy 33 [Suppl I]: A2004

von Herbay A (1999) Anatomie, Entwicklung und Fehlbildungen von Dünn- und Dickdarm. In: Caspary WF, Stein J (eds) Darmkrankheiten. Klinik, Diagnostik und Therapie. Springer, Berlin Heidelberg New York, pp 3–16

Diverticula

A. Van Gossum, M. Keuchel

Acquired Diverticula of the Small Intestine

Definition. Acquired diverticula of the small bowel are pseudodiverticula that protrude through muscular gaps in the mesenteric side of the bowel wall.

Epidemiology. Small bowel diverticula are most commonly located in the duodenum, followed by the jejunum; they are very rarely found in the ileum (Akhrass et al. 1997). Diverticula in the jejunum or ileum occur in 1–5% of the population (Chow et al. 1997).

Clinical Features. Acquired diverticula are usually asymptomatic. They occasionally present with abdominal pain, intestinal bleeding, and less commonly with bowel obstruction (Agnifili et al. 1990; Kouraklis et al. 2001).

Endoscopy. A small diverticular opening is easy to identify by video capsule endoscopy (◘ Figs. 4-2 and 4-3a). With a larger opening, it is very common to find a septum between the mouth of the diverticulum and the bowel lumen (◘ Fig. 4-5), an apparent double lumen (◘ Fig. 4-9a), and folds radiating into the neck of the diverticulum (◘ Fig. 4-3). These features are difficult to distinguish from an acute bend in a normal loop of small bowel. The capsule may linger for some time in the area of the diverticulum (◘ Fig. 4-1) or may enter a larger diverticular pouch. Peridiverticular redness or ulceration are endoscopic signs of diverticulitis (◘ Fig. 4-4b).

Treatment. Most cases do not require treatment (Wilcox and Shatney 1988). Antibiotics may be indicated in patients with diverticulitis or bacterial overgrowth in the diverticular pouch. Surgical treatment is necessary in cases of perforation, bowel obstruction due to volvulus or intussusception, and massive bleeding (Nightingale et al. 2003; Wilcox and Shatney 1990).

Duodenal Diverticulum

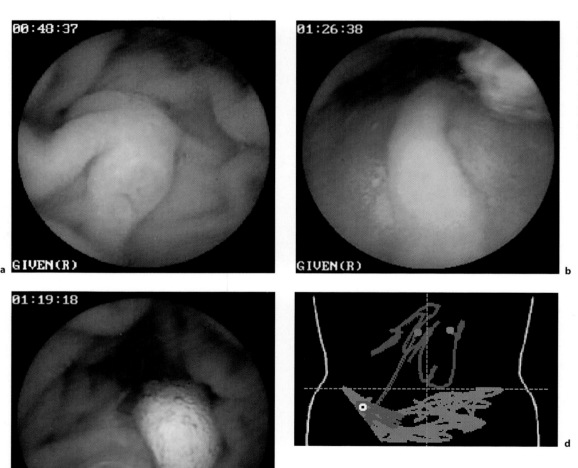

◘ **Fig. 4-1a–e.** Duodenal diverticulum. **a** Papilla. **b** Mouth of the diverticulum. **c** Reappearance of the papilla 31 min later. **d** The localization software shows the capsule remaining in the duodenum for some time (white circle: current capsule position; blue: stomach; green: duodenum). **e** Radiographic view of the diverticulum (courtesy of Christian Müller, M.D.)

Abb. 4-1e

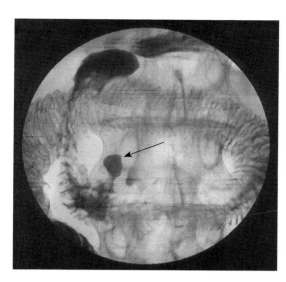

Jejunal Diverticulum

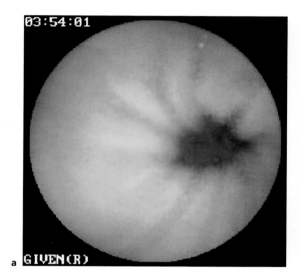

a **GIVEN(R)**

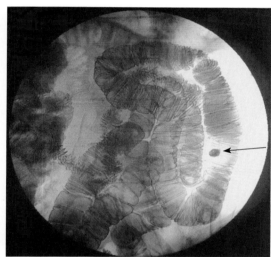

b

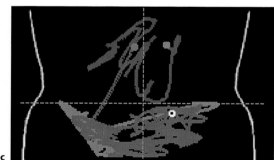

c

□ **Fig. 4-2a–c.** Small jejunal diverticulum showing no sign of irritation. **a** VCE. **b** Enteroclysis (courtesy of Christian Müller, M.D.). **c** Capsule localized to the left mid-horizontal line

4

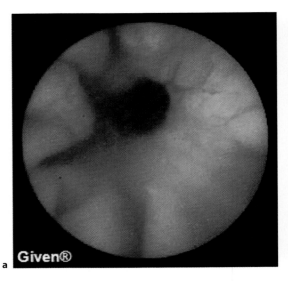

a

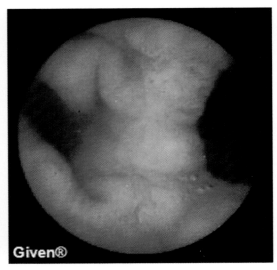

b

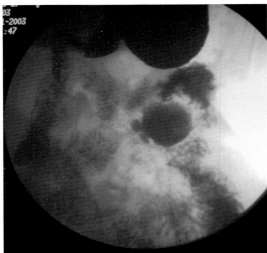

c

Fig. 4-3a, b. Jejunal diverticulum (case courtesy of Markus Oeyen, M.D.). **a** Orifice. **b** Septum and two lumina. **c** Radiographic aspect

Small Intestine Diverticulitis

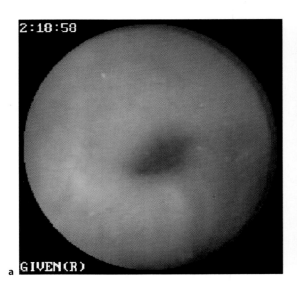

a

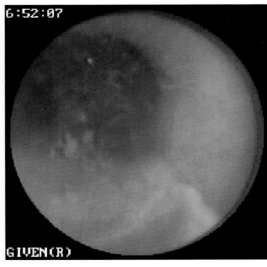

b

Fig. 4-4a, b. Diverticulitis: multiple diverticula in the small bowel (**a**), showing no sign of irritation proximally but showing redness and shallow ulcerations farther distally (**b**). Patient presented clinically with iron deficiency anemia, and iron kinetics indicated occult gastrointestinal bleeding. Enteroclysis was normal

Meckel's Diverticulum

Definition. A Meckel's diverticulum results from an abnormal persistence of the embryonic vitelline (omphalomesenteric) duct. It is the most common gastrointestinal anomaly, with a prevalence of up to 3%. In adults it is typically located on the antimesenteric side of the bowel 60–90 cm oral to the ileocecal valve. In approximately 50% of cases the diverticulum contains ectopic mucosa, usually gastric mucosa (◘ Figs. 4-6–4-8), which may ulcerate (◘ Fig. 4-9) and bleed (◘ Fig. 4-10). Ectopic gastric mucosa can be detected by technetium scanning (◘ Fig. 4-6d; Chap. 2.4).

Clinical Features. The majority of Meckel's diverticula are asymptomatic. If clinical manifestations are present, they usually consist of painless intestinal bleeding (Chiu et al. 2000). Abdominal pain is less commonly present. Diverticulitis, perforation, intussusception, bowel obstruction, and associated tumors are rare.

Treatment. Treatment consists of surgical resection in symptomatic patients. In many cases asymptomatic Meckel's diverticula are removed as a precautionary measure during a surgical procedure for some other indication, although this is not routinely recommended in adults (Stone et al. 2004).

Endoscopy. Video capsule endoscopy can detect diverticula of the middle or lower small bowel, possibly with an associated ulcer (◘ Fig. 4-9) and/or ectopic gastric mucosa (◘ Figs. 4-6–4-8). Larger diverticula may cause a visible indentation of adjacent small bowel loops. There are isolated cases that can be diagnosed only by VCE (Mylonaki et al. 2002). Often it is difficult to distinguish a diverticular septum (◘ Fig. 4-5) from a normal fold in an angled loop of small bowel. An everted diverticulum can mimic a tumor (Dubcenco et al. 2004). Seldom, active bleeding is observed with a Meckel's diverticulum (Tang et al. 2004) (◘ Fig. 4-10). No data are currently available on the sensitivity and specificity of VCE in the diagnosis of Meckel's diverticulum.

❗ The capsule may pause at a diverticulum for some time, causing the same pouch to be imaged more than once.

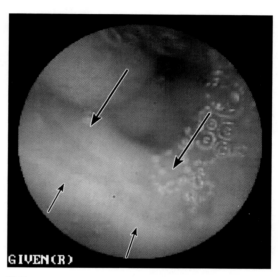

◘ **Fig. 4-5.** Meckel's diverticulum: only part of the diverticular septum (*thick arrow*) is visible. It is slightly thicker than a normal mucosal fold and shows faint red streaks (*thin arrow*). The diagnosis was confirmed at operation. Technetium scanning was negative. The patient presented clinically with iron deficiency anemia

4

Ectopic Gastric Mucosa in a Meckel's Diverticulum

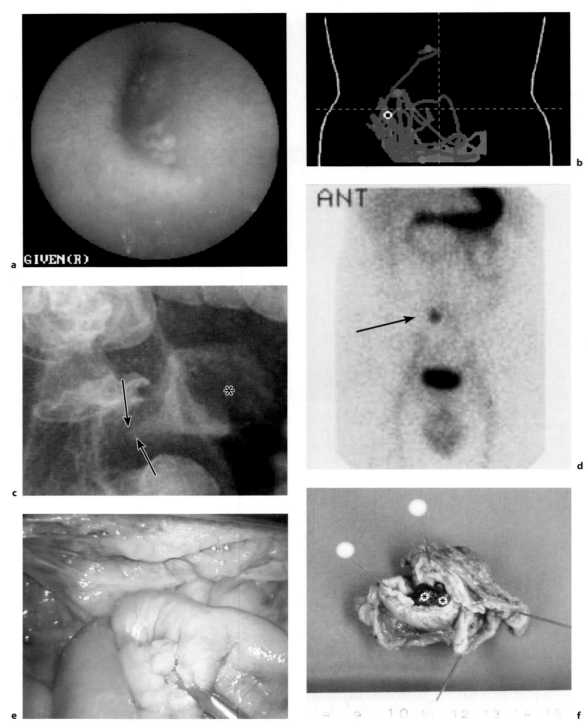

■ **Fig. 4-6a–f.** Meckel's diverticulum. **a** Small, noninflamed diverticular orifice imaged by VCE. **b** Capsule localized (*white circle*) to the right mid-horizontal line. **c** Enteroclysis defines the narrow diverticular orifice (*arrows*) and a filling defect in the diverticulum (*, courtesy of Ernst Malzfeldt, M.D.). **d** Technetium scans show ectopic gastric mucosa (*arrow*) on the right mid-horizontal line (courtesy of Michaela Garn, M.D.). **e** Intraoperative view of the antimesenteric Meckel's diverticulum (courtesy of Wolfgang Teichmann, M.D.). **f** Surgical specimen contains an enterolith (courtesy of Jörg Caselitz, M.D.), which produced the filling defect in the contrast radiograph. The patient presented clinically with gastrointestinal bleeding requiring transfusion

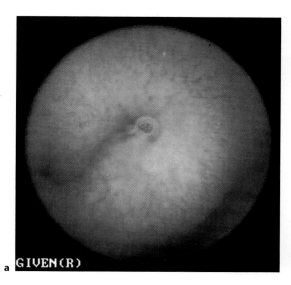

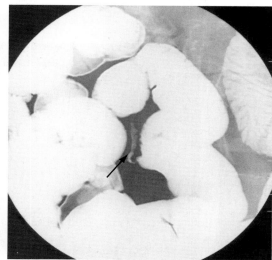

■ **Fig. 4-7a–c.** Meckel's diverticulum.
a Small, noninflamed diverticular orifice.
b Enteroclysis shows a very narrow diverticulum. **c** Histology: Meckel's diverticulum
(➜) with ectopic gastric tissue

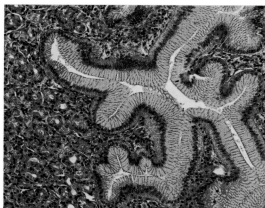

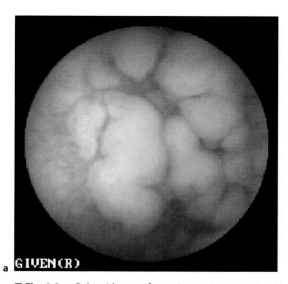

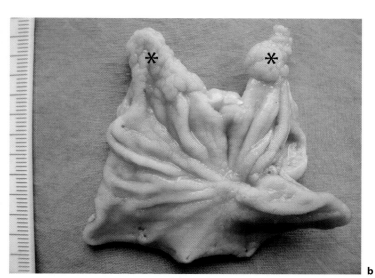

■ **Fig. 4-8. a** Polypoid mass of ectopic gastric mucosa in a Meckel's diverticulum.
b Specimen cut open to show portions of the ectopic gastric mucosa (*, courtesy of Hanns-Olof Wintzer, M.D.). The patient presented clinically with intestinal bleeding requiring transfusion. Technetium scanning was negative

4

Ulcerated Meckel's Diverticulum

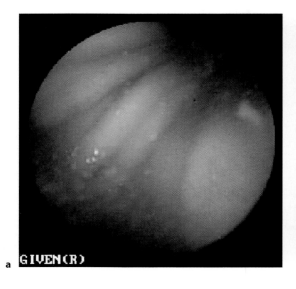
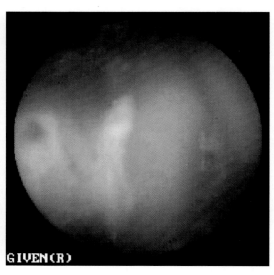

a GIVEN(R)

b

■ **Fig. 4-9a, b.** Ulcerated Meckel's diverticulum: large diverticulum with a septum, radial folds, two lumina (**a**), and a large shallow ulcer at the edge of the diverticulum with a red spot (**b**) (vascular stump?). The diagnosis was confirmed laparoscopically. The patient presented with iron deficiency anemia, and bleeding was detected by ^{59}Fe kinetics. Magnetic resonance enteroclysis and Meckel's scintigraphy were negative (▶ Fig. 9-14)

Bleeding Meckel's Diverticulum

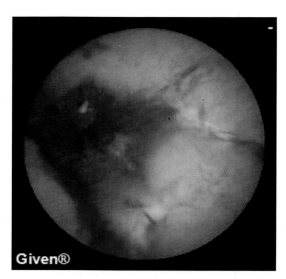

Given®

■ **Fig. 4-10.** Bleeding Meckel's diverticulum (courtesy of Florentin Stachow, M.D.): orifice of diverticulum with blood and ulcers on the edge. Diagnosis was confirmed at surgery

References

Agnifili A, Gola P, Gianfelice F et al (1990) Rare digestive hemorrhage caused by diverticular pathology of the small intestine. Minerva Chir 45:721–724

Akhrass R, Yaffe MB, Fischer C et al (1997) Small-bowel diverticulosis: perceptions and reality. J Am Coll Surg 184:383–388

Dubcenco E, Tang SJ, Streutker CJ, Jeejeebhoy KN, Baker JP (2004) Meckel's diverticulum mimicking small bowel tumor. Gastrointest Endosc 60:263

Chiu EJ, Shyr YM, Su CH et al (2000) Diverticular disease of the small bowel. Hepato-gastroenterology 47:181–184

Chow DC, Babaian M, Taubin HL (1997) Jejunoileal diverticula. Gastroenterologist 5:78–84

Kouraklis G, Mantas D, Glivanou A et al (2001) Diverticular disease of the small bowel: report of 27 cases. Int Surg 86:235–239

Mylonaki M, MacLean D, Fritscher-Ravens A, Swain P (2002) Wireless capsule endoscopic detection of Meckel's diverticulum after nondiagnostic surgery. Endoscopy 34:1018–1020

Nightingale S, Nikfarjam M, Iles L, Djeric M (2003) Small bowel diverticular disease complicated by perforation. Aust N Z J Surg 73:867–869

Stone PA, Hofeldt MJ, Campbell JE, Vedula G, DeLuca JA, Flaherty SK (2004) Meckel diverticulum: ten-year experience in adults. South Med J 97:1038–1041

Tang SJ, Dubcenco E, Kortan P (2004) Bleeding Meckel's diverticulum. Gastrointest Endosc 60:264

Wilcox RD, Shatney CH (1988) Surgical implications of jejunal diverticula. South Med J 81:1386–1391

Wilcox RD, Shatney CH (1990) Surgical significance of acquired ileal diverticulosis. Am Surg 56:222–225

Vascular Diseases of the Small Intestine

5.1   Arteriovenous Diseases

M. Keuchel, M. Pennazio, D.M. Jensen, G.S. Dulai

Angiectasias

Definition. Angiectasia (synonyms: vascular ectasia, angiodysplasia, telangiectasia, arteriovenous malformation or AVM) is a circumscribed dilatation of the capillary vessels in the mucosa or submucosa of the gastrointestinal (GI) tract.

Clinical Features. Angiectasias are the most common lesions identified in the small bowel of patients with obscure GI bleeding, yet they can be missed by capsule endoscopy – especially in the stomach, duodenum, and colon. It should be understood that while angiectasias are commonly seen, they may or may not bleed. Clinical correlation and exclusion of other lesions are therefore required. Certain hereditary, iatrogenic, and acquired conditions can predispose to bleeding from angiectasia, most notably the use of aspirin, nonsteroidal anti-inflammatory drugs (NSAIDs), and anticoagulants.

The **acquired form** of angiectasia is the most common pathologic finding in patients with obscure GI bleeding. An increased incidence is seen in association with aging, hemodialysis, heart failure, aortic stenosis (Heyde's syndrome) (Warkentin et al. 2002), radiation therapy, and von Willebrand's syndrome (Warkentin et al. 2003). Gastric antral vascular ectasia or watermelon stomach is a special case that may be associated with autoimmune disorders (◘ Fig. 6.5-7), liver cirrhosis, or end stage renal disease.

The **hereditary form** is known as hereditary hemorrhagic telangiectasia (HHT) (Osler-Weber-Rendu disease, ◘ Fig. 5.1-2) (van den Driesche et al. 2003). To date, two genetic defects have been identified. A clinical diagnosis can be made when three of the four Curaçao criteria (epistaxis, telangiectasias, visceral vascular lesions, and/or positive family history) are present (Shovlin et al. 2000). Although significant GI hemorrhage occurs in ~one-fifth of patients with HHT, VCE studies have found GI angiectasia in >50% of cases (Ingrosso et al. 2004).

Diagnosis. Diagnostic criteria for the endoscopic appearance of angiectasia are not uniform and have not been validated. For example, a small, flat, clearly demarcated red spot (◘ Fig. 5.1-3a) may be an angiectasia, petechia, effect of bowel preparation, erosion, or inflammation. These red spots should be distinguished from the more characteristic fern-like appearance of an angioma with central vessel (◘ Fig. 5.1-2). Active bleeding in the vicinity of an angiectasia is helpful in confirming the source of bleeding (◘ Fig. 5.1-3). The anatomic distribution and focality of endoscopic lesions are critical for therapeutic decision making.

Radiographic imaging studies are usually unrewarding, but angiography may be diagnostic in rare cases when severe active bleeding is present. **Biopsy** is not recommended for clearly identifiable lesions due to the risk of bleeding, but it can be used to differentiate an atypical-appearing lesion from redness related to inflammation. Histologic examination of larger lesions can show small, distended, lacuna-like vessels with intraluminal red cells (◘ Fig. 5.1-4a); however, most lesions defy histologic diagnosis due to their small size (shrinkage with processing of the specimen, error in targeting biopsy, etc.).

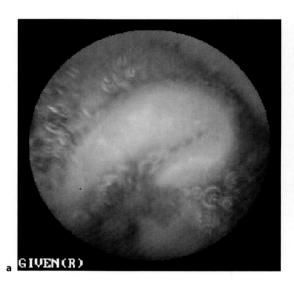

a GIVEN(R)

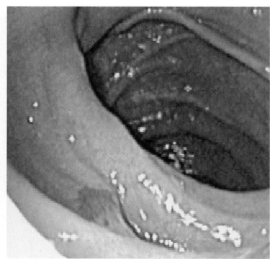

b

◘ **Fig. 5.1-1a, b.** Jejunal angiectasia.
a VCE. **b** Push enteroscopy

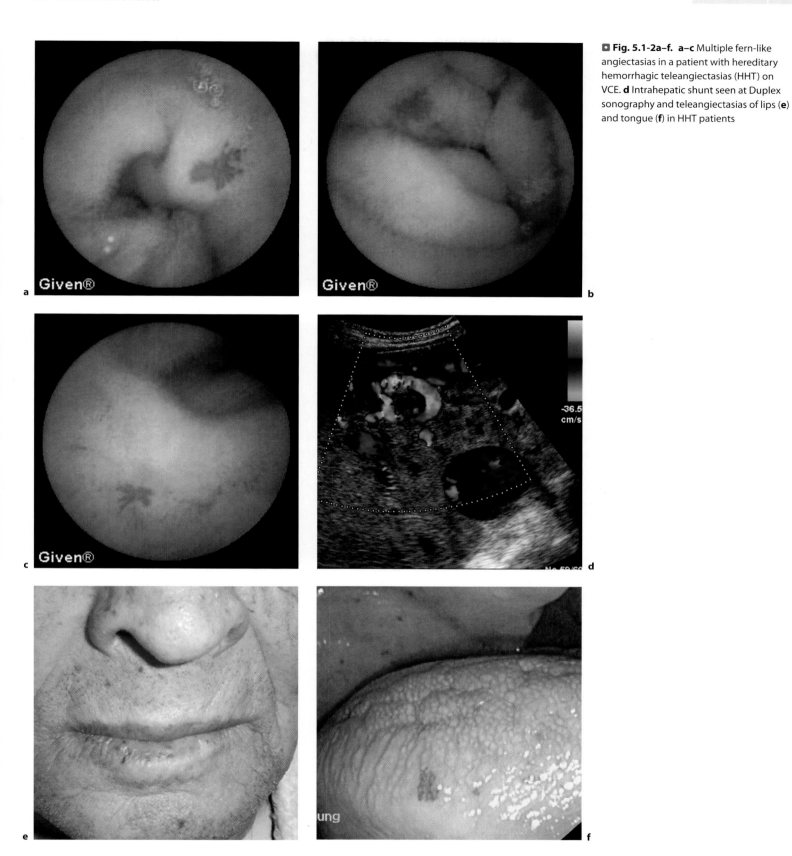

Fig. 5.1-2a–f. **a–c** Multiple fern-like angiectasias in a patient with hereditary hemorrhagic teleangiectasias (HHT) on VCE. **d** Intrahepatic shunt seen at Duplex sonography and teleangiectasias of lips (**e**) and tongue (**f**) in HHT patients

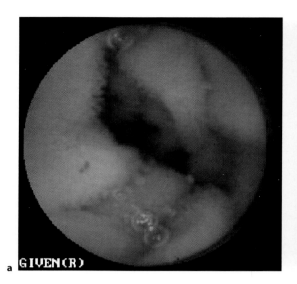

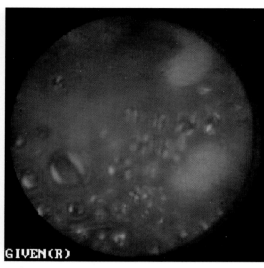

Fig. 5.1-3a, b. Patient with end-stage renal disease and recurrent transfusion-requiring GI bleeding. VCE revealed minute jejunal angiectasias (**a**) and active bleeding (**b**)

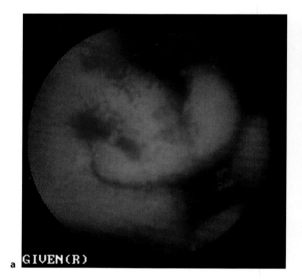

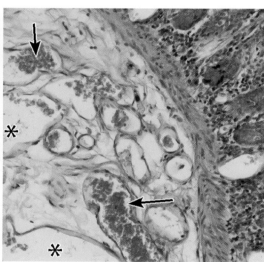

Fig. 5.1-4a, b. 83 year-old man with transfusion-requiring intestinal blood loss. **a** An angiectasia in the middle of the VCE image is poorly visible due to dark blood (**b**). Active bleeding was observed more distally. Intraoperatively, multiple angiectasias of the jejunum were treated by segmental resection. **b** Histology of resected segment from the small intestine*, intraluminal erythrocytes (*arrow*) (H&E stain, courtesy of Jörg Caselitz, M.D.)

Treatment. Treatment should be considered when actively bleeding angiectasias are seen and/or when these are the only potential sources of bleeding identified. There is a clear need for new medical and endoscopic treatment modalities. At present, endoscopic coagulation (■ Fig. 5.1-5) may be done with electrocautery (bipolar, argon plasma), heater probe, or laser (Pavey and Craig 2004). Large focal lesions can be treated surgically by a segmental resection of the small bowel (Steffani et al. 2003). Empiric treatment (iron replacement, Epogen, transfusion, avoidance of platelet aggregation inhibitors such as aspirin or clopidogrel, NSAIDs, anticoagulants) may be considered for cases with diffuse involvement or for rebleeding after endoscopic or surgical treatment (Lewis 1999). Intraoperative treatment of diffuse small bowel lesions is usually ineffective. With the advent of double-balloon endoscopy (Chap. 2.2) it is possible to reach more intestinal lesions without need for surgery. Whether this will change outcome in terms of rebleeding rates has to be seen. Hormonal therapy may be administered, but its benefit has not been confirmed (Junquera et al. 2001). Anecdotal reports have been published on the use of somatostatin analogs (Blich et al. 2003; Rossini et al. 1993) and thalidomide (Shurafa and Kamboj 2003).

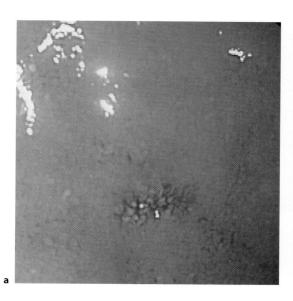
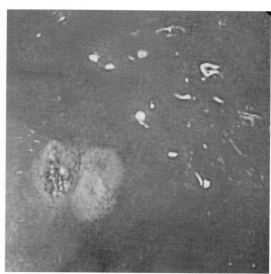

■ **Fig. 5.1-5a, b.** Push enteroscopy: angiectasia before (**a**) and after electrocoagulation (**b**)

a

b

Dieulafoy's Ulcer

Definition. A Dieulafoy's lesion is a protruding large-caliber submucosal artery without ulceration. The lesion may bleed profusely. Rebleeding is common. Arteries may be >2 mm in size. These lesions most commonly occur in the stomach; they are less common in the duodenum and rare in the jejunum or ileum (Lee et al. 2003).

Treatment. Endoscopic hemostasis can be achieved by injection, coagulation, clipping, rubber band ligation, or a combination of these techniques. If endoscopic treatment is ineffectual, a segmental bowel resection is indicated.

Endoscopy. Without active (arterial type) bleeding or other stigmata such as a non-bleeding visible vessel, Dieulafoy's lesions are often difficult to identify. When active bleeding is present, the source may be obscured by blood (■ Fig. 5.1-6). Even when the bleeding stops, the lesion may be missed due to its small size.

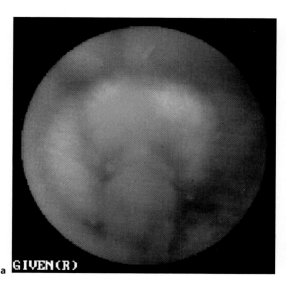
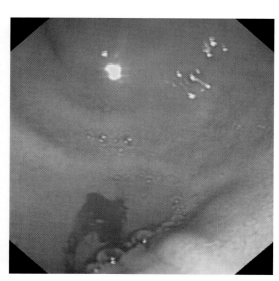

■ **Fig. 5.1-6a, b.** Bleeding jejunal Dieulafoy's lesion (courtesy of Michel Delvaux, M.D. and Gerard Gay, M.D.). **a** VCE. **b** Enteroscopy

a GIVEN(R)

b

Blue Rubber Bleb Nevus Syndrome

Definition. This is a very rare, hereditary syndrome characterized by multiple hemangiomas involving the GI tract (■ Figs. 5.1-7, 5.1-8a, and 7.1-14) and the skin (■ Fig. 5.1-8b).

Endoscopy. Soft, blue, rubbery hemangiomas may be seen throughout the GI tract at endoscopy (Fish et al. 2004)

Treatment. Treatment can be difficult due to the often diffuse distribution of lesions. The principal options are endoscopic coagulation and surgical resection (Shahed et al. 1990).

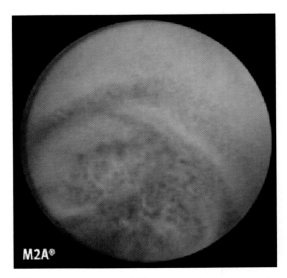

■ **Fig. 5.1-7.** Blue rubber bleb nevus syndrome: hemangiomas of the small bowel [courtesy of Jürgen Riemann, M.D., reprinted from Hahne and Riemann (2002) with permission of Given Imaging]

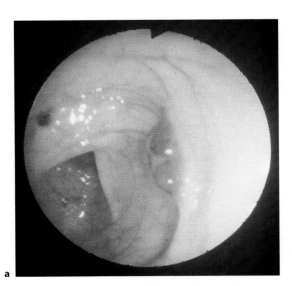

a

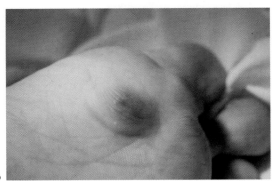

b

■ **Fig. 5.1-8a, b.** Blue rubber bleb nevus syndrome: hemangioma of colon (**a**) and skin (**b**)

Venous Ectasias, Varices

Endoscopy. Large veins are frequently seen during capsule endoscopy of the normal small bowel. It is not unusual to find small venous ectasias (■ Fig. 5.1-9), which generally do not bleed. However, if varices

(■ Figs. 5.1-10 and 5.1-11) or venous ectasias with an eroded surface (■ Fig. 5.1-12) are found, they should be considered a potential bleeding source (Ostrow and Blanchard 1984; Tang et al. 2004).

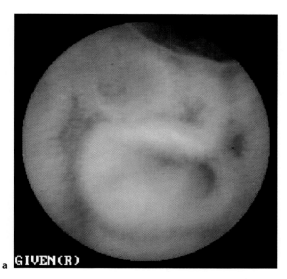

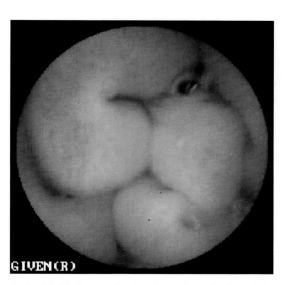

■ **Fig. 5.1-10.** Duodenal varices in a patient with liver cirrhosis who had recurrent transfusion-requiring bleeding episodes

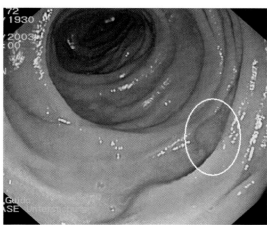

■ **Fig. 5.1-9a, b.** Venectasias: nonbleeding, incidental findings on VCE (**a**) and push enteroscopy (**b**)

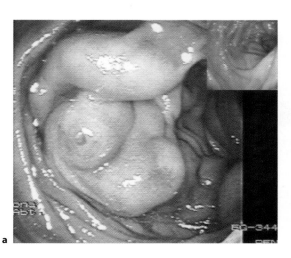

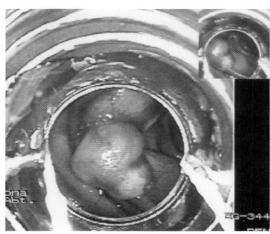

■ **Fig. 5.1-11a, b.** Large convolution of varices in the deep duodenum with hematocystic spot (**a**) due to liver cirrhosis. Hemorrhagic shock. After rubber band ligation (**b**) no further bleeding

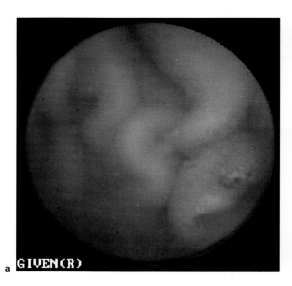

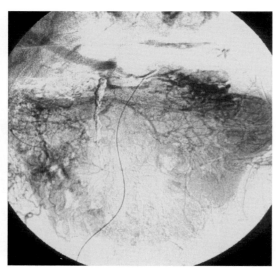

a GIVEN(R)   b

▫ Fig. 5.1-12a, b. Venous bleeding. **a** Venectasia with small mucosal defect. Active bleeding at another small bowel segment not shown. Angiography (**b**) reveals residual convoluted venous structure after mesenteric vein thrombosis (courtesy of Uwe Peters, M.D.)

Portal Hypertensive Enteropathy

Definition. Enteropathic lesions develop secondarily to portal hypertension caused by hepatic cirrhosis or portal vein thrombosis with congestion of the mesenteric veins.

Clinical Features. The clinical significance of the enteropathic lesions is difficult to assess (Viggiano and Gostout 1992), particularly since they often coexist with esophageal varices and/or portal hypertensive gastropathy (Desai et al. 2004; Misra et al. 2004).

Endoscopy. Patchy redness of the mucosa (Evrard et al. 2004) and diffuse venous ectasias, possibly accompanied by small, superficial mucosal defects, are nonspecific findings (▫ Figs. 5.1-13 and 5.1-14). Small bowel varices may be found in rare cases (▫ Figs. 5.1-10 and 5.1-11) (Tang et al. 2004).

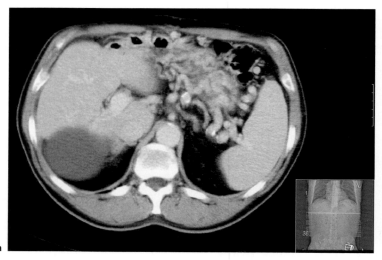

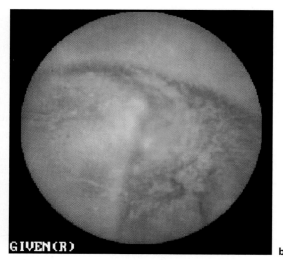

a   b

▫ Fig. 5.1-13a, b. Splenic vein thrombosis. **a** CT shows collaterals, state after partial liver resection (courtesy of Ernst Malzfeldt, M.D.). **b** VCE reveals red spots in the jejunum

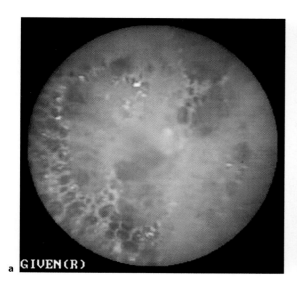
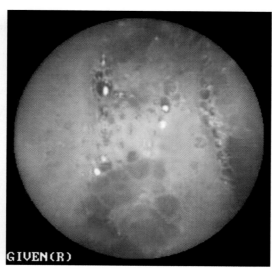

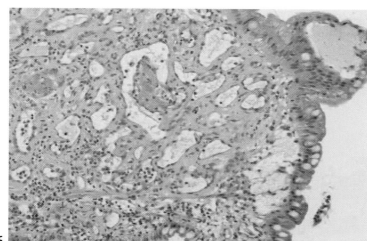

◨ **Fig. 5.1-14a–c.** Portal hypertensive enteropathy in a cirrhotic patient (courtesy of Andrè Van Gossum, M.D.). VCE shows elevated red bumps in the terminal ileum (**a**, **b**). Biopsy shows vascular dilation (**c**)

Ischemic Enteropathy

Definition. Ischemic enteropathy is an acute or chronic occlusion of the celiac trunk, the superior mesenteric artery, or systemic low-flow state (e.g., shock, sepsis, bypass, etc.) with or without small vessel disease. The chronic form is almost always atherosclerosis-related and is rarely symptomatic due to the development of a collateral supply. Acute and chronic ischemic lesions can also result from the angiographic embolization of small bowel segmental arteries done for purposes of hemostasis.

Clinical Features. Postprandial abdominal pain, diarrhea, and weight loss are the clinical hallmarks of chronic ischemia of the small bowel (Brandt and Boley 2000). The acute form may be characterized by abdominal pain, acute abdomen, bleeding, and even rare instances of perforation, depending on the extent of the infarction.

Diagnosis. The mainstays in the diagnosis of ischemic enteropathy are arterial (subtraction) angiography and color Doppler sonography. Endoscopy has a confirmatory role in cases where there is clinical suspicion of acute ischemia, and it can demonstrate the presence of residual strictures. Acute intestinal ischemia may be associated with edema and bleeding (◘ Fig. 5.1-15). Ulcers of the small bowel are frequently segmental and circumferential (◘ Fig. 5.1-16).

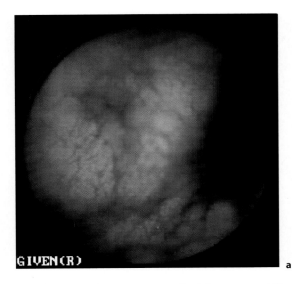

a

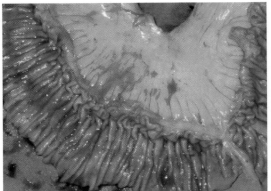

b

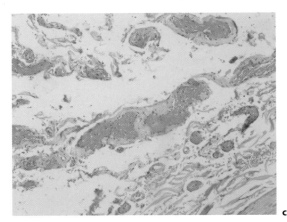

c

◘ **Fig. 5.1-15a–c.** Patient with acute mesenteric ischemia due to cardiogenic shock. **a** VCE revealed edematous swelling of a long segment with dark blood. **b** Resection of an ischemic jejunal segment after intraoperative enteroscopy because of hemorrhagic shock. **c** Histology shows ischemia (case courtesy of Michel Delvaux, M.D. and Gerard Gay, M.D.)

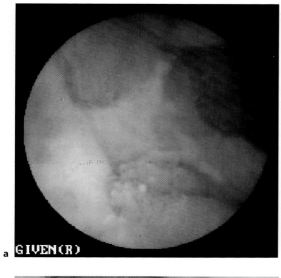

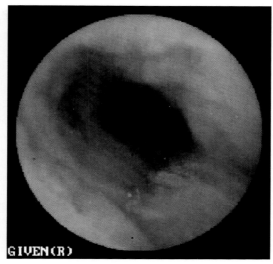

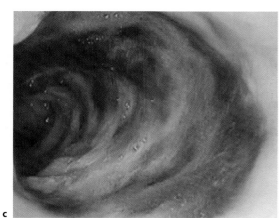

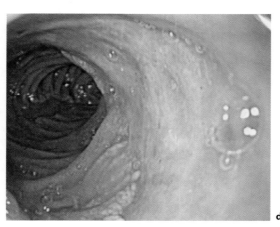

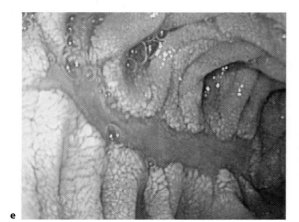

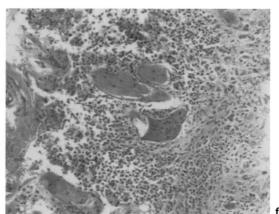

Fig. 5.1-16a–f. Ischemic enteritis: on VCE longitudinal (**a**) and circular (**b**) jejunal ulcers. Push enteroscopy initially reveals dark jejunal ulceration (**c**), healing ulcers at follow-up (**d**), and »snail track«-like appearance of a healed ischemic ulcer (**e**). Histology (**f**) demonstrates ischemic enteritis with complete necrosis and hyaline thrombi (H&E, courtesy of Jörg Caselitz, M.D.). A 63-year-old man with abdominal pain, inflammatory signs, compensated stenosis of the celiac trunk, microangiopathy and state after »spontaneous« duodenal perforation

Internet

www.hht.org: HHT Foundation International (Scientific Advisory Board)

References

Blich M, Fruchter O, Edelstein S, Edoute Y (2003) Somatostatin therapy ameliorates chronic and refractory gastrointestinal bleeding caused by diffuse angiodysplasia in a patient on anticoagulation therapy. Scand J Gastroenterol 38:801–803

Brandt LJ, Boley SJ (2000) AGA technical review on intestinal ischemia. Gastroenterology 118:954–968

Desai N, Desai D, Pethe V (2004) Portal hypertensive jejunopathy: a case control study. Indian J Gastroenterol 23:99–101

Evrard S, Le Moine O, Devière J, Yengue P, Nagy N, Adler M, Van Gossum A (2004) Unexplained digestive bleeding in a cirrhotic patient. Gut 53:1771

Fish L, Fireman Z, Kopelman Y, Sternberg A (2004) Blue rubber bleb nevus syndrome: small-bowel lesions diagnosed by capsule endoscopy. Endoscopy 36:836

Hahne M, Riemann J (2002) Vascular abnormalities. In: Halpern M, Jacob H (eds) Atlas of capsule endoscopy. Given Imaging, Norcross, GA, USA, pp 73–80

Ingrosso M, Sabba C, Pisani A et al (2004) Evidence of small-bowel involvement in hereditary hemorrhagic telangiectasia: a capsule-endoscopic study. Endoscopy 36:1074–1079

Junquera F, Feu F, Papo M et al (2001) A multicenter, randomized, clinical trial of hormonal therapy in the prevention of rebleeding from gastrointestinal angiodysplasia. Gastroenterology 121:1073–1079

Lee YT, Walmsley RS, Leong RWL, Sung JJS (2003) Dieulafoy's lesion. Gastrointest Endosc 58:236-243

Lewis BS (1999) Medical and hormonal therapy in occult gastrointestinal bleeding. Semin Gastrointest Dis 10:71–77

Misra SP, Dwivedi M, Misra V, Gupta M (2004) Ileal varices and portal hypertensive ileopathy in patients with cirrhosis and portal hypertension. Gastrointest Endosc 60:778–783

Ostrow B, Blanchard RJ (1984) Bleeding small-bowel varices. Can J Surg 27:88–89

Pavey DA, Craig PI (2004) Endoscopic therapy for upper-GI vascular ectasias. Gastrointest Endosc 59:233–238

Rossini FP, Arrigoni A, Pennazio M (1993) Octreotide in the treatment of bleeding due to angiodysplasia of the small intestine. Am J Gastroenterol 88:1424–1427

Shahed M, Hagenmüller F, Rösch T et al (1990) A 19-year-old female with blue rubber bleb naevus syndrome. Endoscopic laser photocoagulation and surgical resection of gastrointestinal angiomata. Endoscopy 22:54–56

Shovlin CL, Guttmacher AE, Buscarini E et al (2000) Diagnostic criteria for hereditary hemorrhagic telangiectasia (Rendu-Osler-Weber syndrome). Am J Med Genet 91:66–67

Shurafa M, Kamboj G (2003) Thalidomide for the treatment of bleeding angiodysplasias. Am J Gastroenterol 98:221–222

Steffani KD, Eisenberger CF, Gocht A et al (2003) Recurrent intestinal bleeding in a patient with arterio-venous fistulas in the small bowel, limited mesenteric varicosis without portal hypertension and malrotation type I. Z Gastroenterol 41:587–590

Tang SJ, Zanati S, Dubcenco E et al (2004) Diagnosis of small-bowel varices by capsule endoscopy. Gastrointest Endosc 60:129–135

van den Driesche DS, Mummery CL, Westermann CJ (2003) Hereditary hemorrhagic telangiectasia: an update on transforming growth factor beta signaling in vasculogenesis and angiogenesis. Cardiovasc Res 58:20–31

Viggiano TR, Gostout CJ (1992) Portal hypertensive intestinal vasculopathy: a review of the clinical, endoscopic, and histopathologic features. Am J Gastroenterol 87:944–954

Warkentin TE, Moore JC, Anand SS et al (2003) Gastrointestinal bleeding, angiodysplasia, cardiovascular disease, and acquired von Willebrand syndrome. Transfus Med Rev 17:272–286

Warkentin TE, Moore JC, Morgan DG (2002) Gastrointestinal angiodysplasia and aortic stenosis. N Engl J Med 347:858–859

5.2   Intestinal Lymphangiectasia

E. Tóth, M. Keuchel, J.F. Riemann

Clinical Features

Endoscopically, the villi of the small bowel in intestinal lymphangiectasia typically appear white and may be swollen (Asakura et al. 1981; Riemann and Schmidt 1981). Less commonly, tiny white spots are visible in the mucosa (◘ Fig. 5.2-1). The whitish discoloration of the villi is caused by chylomicrons, which accumulate in and obstruct the dilated lymphatic capillaries. These changes can also be demonstrated histo-

logically. Lymphangiectasia is characterized endoscopically as localized, patchy, or diffuse. Diffuse lymphangiectasia causes the mucosa to appear »snow-covered« or »dusted with powdered sugar« at endoscopy.

Functional lymphangiectasia appears to have no pathologic significance (Barnes and deRidder 1993). **Secondary** lymphangiectasia is an accompanying feature of many underlying intestinal and extraintestinal diseases (Fürstenau et al. 1977). There is also the very rare **primary** form (also called idiopathic or essential) with severe exudative enteropathy. White, swollen villi are occasionally found in a localized area (**focal lymphangiectasia**); this form has not been shown to have pathologic significance (◘ Fig. 5.2-1). **Cystic lymphangiectasia** is also a harmless finding unless the lesions are exceptionally large or eroded (Chap. 7.1).

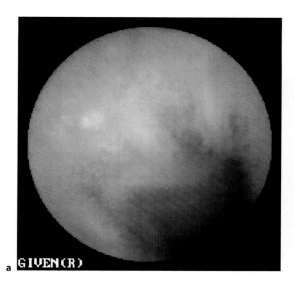

a GIVEN(R)

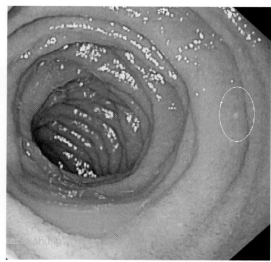

b

◘ Fig. 5.2-1a, b. Biopsy-confirmed circumscribed lymphangiectasia: tiny white nodule on normal mucosa. **a** VCE (courtesy of Bernd Falke, M.D.). **b** Push enteroscopy

Secondary Lymphangiectasia

The causes of secondary lymphangiectasia should be investigated based on the history and clinical examination, and if necessary by performing microbiologic tests and imaging studies [ultrasound, computed tomography (CT), magnetic resonance imaging (MRI)]. In cases with concomitant diarrhea and malabsorption, it is advisable to proceed with an endoscopic biopsy of the small bowel.

Etiology of secondary lymphangiectasia:

- Infections (e.g., Whipple's disease, ◘ Fig. 5.2-3)
- Inflammations (e.g., Crohn's disease, ◘ Figs. 5.2-2, 5.2-4, and 5.2-5)
- Intra-abdominal tumors (◘ Fig. 5.2-8)
- Radiation enteritis (◘ Fig. 5.2-6)
- Right heart failure, ischemia (◘ Fig. 5.2-7)

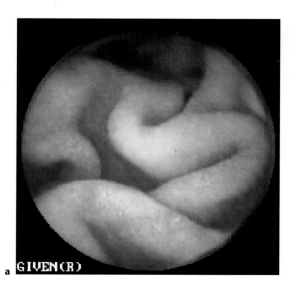

a GIVEN(R)

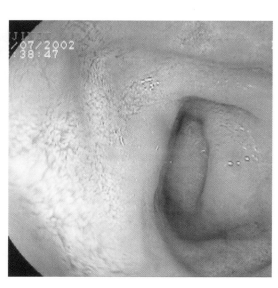

b

◘ Fig. 5.2-2a, b. Inflammation in a 74-year-old dialysis patient with unexplained bleeding: moderate, diffuse white discoloration of the duodenal villi (**a**). No evidence of a bleeding source in the small bowel. Corresponding video endoscopic image, which additionally shows faint patchy redness (**b**). Histology revealed nonspecific duodenitis

5

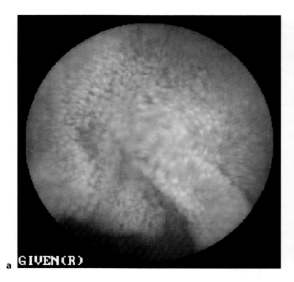

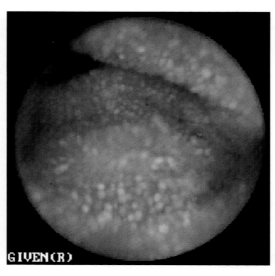

■ **Fig. 5.2-3a, b.** Infection: diffuse lymphangiectasia in human immunodeficiency virus infection (**a**) and atypical mycobacteriosis (**b**, pseudo-Whipple's disease)

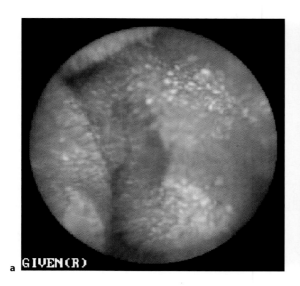

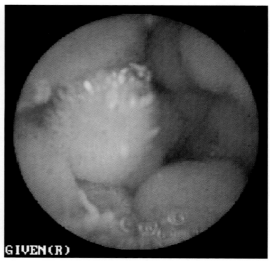

■ **Fig. 5.2-4a, b.** Crohn's disease. **a** Diffuse lymphangiectasia with circumscribed loss of villi proximal to ulcerations (not shown). **b** Circumscribed lymphangiectasia on polypous mucosa

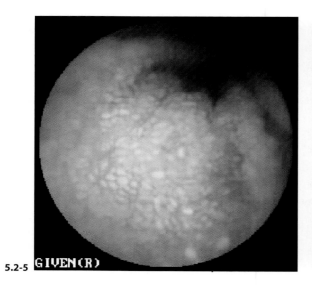

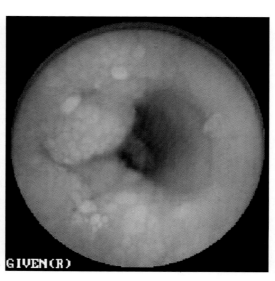

■ **Fig. 5.2-5.** Villous atrophy: villi are again seen in the distal small bowel but are still irregular, white, and broadened

■ **Fig. 5.2-6.** Radiation enteritis: fibrous thickening of the mucosa with stenosis and patches of white, broadened villi. The capsule passed spontaneously through the stenosis

5.2-5

5.2-6

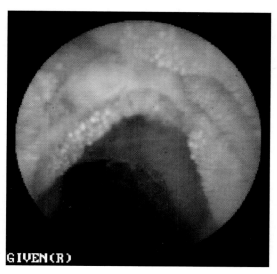

❗ Uncharacteristic lymphangiectasias and specific features of the underlying disease may occur in small intestinal segments that are widely separate from each other.

◼ Fig. 5.2-7. Ischemic enteritis with semi-circumferential ulcers and diffuse lymphangiectasia

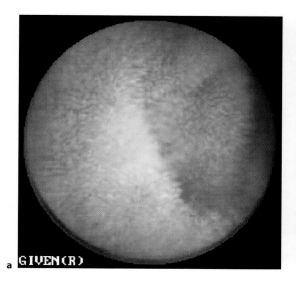 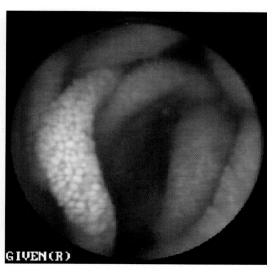

◼ Fig. 5.2-8a, b. Diffuse lymphangiectasia distant from small bowel tumors: carcinoid (**a**) and adenocarcinoma (**b**)

Primary Lymphangiectasia

Occurrence. Primary lymphangiectasia (Waldmann disease; Waldmann et al. 1961) is a very rare, presumably hereditary disease that predominantly affects children and adolescents.

Clinical Features. Typical features are diarrhea, exudative enteropathy with malassimilation, protein deficiency edema, and lymphocytopenia.

Endoscopy. Primary lymphangiectasia (◼ Figs. 5.2-9 and 5.2-10) may appear more pronounced at endoscopy and involve a longer intestinal segment than the secondary form. Additionally, the mucosa itself may have a whitish appearance (Aoyagi et al. 1997) as if covered by a thin blanket of snow (◼ Fig. 5.2-9a, b). Biopsy confirmation (◼ Fig. 5.2-10e) is advised.

Treatment. First the patient should be placed on a low-fat diet with medium-chain fatty acids (Munck et al. 2002). Somatostatin has been tried as an experimental therapy (Kuroiwa et al. 2001).

5

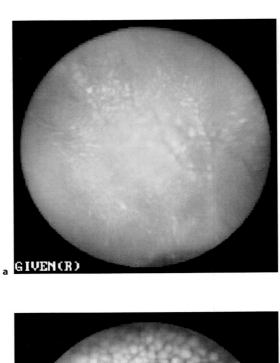

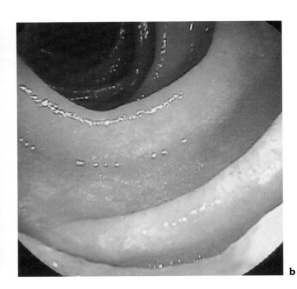

Fig. 5.2-9a, b. Primary lymphangiectasia in a 43-year-old man with severe exudative enteropathy: white, slightly thickened villi and patchy white areas that give the mucosa a »snow-covered« or »powdered sugar« appearance. **a** VCE. **b** Corresponding push enteroscopy image. The serum albumin level normalized in response to somatostatin therapy

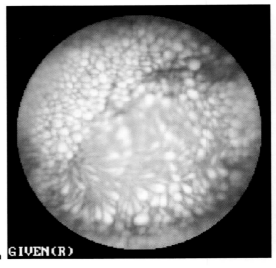

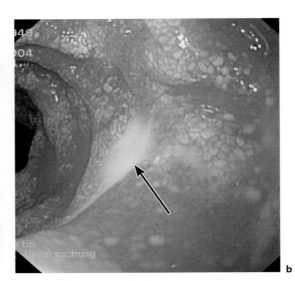

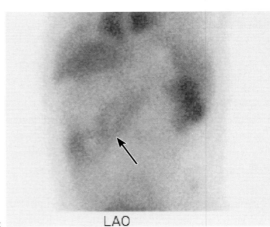

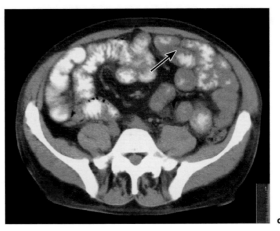

Fig. 5.2-10a–e. Diffuse intestinal lymphangiectasia. **a** Massive thickening of the villi in the jejunum and ileum, with a normal-appearing duodenum (courtesy of Sönke Martens, M.D.). **b** Push enteroscopy additionally shows white lymphatic exudate (*arrow*). **c** Radionuclide scans document intestinal protein loss (*arrow*; courtesy of Michaela Lürken, M.D.). **d** CT demonstrates thickened loops of small bowel (courtesy of Ernst Malzfeldt, M.D.). **e** Histologic section shows pronounced lymphangiectasia (*arrow*; courtesy of Jörg Caselitz, M.D.). The patient presented clinically with iron deficiency anemia and abnormal α_1-antitrypsin clearance

Lymphangiectasia as Part of a Syndrome

Intestinal lymphangiectasia may occur together with other syndromes.

The **yellow nail syndrome** comprises dystrophic yellow nails, lymphedema, pleural effusion, and intestinal lymphangiectasia (◘ Fig. 5.2-11) (Danielsson et al. 2006; Malek et al. 1996). **Hennekam**

syndrome, an autosomal recessive inherited disorder, includes intestinal lymphangiectasia and lymphedema, together with facial anomalies and mental retardation (Hennekam et al. 1989). **Noonan's syndrome** may occur as an autosomal dominant inherited condition or sporadically. Abnormalities of the face, neck, sternum, and heart such as pulmonic stenosis may be accompanied by intestinal lymphangiectasia (Keberle et al. 2000).

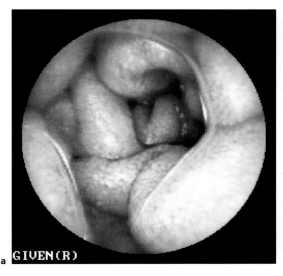
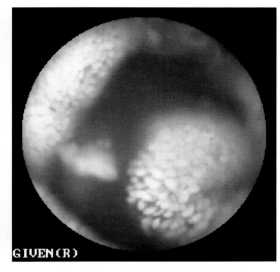
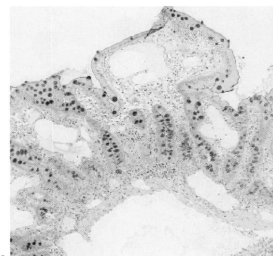
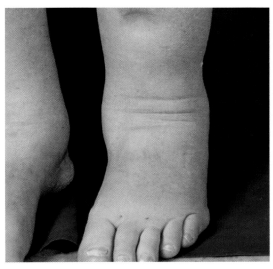

◘ **Fig. 5.2-11a–d.** Yellow nail syndrome. VCE reveals swollen mucosa with thick and short villi covered with opalescent »milky« fluid in the jejunum (**a**) and ileum (**b**) (case of Ervin Tóth, M.D. and Henrik Thorlacius, M.D.). Duodenal biopsy shows lymphangiectasia (**c**). This patient presented with hypoalbuminemia, bilateral lower limb edema, and slowly growing, dystrophic yellow nails (**d**) (**c** and **d** courtesy of Åke Danielsson, M.D.)

References

Aoyagi K, Iida M, Yao T et al (1997) Characteristic endoscopic features of intestinal lymphangiectasia: correlation with histological findings. Hepatogastroenterology 44:133–138

Asakura H, Miura S, Morishita T et al (1981) Endoscopic and histopathological study on primary and secondary intestinal lymphangiectasia. Dig Dis Sci 26:312–320

Barnes RE, deRidder PH (1993) Fat absorption in patients with functional intestinal lymphangiectasia and lymphangiectic cysts. Am J Gastroenterol 88:887–890

Danielsson A, Tóth E, Thorlacius H (2006) Capsule endoscopy in the management of a patient with a rare syndrome – yellow nail syndrome with intestinal lymphangiectasia. Gut 55:233

Fürstenau M, Kratzsch KH, Zimmermann S, Büttner W (1977) Fiberendoskopischer Nachweis, Häufigkeit und klinische Bedeutung der intestinalen Lymphangiektasie. Z Gesamte Inn Med 32:638–640

Hennekam RC, Geerdink RA, Hamel BC et al (1989) Autosomal recessive intestinal lymphangiectasia and lymphedema, with facial anomalies and mental retardation. Am J Med Genet 34:593–600

Keberle M, Mork H, Jenett M et al (2000) Computed tomography after lymphangiography in the diagnosis of intestinal lymphangiectasia with protein-losing enteropathy in Noonan's syndrome. Eur Radiol 10:1591–1593

Kuroiwa G, Takayama T, Sato Y et al (2001) Primary intestinal lymphangiectasia successfully treated with octreotide. J Gastroenterol 36:129–132

Malek NP, Ocran K, Tietge UJ et al (1996) A case of the yellow nail syndrome associated with massive chylous ascites, pleural and pericardial effusions. Z Gastroenterol 34:763–766

Munck A, Sosa VG, Faure C et al (2002) Suivi de long cours des lymphangiectasies intestinales primitives de l'enfant. À propos de six cas. Arch Pediatr 9:388–391

Riemann JF, Schmidt H (1981) Synopsis of endoscopic and other morphological findings in intestinal lymphangiectasia. Endoscopy 13:60–63

Waldmann TA, Steinfeld JL, Dutcher TF et al (1961) The role of the gastrointestinal system in idiopathic hypoproteinemia. Gastroenterology 41:197–207

Inflammatory and Systemic Diseases

6.1 Crohn's Disease

W. Voderholzer, A. Kornbluth, P.E. Legnani, J.A. Leighton

Definition. Crohn's disease (CD) is a chronic inflammatory bowel disease (IBD) characterized by mucosal and transmural inflammation. Although CD can affect the entire gastrointestinal (GI) tract, in about 70% of patients it involves the small intestine (SI). The ileocolonic region is the most common location in 40% of patients, whereas the colon alone is involved in 25% of patients. Other areas of the GI tract, such as the stomach or esophagus, are involved in 5% of patients. As many as 30–40% of patients with CD have lesions limited to the SI, usually the ileum. The diagnosis of CD in these patients can be difficult compared with the diagnosis of CD in patients who also have colonic involvement. The disease usually takes an alternating relapsing and remitting course.

Etiology. The pathogenesis of CD is thought to involve genetic, environmental, and immune system factors. A genetic predisposition is associated with chromosomes 6, 12, and 16. NOD2 (CARD15) was identified as the first disease gene on chromosome 16. Environmental influences such as the Western lifestyle, modern hygienic standards, and smoking also have causal significance. The pathogenesis apparently involves an inappropriately activated immune system that most likely responds to commensal flora with uncontrolled inflammation in the GI tract. The specific precipitating factors are still unclear.

Clinical Features. Typical symptoms are bouts of colicky abdominal pain and diarrhea, frequently associated with low-grade fever and weight loss. In the two-thirds of patients with ileocecal involvement, a palpable mass, corresponding to inflamed bowel loops, mesentery, or intra-abdominal abscess may be noted in the right lower abdomen. In these patients with colonic involvement, one-half of patients have bloody stools and one-third show involvement of the anus and surrounding tissue (fistulae, fissures, strictures, incontinence). Extensive involvement of the small bowel can lead to malabsorption; however, the most common cause for malabsorption in CD is the consequence of small intestinal surgical resection. Due to the transmural nature of the inflammatory process, fistulae, strictures, and abscesses may occur throughout the GI tract.

Extraintestinal Symptoms. Various extraintestinal symptoms may occur such as peripheral arthropathy (15–20%), sacroiliitis (10%), ocular manifestations (6%) such as episcleritis and uveitis, and skin manifestations such as pyoderma gangrenosum (rare) and erythema nodosum (15%). CD also predisposes to gallstone formation (25%) and primary sclerosing cholangitis (4%).

Histology. Mucosal biopsies can establish the diagnosis of CD and may help differentiate CD from ulcerative colitis. There is no single diagnostic pathologic criterion that can definitively make an IBD diagnosis. Several features suggest chronicity (indicating IBD rather than an acute colitis) such as architectural distortion with crypt distortion and basal plasma cell infiltration. The presence of granulomas (■ Fig. 6.1-1) suggests CD, but the frequency of granuloma formation is variable and is reported to be in 50–63% of surgically resected specimens, in 20–38% of regional lymph nodes, and in 15–36% of biopsy specimens obtained with an endoscope (Ramzan et al. 2002). In addition, other diseases can be associated with granulomas such as tuberculosis, fungal and

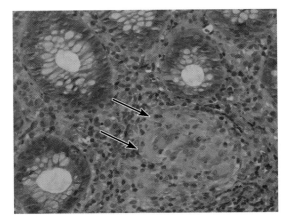

■ **Fig. 6.1-1.** Typical epithelioid cell granuloma (courtesy of Wilko Weichert, M.D.)

bacterial infections, diversion colitis, and sarcoidosis, as well as the infrequent patient with nonspecific foreign body granulomas, especially in the colon.

Treatment. Active CD can be treated with several different medications. The 5-aminosalicylic acid (ASA) agents are often useful for mild to moderate disease, especially in the colon. For moderate disease involving the ileum and ascending colon, budesonide an oral, topically active corticosteroid with extensive first-pass hepatic metabolism is effective. In patients with more severe disease oral and i.v. corticosteroids are useful for inducing a remission, but are not effective as maintenance medications and are associated with frequent and potentially serious toxicity. Antibiotics such as metronidazole and/or ciprofloxacin are useful for mild to moderate symptoms and in cases with mild perianal disease. Immunomodulatory drugs such as 6-mercaptopurine (MP), azathioprine, or methotrexate should be used in chronic active cases as steroid-sparing agents, or when 5-ASA medication, antibiotics or budesonide are not controlling symptoms. The anti-tumor necrosis factor (TNF) alpha antibody infliximab should be used in cases that do not respond to standard treatments. For maintaining remission, azathioprine, 6-MP, methotrexate, and infliximab have all demonstrated efficacy. 6-MP/azathioprine and metronidazole may retard relapse after surgical remission. Endoscopic balloon dilatation (■ Fig. 6.1-14) may be used in selected patients with strictures due to CD.

Indications for surgical treatment of CD:

- Symptomatic obstructing strictures
- Massive bleeding
- Perforation
- Intractable obstruction or symptomatic fistulae
- High-grade dysplasia or carcinoma
- Medically refractory inflammatory disease
- Medically refractory perianal disease

Endoscopy. Endoscopy is useful in the diagnosis and management of CD in accessible areas. In addition, it can provide valuable information regarding anatomic extent and severity of the mucosal inflammation. Endoscopy also aids in obtaining mucosal biopsies, performing cancer surveillance in high-risk individuals, and examining and dilating strictures. Because of the difference in distribution and pattern of inflammation, endoscopy can also help differentiate between ulcerative colitis and CD.

Classic lesions seen at endoscopy are notched (■ Fig. 6.1-2b) or shallow aphthae (■ Figs. 6.1-4 and 6.1-5), fissural ulcers (■ Figs. 6.1-7 and 6.1-8), crater-like ulcers (■ Figs. 6.1-9 and 6.1-10), which may actively bleed (■ Fig. 6.1-12b), and fistulae (■ Figs. 6.1-13e and 6.1-15). The lesions typically show a discontinuous pattern of involvement with normal mucosa intervening between diseased segments (»skip lesions«). The endoscopic appearance of strictures is not a definite indicator of whether the capsule can pass through (■ Figs. 6.1-11 and 6.1-12b) or not (■ Fig. 6.1-12a). VCE in an early stage of CD may demonstrate circumscribed lesions such as villous denudation (■ Figs. 6.1-2a and 6.1-3), which apparently are precursors to the typical aphthous lesions (Mitty et al. 2002). Patients with superficial lesions may present with normal findings in small bowel follow through or computed tomography (CT) enteroclysis (■ Figs. 6.1-6a and 6.1-4c).

Endoscopic findings in Crohn's disease:

- Erythema
- Loss of vascular pattern
- Granularity
- Notched or shallow aphthae
- Fissural and crater-like ulcers
- Strictures
- Fistulae

Differential Diagnosis. The differentiation of small bowel CD from the conditions listed below which are part of a large number of alternative diagnoses must be based on an overall evaluation of the clinical picture, pattern of involvement, histologic findings, and serologic data. It cannot be accomplished with endoscopic findings alone (Lo 2004).

Frequent differential diagnosis of small intestinal Crohn's disease:

- Drug-related enteropathy (nonsteroidal anti-inflammatory drugs)
- Tuberculosis
- Vasculitis/ischemic bowel disease
- Lymphoma
- Infectious enteritis

Role of VCE. Video capsule endoscopy (VCE) is a technique that provides an opportunity for the complete endoscopic evaluation of the entire SI mucosa. It has the potential to provide a more accurate way of diagnosing and evaluating the severity of CD by examining the degree, location, and extent of inflammation, particularly in patients with mild to moderate disease who have normal findings on small bowel follow through (SBFT). In fact, multiple studies have shown VCE to be superior to SBFT for detecting lesions in the SI. It also appears to be superior to SBFT for diagnosing CD, and it may be superior as well to enteroclysis (Eliakim et al. 2004; Fireman et al. 2003; Herrerias et al. 2003). This particularly applies to small lesions such as aphthae and small erosions

(Voderholzer et al. 2005). It should be added, however, that pathologic findings, specifically »mucosal breaks,« are noted in up to 14% of healthy subjects (Goldstein et al. 2005). Enteroclysis, CT, magnetic resonance imaging (MRI), and ultrasound also have their role in the diagnosis of complications such as strictures, fistulae, abscesses, and perforations.

Given the paucity of data and the risk of capsule retention, it is best at present to use VCE in patients with known CD only after the possibility of stricture has been excluded by other preceding imaging studies or within the framework of clinical studies, e.g., to assess the value of early aggressive treatment in healing mucosal lesions (Rey et al. 2004). It remains to be seen whether a more precise knowledge of involvement patterns will have therapeutic and prognostic implications and whether VCE can provide an effective method of surveillance.

Suspected Crohn's disease*

Patients with at least two of the following criteria:

- Abdominal pain or diarrhea
- Iron deficiency anemia
- Elevated ESR or CRP
- Hypoalbuminemia
- Extraintestinal manifestations
- Family history of IBD
- Abnormal serologies

---

* Suggested criteria for evaluation in further studies (ICCE consensus, Kornbluth et al. 2005)

Strictures. Strictures are described in one-third of patients with CD and increase with duration of disease. GI tract strictures may complicate CD or may be seen postoperatively. They may be asymptomatic or cause obstructive symptoms. Strictures may be fibrotic, inflammatory, occur at previous anastomoses, or be malignant. Endoscopy, when possible, is indicated for assessment and biopsy. In cases of chronic fibrotic strictures associated with obstructive symptoms, endoscopy with balloon dilation may relieve symptoms in open-label series (Saunders et al. 2004). Local steroid injection along with balloon dilation may improve outcome. Surgery is indicated when there is a high suspicion of malignancy or intractable obstructive symptoms.

Strictures are associated with an increased risk of capsule retention. Higher-grade strictures can be detected in standard radiological studies. Nevertheless, the majority of strictures that cause capsule retention or impaction are not detected radiographically prior to VCE (■ Fig. 6.1-12a). A test device called the »Patency Capsule« (Chap. 1.5) may be helpful for this purpose. If the capsule endoscope is retained by an inflammatory stricture, high doses of intravenous steroids administered for several days may restore passage (Voderholzer et al. 2005). Balloon dilatation can be used on strictures in the terminal ileum (■ Fig. 6.1-14) or proximal small bowel.

❶ Long-segment strictures (>15 cm) pose a particularly high risk of obstruction during capsule endoscopy (Boivin et al. 2005).

6

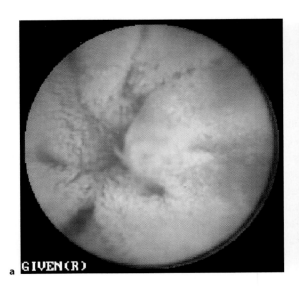

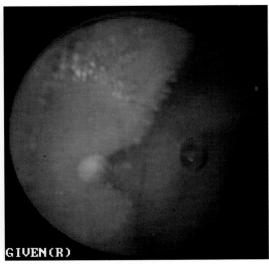

Fig. 6.1-2a, b. Circumscribed villous denudation – this is a nonspecific finding (**a**); additionally notched ulcer (**b**)

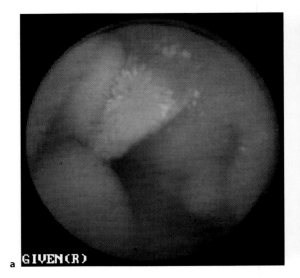

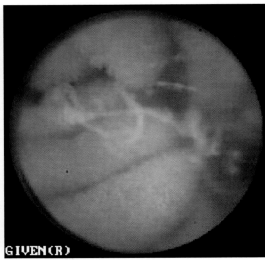

Fig. 6.1-3a, b. Circumscribed erythema and villous denudation

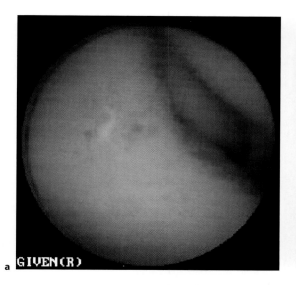

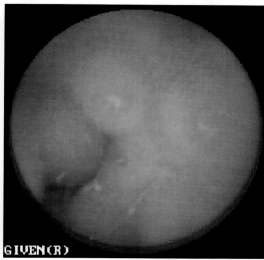

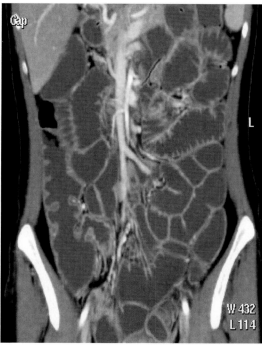

■ **Fig. 6.1-4a–c. a–b** VCE shows aphthae in the jejunum. **c** Negative CT-enteroclysis in the same patient (**c** courtesy of Patrik Rogalla, M.D.)

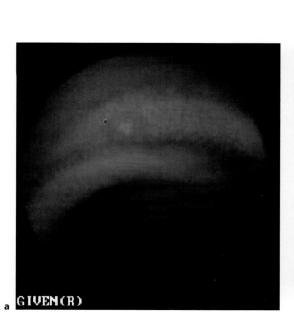

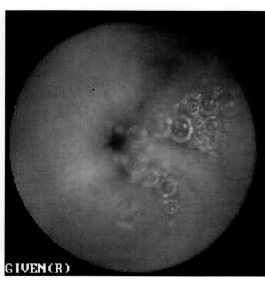

■ **Fig. 6.1-5a, b.** Aphthous ulcers that were found throughout the small intestine

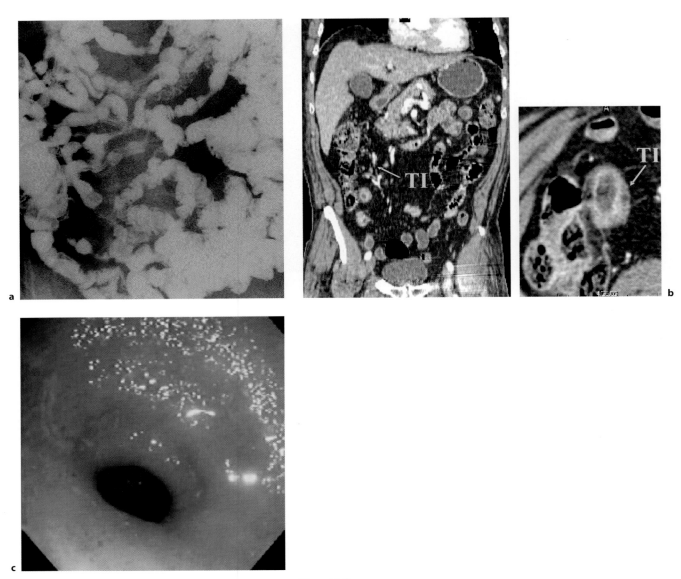

▫ Fig. 6.1-6a–c. Same patient as in Fig. 6.1-5a, b: negative small bowel follow through (**a**) and mild terminal ileal inflammation seen at CT enterography (**b**). Ileocolonoscopy of the same patient showed terminal ileal erythema (**c**)

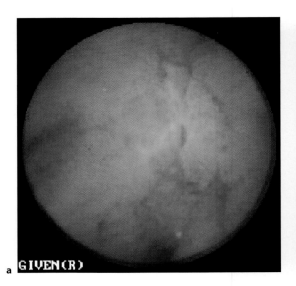

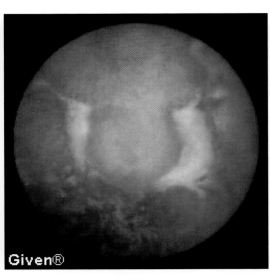

▫ Fig. 6.1-7a, b. Linear ulcers in the jejunum (**a**) and ileum (**b**)

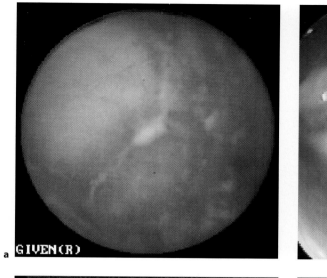

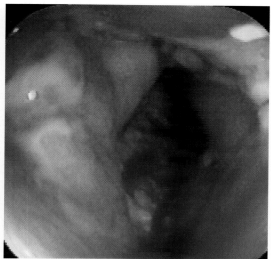

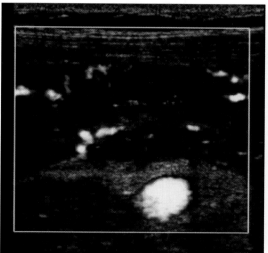

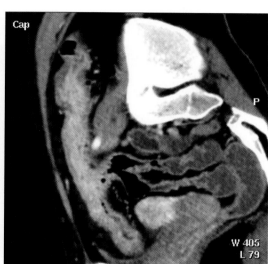

Fig. 6.1-8. a Linear ulcer in the ileum.
b Ileocolonoscopic view of the same
patient showing ulceration and edema.
c Ultrasound view (power Doppler) of the
same patient. **d** CT enteroclysis view of the
same patient

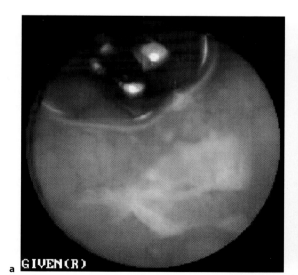

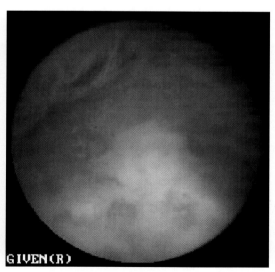

Fig. 6.1-9a, b. Ulcers in the ileum

6

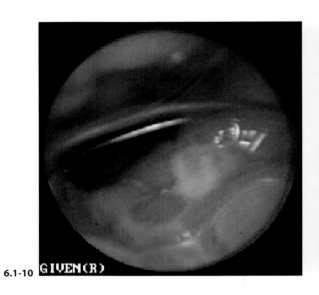

6.1-10

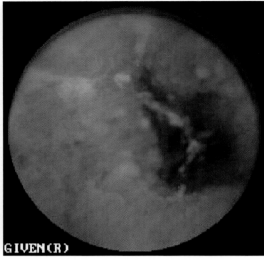

6.1-11

 Fig. 6.1-10. Ulcer in the jejunum

Fig. 6.1-11. Stricture in the ileum

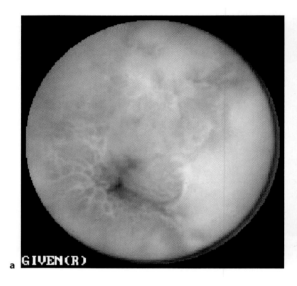

a

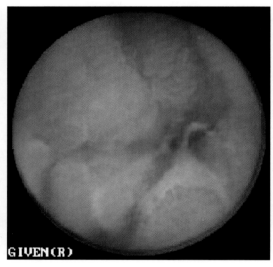

b

Fig. 6.1-12a, b. Inflammatory jejunal stricture with an ulcer not seen on CT enteroclysis with ultimate capsule retention (**a**). Inflammatory ileal stenosis with ulcer and with active bleeding. The capsule passed (**b**)

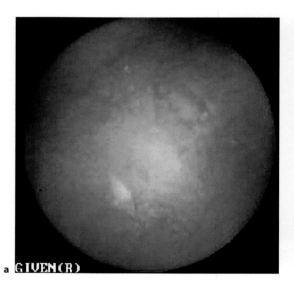

a

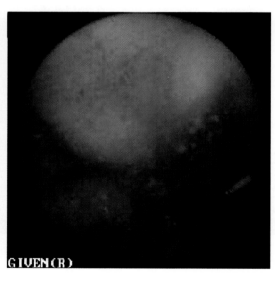

b

Fig. 6.1-13a, b. Patient with ileal disease. Erythema and erosions (**a**, **b**)

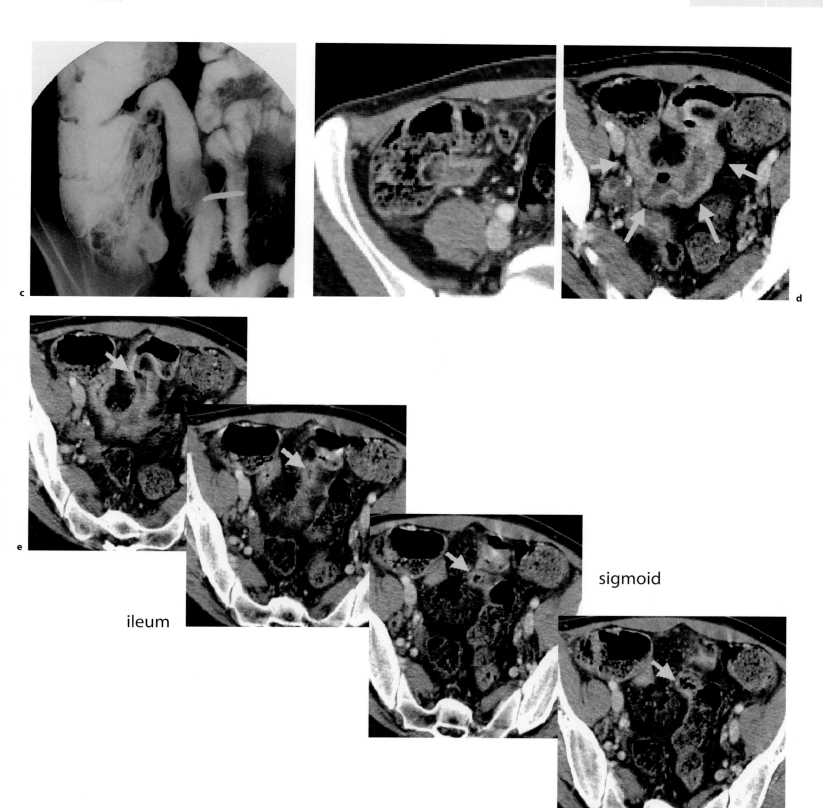

ileum

sigmoid

□ **Fig. 6.1-13c–e.** Patient with ileal disease. Terminal and ileal stenosis (**c**), and CT enteroclysis showing more extensive disease and enterocolic fistula (**d**, **e**)

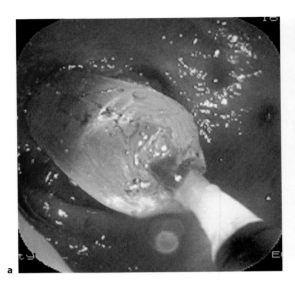
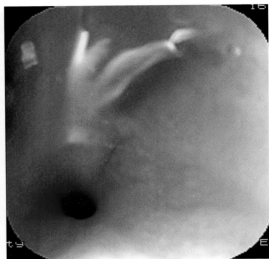

Fig. 6.1-14a, b. Balloon dilatation of narrow neoterminal ileal stenosis

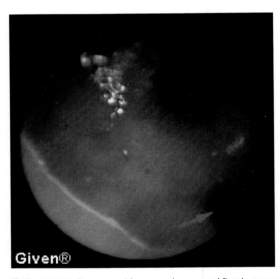

Fig. 6.1-15. Stricture with narrow lumen and fistula, seen as second smaller orifice

Internet

www.ccfa.org: The Crohn's and Colitis Foundation of America
www.efcca.org: European Federation of Crohn's and Ulcerative Colitis Association

References

Boivin ML, Lochs H, Voderholzer W (2005) Does passage of the patency capsule indicate small bowel patency? A prospective clinical evaluation. Endoscopy 37:808–815

Eliakim R, Suissa A, Yassin K et al (2004) Wireless capsule video endoscopy compared to barium follow-through and computerised tomography in patients with suspected Crohn's disease – final report. Dig Liver Dis 36:519–522

Fireman Z, Mahajna E, Broide E et al (2003) Diagnosing small bowel Crohn's disease with wireless capsule endoscopy. Gut 52:390–392

Goldstein JL, Eisen G, Lewis B et al (2005) Video capsule endoscopy to prospectively assess small bowel injury with celecoxib, naproxen plus omeprazole, and placebo. Clin Gastroenterol Hepatol 3:133–141

Herrerias JM, Caunedo A, Rodriguez-Tellez M et al (2003) Capsule endoscopy in patients with suspected Crohn's disease and negative endoscopy. Endoscopy 35:564–568

Kornbluth A, Colombel JF, Leighton JA, Loftus E (2005) ICCE consensus for inflammatory bowel disease. Endoscopy 37:1051–1054

Lo SK (2004) Capsule endoscopy in the diagnosis and management of inflammatory bowel disease. Gastrointest Endosc Clin N Am 14:179–193

Mitty R, Cave DR, Brighton MA (2002) Focal villous denudation: a precursor to aphthoid ulcers in Crohn's disease as detected by video capsule endoscopy. Gastroenterology 122 [Suppl]:A217

Ramzan NN, Leighton JA, Heigh RI, Shapiro MS (2002) Clinical significance of granuloma in Crohn's disease. Inflamm Bowel Dis 8:168–173

Rey JF, Gay G, Kruse A, Lambert R (2004) European Society of Gastrointestinal Endoscopy guideline for video capsule endoscopy. Endoscopy 36:656–658

Saunders BP, Brown GJ, Lemann M, Rutgeerts P (2004) Balloon dilation of ileocolonic strictures in Crohn's disease. Endoscopy 36:1001–1007

Voderholzer W, Beinhoelzl J, Rogalla P et al (2005) Small bowel involvement in Crohn's disease. A prospective comparison of wireless capsule endoscopy and CT enteroclysis. Gut 54:385–387

6.2 Villous Atrophy

D. Schuppan, M. Keuchel, J.A. Murray

Villous atrophy results from the inflammatory destruction of villi. The most frequent cause is celiac sprue; other etiologies are rare (combined immunodeficiency states, radiation damage, recent chemotherapy, graft-versus-host disease), due to infection (giardiasis, tropical sprue), or appear to be rare (pre-) malignant consequences of long-term untreated celiac sprue (refractory sprue, ulcerative jejunitis, intestinal T-cell lymphoma).

Celiac Sprue

Etiology. Celiac sprue (synonyms: gluten-sensitive enteropathy, non-tropical sprue, celiac disease) is a relatively common autoimmune disease (prevalence 1%, except East Asia) with a genetic predisposition (HLA-DQ2 or HLA-DQ8, prevalent in 30–35% of the population). The ingestion of gluten from grains (wheat, barley, and rye) damages the proximal small intestine, by activating mucosal T cells, causes villous atrophy and crypt hyperplasia, and triggers a reaction to the autoantigen tissue transglutaminase (tTG, the autoantigen of endomysial antibodies, EMA). Celiac sprue is associated with the skin disease dermatitis herpetiformis and other autoimmune diseases such as type 1 diabetes or autoimmune thyroiditis (Ciclitira et al. 2001; Dieterich et al. 2003; Farrell and Kelly 2002; Collin and Reunala 2003).

Prevalence. The prevalence of clinically manifest celiac sprue in the West, North Africa, and the Near and Middle East is 1:1000 to 1:4000, with regional variations (Murray at al. 2003). Oligosymptomatic (e.g., iron deficiency anemia, osteoporosis), asymptomatic, or atypical forms (e.g., associated autoimmunity), as detected by autoantibody screening (IgA anti-tTG, EMA) and confirmed by biopsy, are much more common (prevalence 1:80 to 1:200) (Schuppan and Esslinger 2003; Fasano et al. 2003).

Clinical Features. Symptoms of classic celiac sprue are diarrhea, malabsorption, and abdominal pain. However, the majority of patients have minor or atypical symptoms (see above). Some may have no symptoms whatsoever.

Diagnosis. IgA autoantibodies to tTG or endomysium (EMA) are highly predictive for celiac sprue (sensitivity above 90%, specificity above 97%) (Wong et al. 2003). Confirmation is by duodenoscopy (Tursi et al. 2002) with duodenal biopsy. Patients with IgA deficiency may have false-negative tests, but display high IgG anti-tTG titers.

Histology. The histologic hallmarks of sprue are villous atrophy, crypt hyperplasia, and lymphocytic infiltration of the small bowel mucosa. A modified version of the Marsh classification is used to describe findings (Marsh 1992; Oberhuber et al. 2001), with partial, subtotal, and total villous atrophy being pathognomonic when combined with positive serology for celiac autoantibodies (Marsh lesions IIIa, b, and c, respectively).

Marsh classification:

0 Normal (refers only to patients with celiac sprue treated by diet)

I Infiltrative type (more than 40 intraepithelial lymphocytes (IEL)/100 epithelial cells)

II Hyperplastic type (more than 40 IEL/100 epithelial cells and crypt hyperplasia)

III Destructive type (villous atrophy)
   IIIa mild
   IIIb subtotal
   IIIc total

IV Hypoplastic type (villous atrophy but no crypt hyperplasia)

Endoscopy. Villous atrophy can be diagnosed endoscopically by VCE (Petroniene et al. 2004). At present, VCE is not recommended as a primary diagnostic study due to its high cost and inability to furnish a biopsy sample. VCE can be helpful for assessing the extent and severity of small bowel involvement (Murray et al. 2004a), confirming refractory sprue or lymphoma, and in cases where symptoms recur despite a strictly gluten-free diet. Celiac disease may rarely be associated with strictures or malignancies in the proximal intestine and occasionally motility disturbances that might impede the passage of the capsule (Schweiger and Murray 1998) (▣ Fig. 6.2-11)

Little has been published on capsule endoscopy in the treated patient. Personal experience is that celiac disease changes are diminished in extent and severity after 6 months of a gluten-free diet (Murray et al. 2004b). In patients who are continuing to have symptoms occasionally erosions and atrophic changes may be seen to persist (▣ Figs. 6.2-5 and 6.2-6).

Endoscopic features of celiac disease:

- Absent or shortened villi (▣ Figs. 6.2-1, 6.2-2, and 6.2-3a)
- Mosaic mucosal pattern (▣ Fig. 6.2-1)
- Scalloped valvulae conniventes (▣ Fig. 6.2-1)
- Mucosal fissures (▣ Figs. 6.2-1, 6.2-4, and 6.2-5)
- Effaced folds (▣ Fig. 6.2-2)
- Involvement of the proximal small bowel (▣ Fig. 6.2-3)
- Occasional tiny erosions (▣ Figs. 6.2-6 and 6.2-8b)
- Patchy atrophy with preserved villi in treated celiac disease
- Steatorrhea in colon (▣ Fig. 6.2-7)

---

❶ Villous atrophy may occasionally be confined to focal areas (Hurlstone and Sanders 2003).

Prognosis. Symptoms improve in about 70% of patients within 2 weeks after institution of a gluten-free diet, with mucosal recovery, while varying degrees of villous atrophy can persist (Collin et al. 2004; Lee et al. 2003). Possible late complications of untreated celiac sprue include osteoporosis and apparently the development of refractory sprue and malignancies such as enteropathy-associated T-cell lymphoma (EATL; ▣ Figs. 6.6-10 and 7.2-23) and small intestinal carcinoma (▣ Fig. 6.2-11).

6

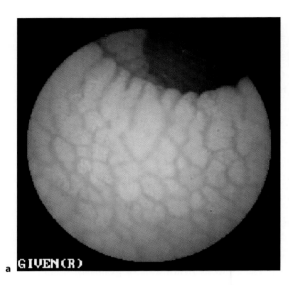

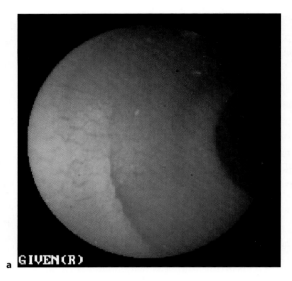

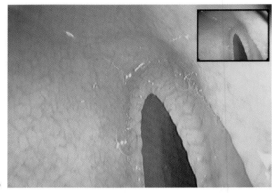

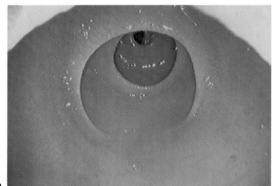

⬛ **Fig. 6.2-1a, b.** Scalloped valvulae conniventes (crest of fold), fissures, and a mosaic mucosal pattern. **a** VCE. **b** Push enteroscopy

⬛ **Fig. 6.2-2a, b.** Effaced valvulae conniventes. **a** VCE. **b** Push enteroscopy

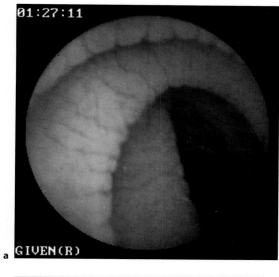

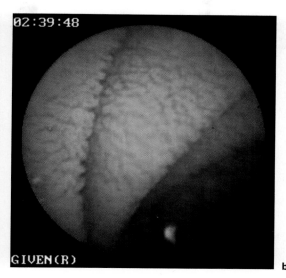

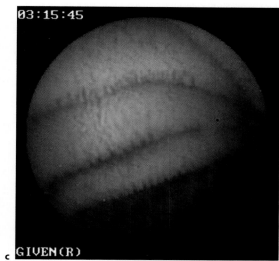

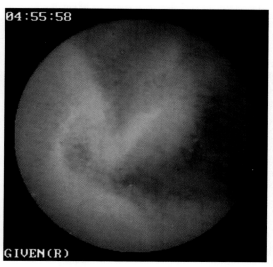

◨ Fig. 6.2-3a–d. Villous atrophy, decreasing from proximal to distal. **a** Subtotal – total atrophy (corresponding to Marsh IIIb-c). **b** Mild atrophy (corresponding to Marsh IIIa) **c, d** Fairly normal. Patient had a long history of sprue despite of dietary modification

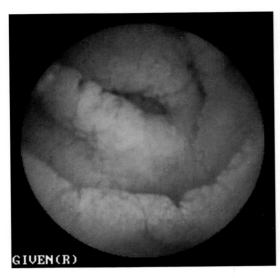

Fig. 6.2-4. Deep fissuring

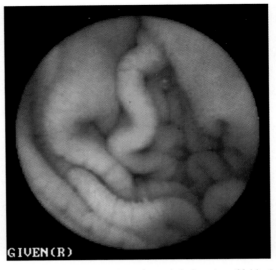

Fig. 6.2-5. Some persistent but subtle fissuring of folds. Compliant patient on a gluten-free diet for 6 months

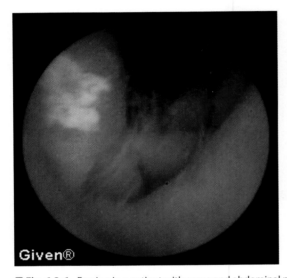

Fig. 6.2-6. Erosion in a patient with sprue and abdominal pain despite treatment

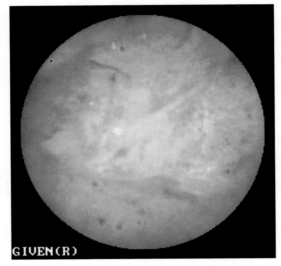

Fig. 6.2-7. Steatorrhea in colon of an untreated celiac patient

Tropical Sprue

This is now rarely seen in travelers returning from the tropics, but more frequently in inhabitants of tropical areas. Tropical sprue has an infectious etiology, but the causative organisms remain ill defined. It has the same endoscopic appearance as nontropical sprue and clinical manifestations are diarrhea and vitamin (especially folate) deficiency. Patients improve on long-term antibiotic therapy (usually tetracyclines) and folic acid replacement (Lim 2001). Studies on tropical sprue using VCE have not been performed.

Autoimmune Enteropathy

This is a very rare disorder of unknown etiology, characterized by villous atrophy (◻ Fig. 6.2-8) and enterocyte antibodies (Ciccocioppo et al. 2002). Gluten is not the trigger and no antibodies to tTG are found. Treatment with steroids and immunosuppressants is of variant efficacy (Daum et al. 2003).

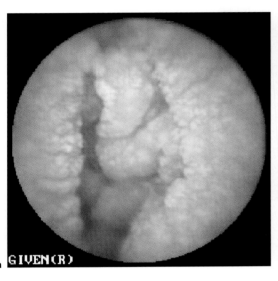
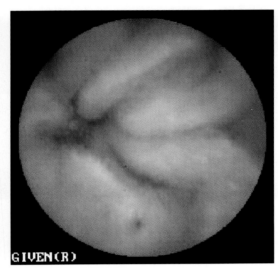
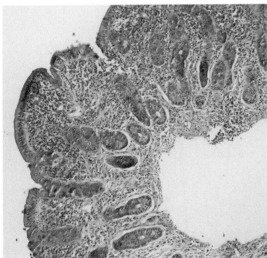
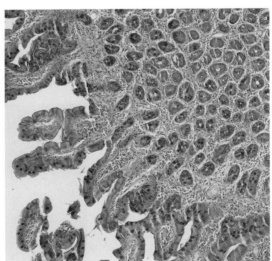

◻ **Fig. 6.2-8a–d.** Villous atrophy in autoimmune enteropathy. **a** Initial finding at VCE, **b** After 20 months of low-dose steroids, the villi appear normal with small erosions. **c** Initial histology showed villous atrophy, crypt hyperplasia, and (polyclonal) lymphocytic infiltration. **d** Essentially normal findings after treatment (courtesy of Jörg Caselitz, M.D.)

Refractory Sprue

Refractory sprue can develop in up to 5% of adults with long-standing (often previously undetected) celiac sprue. Patients do not respond to or relapse while on a strictly gluten-free diet. Small bowel involvement is often extensive (◘ Fig. 6.2-9) and there is growth of monoclonal in-

testinal T-cell populations which can be detected by polymerase chain reaction (PCR) for T-cell receptors from biopsies. Refractory sprue type I is responsive to steroids and immunosuppressants, while refractory sprue type II evolves into overt T-cell lymphoma (see below) (Cellier et al. 2000; Wahab et al. 2002).

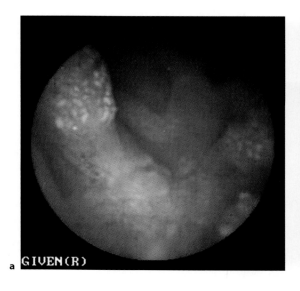
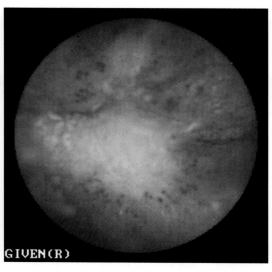

◘ Fig. 6.2-9a, b. Refractory sprue type II. **a** Lymphangiectatic changes. **b** Mucosal hemorrhage in the distal small bowel

Intestinal Lymphoma

This is an initially intraepithelial enteropathy-associated T-cell lymphoma (EATL) which appears to develop from refractory sprue (Foss et al. 2000; ◘ Figs. 6.2-10 and 7.2-23.

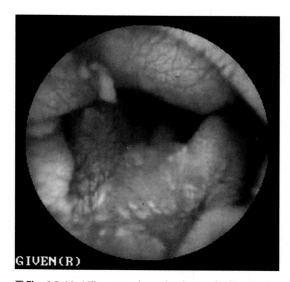

◘ Fig. 6.2-10. Villous atrophy and red area of infiltrative lymphoma

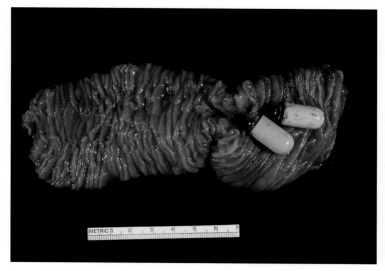

◘ Fig. 6.2-11. Retained capsules at site of unexpected adenocarcinoma of the jejunum complicating sprue

Internet

http://digestive.niddk.nih.gov/ddiseases/pubs/celiac
www.celiac.org: Celiac Disease Foundation
www.csaceliacs.org: Celiac Sprue Association (USA)
www.gluten.net: Gluten Intolerance Group
http://bidmc.harvard.edu/display.asp?node_id=5449: Celiac Center of Harvard
    Medical School (USA)

References

Cellier C, Delabesse E, Helmer C et al (2000) Refractory sprue, coeliac disease, and
    enteropathy-associated T-cell lymphoma. French Coeliac Disease Study Group.
    Lancet 356:203–208
Ciclitira PJ, King AL, Fraser JS (2001) AGA technical review on Celiac Sprue. American
    Gastroenterological Association. Gastroenterology 120:1526–1540
Ciccocioppo R, d'Alo S, di Sabatino A et al (2002) Mechanisms of villous atrophy in
    autoimmune enteropathy and coeliac disease. Clin Exp Immunol 128:88–93
Collin P, Mäki M, Kaukinen K (2004) Complete small intestinal mucosal recovery is
    obtainable in the treatment of celiac disease. Gastrointest Endosc 59:158–159
Collin P, Reunala T (2003) Recognition and management of the cutaneous manifesta-
    tions of celiac disease: a guide for dermatologists. Am J Clin Dermatol 4:13–20
Daum S, Sahin E, Jansen A et al (2003) Adult autoimmune enteropathy treated
    successfully with tacrolimus. Digestion 68:86–90
Dieterich W, Esslinger B, Schuppan D (2003) Pathomechanisms in celiac disease. Int
    Arch Allergy Immunol 132:98–108
Fasano A, Berti I, Gerarduzzi T, Not T, Colletti RB, Drago S, Elitsur Y, Green PHR,
    Guandalini S, Hill I, Pietzak M, Ventura A, Thorpe M, Kryszak D, Fornaroli F,
    Wasserman SS, Murray JA, Horvath K (2003) Prevalence of celiac disease in at-risk
    and not-at-risk groups in the United States: a large multicenter study. Arch Intern
    Med 163:286–292
Farrell RJ, Kelly CP (2002) Celiac sprue. N Engl J Med 346:180–188
Foss HD, Coupland SE, Stein H (2000) Klinisch-pathologische Formen peripherer
    T- und NK-Zell-Lymphome. Pathologe 21:137–146

Hurlstone DP, Sanders DS (2003) High-magnification immersion chromoscopic
    duodenoscopy permits visualization of patchy atrophy in celiac disease: an
    opportunity to target biopsies of abnormal mucosa. Gastrointest Endosc
    58:815
Lee SK, Lo W, Memeo L et al (2003) Duodenal histology in patients with celiac disease
    after treatment with a gluten-free diet. Gastrointest Endosc 57:187–191
Lim ML (2001) A perspective on tropical sprue. Curr Gastroenterol Rep 3:322–327
Marsh MN (1992) Gluten, major histocompatibility complex, and the small intestine:
    a molecular and immunobiologic approach to the spectrum of gluten sensitiv-
    ity (›celiac sprue‹). Gastroenterology 102:330–354
Murray JA, van Dyke C, Plevak MF, Dierkhising, Zinsmeister AR, Melton LJ III (2003)
    Trends in the identification and clinical features of celiac disease in a North
    American community 1950-2001. Clin Gastroenterol Hepatol 1:19–27
Murray JA, Brogan D, Van Dyke C, Knipschield MA, Gostout CJ (2004a) Mapping
    the extent of untreated celiac disease with capsule enteroscopy. Gastrointest
    Endosc 59:AB101
Murray JA, Watson T, Clearman B, Mitros F (2004b) Effect of a gluten-free diet on
    gastrointestinal symptoms in celiac disease. Am J Clin Nutr 79:669–673
Oberhuber G, Caspary WF, Kirchner T et al (2001) Arbeitsgemeinschaft für Gastro-
    enterologische Pathologie der Deutschen Gesellschaft für Pathologie. Empfeh-
    lung zur Zöliakie-/Spruediagnostik. Z Gastroenterol 39:157–168
Petroniene R, Dubcenco E, Baker J et al (2004) Given capsule endoscopy in celiac
    disease. Gastrointest Endosc Clin N Am 14:115–127
Schuppan D, Esslinger B (2003) Einheimische Sprue (Zöliakie) – Diagnostik, asso-
    ziierte Erkrankungen und Therapie. Dtsch Med Wochenschr 128 [Suppl 2]:
    S69–S71
Schweiger GD, Murray JA (1998) Post-bulbar duodenal ulceration and stenosis
    associated with celiac disease. Abdom Imaging 23:347–349
Tursi A, Brandimarte G, Giorgetti GM, Gigliobianco A (2002) Endoscopic features of
    celiac disease in adults and their correlation with age, histological damage, and
    clinical form of the disease. Endoscopy 34:787–792
Wahab PJ, Meijer JW, Goerres MS, Mulder CJ (2002) Coeliac disease: changing views
    on gluten-sensitive enteropathy. Scand J Gastroenterol Suppl 236:60–65
Wong RC, Steele RH, Reeves GE et al (2003) Antibody and genetic testing in coeliac
    disease. Pathology 35:285–304

6.3 Eosinophilic Enteritis

E.G. Seidman, M.H. Dirks

Definition. Primary eosinophilic gastrointestinal (GI) diseases are defined as disorders that selectively affect segments of the GI tract with eosinophil-rich inflammation, in the absence of other known causes (e.g., drug reactions, parasitic infections, and malignancy).

Etiology. Both genetic and environmental factors are incriminated. An allergic etiology is presumed to be involved in many cases, usually implicating food or other environmental allergens. Studies have identified a contributory role for T-helper cell type 2 (Th2) cytokines such as interleukin (IL)-5 and chemokines such as eotaxin (Rothenberg 2004).

Clinical Features. The disease is relatively uncommon, predominantly affecting males, typically young adults or children. Signs and symptoms are related to the site, extent, and layer of the GI wall involved (Baehler and Seidman 2002). The most common form of eosinophilic gastroenteritis is mucosal disease, with involvement of the stomach (most often the antrum), small intestine, and sometimes the esophagus or colon (Lake 2004; Potter et al. 2004). With mucosal involvement of the small bowel, the dominant symptoms are diarrhea and malabsorption. Patients frequently present with iron deficiency anemia and may have peripheral edema due to the protein-losing enteropathy. This condition may be confused with irritable bowel syndrome or dyspepsia (Daneshjoo and Talley 2002).

Involvement of the muscularis layer results in wall thickening and variable degrees of obstruction, with gastric outlet stenosis being most common. Symptoms, such as postprandial vomiting, resemble pyloric stenosis. Stenotic lesions elsewhere in the gut may mimic Crohn's strictures. Serosal involvement is rare, resulting in the insidious appearance of eosinophilic ascites, usually without significant GI symptoms. Pericardial or even pleural effusions may occur in a polyserositis-like presentation. Tissue eosinophilia also rarely may involve extraintestinal organs such as the peritoneum, gallbladder, spleen, pancreas, urinary bladder, and even pericardium. One-third or more of patients have a history of atopic disease (e.g., urticaria, eczema, asthma) and/or environmental or food allergies, with positive allergen-specific IgE antibodies or positive skin prick tests.

Diagnosis. The diagnosis is based on the histological demonstration of tissue eosinophilia, in the absence of other causes. The dilemma for clinicians, in the era prior to video capsule endoscopy, was that the small bowel lesions are focal and often inaccessible to endoscopic biopsy. Random biopsies of the upper and lower GI tract obtained by gastroscopy and colonoscopy often failed to demonstrate the histological findings.

Video Capsule Endoscopy. The typical small intestinal endoscopic findings are sharply demarcated foci of severe villous atrophy and marked erythema (◘ Fig. 6.3-1a) (Sant'Anna et al. 2005). Focal shallow ulcers can also be seen. Gastric inflammatory polyps are found in some cases (◘ Fig. 6.3-1b). Strictures may occur (◘ Fig. 6.3-1c), which may cause capsule retention (Sant'Anna et al. 2005; Seidman et al. 2004).

Treatment. Treatment consists of an elimination diet in cases with food allergies. In rare cases with multiple food allergies, an amino acid diet may be required (Justinich et al. 1996). Oral corticosteroids are indicated for more severe or refractory cases (Caldwell 2002; Rothenberg 2004). Locally acting corticosteroids with less risk of adrenal suppression (budesonide, fluticasone) may be substituted in some cases, although controlled trials are lacking. Promising new drugs for this condition include montelukast, a selective leukotriene receptor antagonist, and suplaplast tosilate, a selective Th2 cytokine inhibitor with inhibitory effects on allergy-induced eosinophilic infiltration and IgE production (Daneshjoo and Talley 2002).

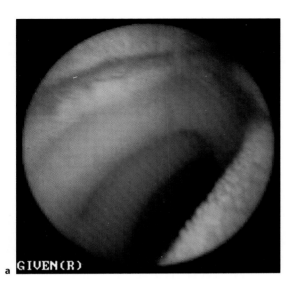

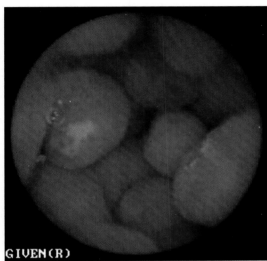

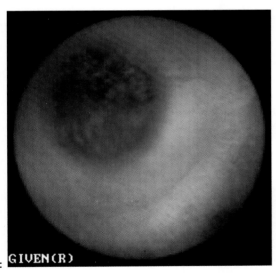

Internet

http://c4isr.com/NEED: The National Eosinophilic Disease Foundation (USA)

References

Baehler P, Seidman EG (2002) Gastrointestinal manifestations of food-protein-induced hypersensitivity; eosinophilic gastroenteritis. In: Rudolph CD et al (eds) Rudolph's pediatrics, 21st edn. McGraw Hill, New York, Chap. 17.21, pp 1444–1447

Caldwell JH (2002) Eosinophilic gastroenteritis. Curr Treat Options Gastroenterol 5:9–16

Daneshjoo RJ, Talley N (2002) Eosinophilic gastroenteritis. Curr Gastroenterol Rep 4:366–372

Justinich C, Katz A, Gurbindo C et al (1996) Elemental diet improves steroid-dependent eosinophilic gastroenteritis and reverses growth failure. J Pediatr Gastroenterol Nutr 23:81–85

Lake AM (2004) Allergic bowel disease. Adolesc Med Clin 15:105–117

Potter JW, Saeian K, Staff D et al (2004) Eosinophilic esophagitis in adults: an emerging problem with unique esophageal features. Gastrointest Endosc 59:355–361

Rothenberg ME (2004) Eosinophilic gastrointestinal disorders (EGID). J Allergy Clin Immunol 113:11–28

Sant'Anna AMGA, Dubois J, Miron MJ et al (2005) Wireless capsule endoscopy for obscure small bowel disorders: final results of the first pediatric controlled trial. Clin Gastroenterol Hepatol 3:264–270

Seidman EG, Sant'Anna AMGA, Dirks MH (2004) Potential applications of wireless capsule endoscopy in the pediatric age group. Gastrointest Endosc Clin N Am 14:207–217

◘ Fig. 6.3-1a–c. Video capsule endoscopic image showing the characteristic focal nature of the mucosal lesions in eosinophilic gastroenteropathy. **a** The patient is an adolescent who presented with a protein-losing enteropathy and an iron deficiency anemia. A typically sharply demarcated area of complete villous atrophy with marked erythema is seen alongside an area with villi. **b** Same case as in **a**, showing inflammatory polyps in the gastric corpus. **c** One of two small bowel strictures observed by video capsule endoscopy in a patient with eosinophilic gastroenteritis. Neither stricture was detected by a recent barium examination of the small bowel. Treatment with corticosteroids successfully relieved the inflammatory stenosis, with uncomplicated, delayed passage of the capsule (reprinted from Seidman et al. 2004 with permission from Elsevier)

6.4   Infectious Diseases of the Small Intestine

M. Keuchel, J. Soares, D. Reddy

Introduction

Most infections that involve the small bowel are self-limiting. There is no need for endoscopic examination in these cases. Suspicion of microbial enteritis can be confirmed by stool cultures and if necessary by toxin or antigen determination. Cases with persistent diarrhea and associated symptoms such as weight loss, fever, arthralgia, neurologic deficits, or findings such as anemia, inflammatory signs, eosinophilia, or signs of malabsorption warrant further investigation. Besides microscopic stool examination, the main tool for this purpose is flexible endoscopy with tissue sampling from the duodenum, terminal ileum, and colon. Video capsule endoscopy can sometimes reveal changes in the jejunum or ileum. Its usefulness is greatly limited by an inability to obtain biopsies, however.

Whipple's Disease

Clinical Features. This is a very rare disease characterized by diarrhea, malassimilation, arthritis, neurologic deficits, and psychiatric changes.

Etiology. The causative organism of Whipple's disease is *Tropheryma whippelii* (Bentley et al. 2003). Affected individuals probably also have a cellular immune defect (Fenollar and Raoult 2003).

Diagnosis. The diagnosis is based on a small bowel biopsy with the detection of PAS-positive macrophages. It can be confirmed by a polymerase chain reaction (PCR) assay in an intestinal biopsy.

Endoscopy. Endoscopy may reveal a glassy-gelatinous edema, lymphangiectasia (▢ Fig. 6.4-1), erosions, ulcers, and diffuse hemorrhage (▢ Fig. 6.4-2) (Fritscher-Ravens et al. 2004; Gay et al. 2005). Similar findings may be noted in intestinal histoplasmosis or atypical mycobacteriosis (Ratnaike 2000).

Treatment. Initial treatment is with an intravenous antibiotic that will enter the subarachnoid space. This should be followed by at least a 12-month course of trimethoprim-sulfamethoxazole or a similar antibiotic.

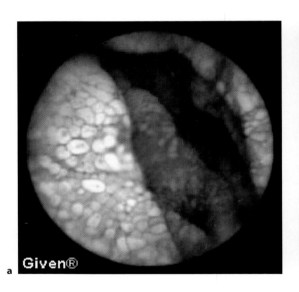
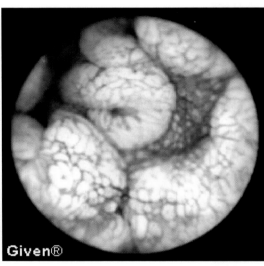

▢ **Fig. 6.4-1a, b.** Whipple's disease. Diffuse lymphangiectasia with swollen whitish, club-shaped villi (**a**) and additionally diffuse edema (**b**) (courtesy of Ingo Franke, M.D.)

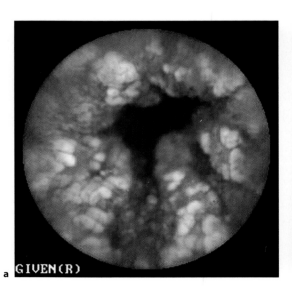
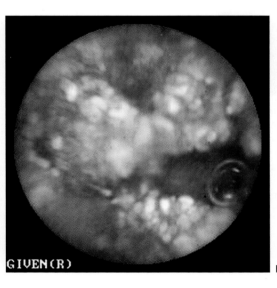

▢ **Fig. 6.4-2a, b.** Whipple's disease. VCE shows edema, severe diffuse lymphangiectasia (**a**) and additionally distinct bleeding (**b**) (courtesy of Anette Fritscher-Ravens, M.D., reprinted from Fritscher-Ravens et al. 2004 with permission from Georg Thieme Verlag)

Infection with *Mycobacterium avium-intracellulare*

Clinical Features. Intestinal involvement by *Mycobacterium avium-intracellulare* is known to occur in addition to pulmonary and cutaneous involvement (Pantongrag-Brown et al. 1998). The infection may take an asymptomatic course or may become disseminated, especially in immunocompromised patients.

Etiology. The infection is caused by atypical mycobacteria, usually *Mycobacterium avium-intracellulare* (MAI).

Diagnosis. Diagnosis is based on the histologic detection of acid-fast rods in biopsy material, PCR assay, or by culturing the organism from blood, bone marrow, biopsies, or sputum. Due to the ubiquitous occurrence of MAI, detection of the organism in normally sterile materials is the most accurate test.

Endoscopy. The endoscopic resemblance of small bowel involvement to Whipple's disease has given rise to the term »pseudo-Whipple's disease« (■ Fig. 6.4-3).

Treatment. If treatment is necessary, it consists of an antimycobacterial combination regimen based on sensitivity testing and often including clarithromycin or azithromycin. The course of treatment may be prolonged, depending on the patient's immune status.

6

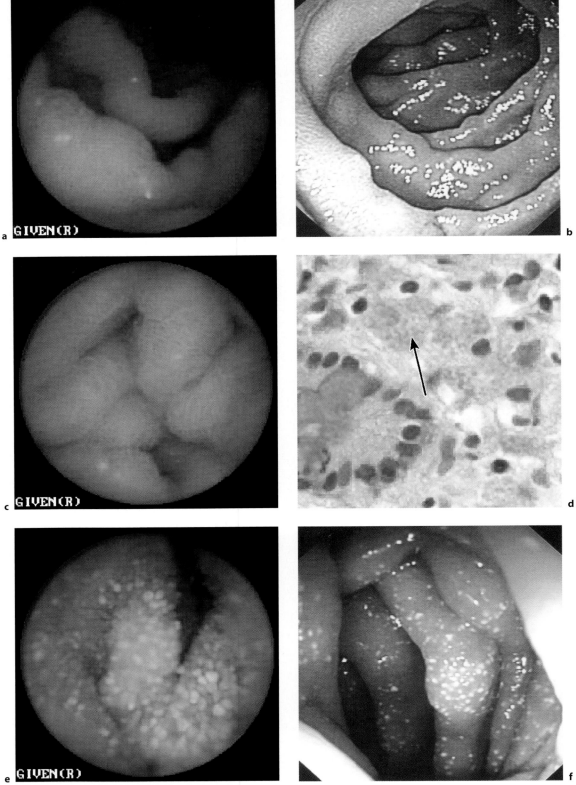

Fig. 6.4-3a–f. »Pseudo-Whipple's disease« in a young man with chronic diarrhea, malassimilation, and lymphadenopathy. *Mycobacterium avium-intracellulare* was isolated from lymph nodes. The patient was HIV-negative. **a, c** Examination of the jejunum shows diffuse, glassy edema with indistinct villi and luminal narrowing (VCE). The capsule passed through the lumen without impediment. **d** Histology revealed weakly PAS-positive macrophages (courtesy of Axel von Herbay, M.D.). **e** Edema diminishes farther distally, but diffuse lymphangiectasia is more pronounced (VCE). **b, f** Corresponding images in push enteroscopy (courtesy of Wolfgang Cordruwisch, M.D.)

Tuberculosis

Etiology. Gastrointestinal tuberculosis most frequently involves the small intestine and ileocecum (Collado et al. 2005). Gastrointestinal tuberculosis may occur as a primary infection with *Mycobacterium bovis* or may be secondary to pulmonary infection with *Mycobacterium tuberculosis*.

Diagnosis. The diagnosis can be established by the biopsy detection of caseating granulomas and acid-fast rods and also by genetic testing (PCR) and culture studies.

Endoscopy. Edematous swelling and patchy redness are typical findings in affected mucosa. Ulcers are most commonly found in the ileocecal region (■ Fig. 6.4-4). Strictures may develop. Differentiation is required from Crohn's disease (Reddy et al. 2003).

Treatment. Treatment consists of a combination regimen like that used for pulmonary tuberculosis (Greinert and Zabel 2003; Kim et al. 2003).

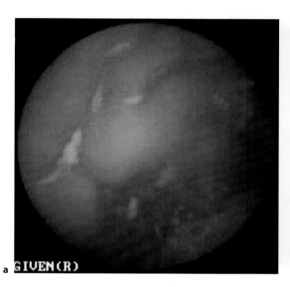

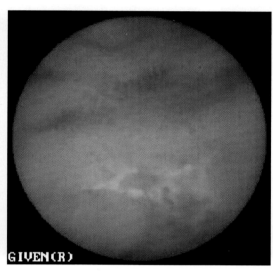

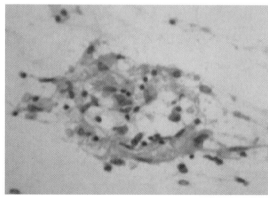

■ **Fig. 6.4-4a–c.** Intestinal tuberculosis. **a, b** Edema and ulcers in the ileum (reprinted from Reddy et al. 2003 with permission from Georg Thieme Verlag). **c** Biopsy from the terminal ileum shows portions of a granuloma with epithelioid and giant cells, consistent with tuberculosis

Cytomegalovirus Enteritis

Etiology. The causative organism of this enteritis is the cytomegalovirus (CMV) from the group of herpesviruses. Owing to the persistence of the virus, the infection may be (re)activated due to acquired immunodeficiency syndrome (AIDS), for example, or by pharmacologic immunosuppression following organ or stem cell transplantation.

Clinical Features. The disease often takes an asymptomatic course. Complications may affect the lungs, CNS, retina, liver, biliary tract, and all portions of the gastrointestinal tract. Ulcers, perforations, and bleeding have been described in the small bowel (Chamberlain et al. 2000).

Diagnosis. The diagnosis is based on the biopsy detection of typical cytomegalic cells (»owl's-eye« cells, ◘ Fig. 6.4-5e), antigen detection in biopsy samples (◘ Fig. 6.4-5f), and PCR assay in peripheral blood lymphocytes. IgM antibodies may be absent in immunosuppressed patients.

Endoscopy. CMV ulcers often show no inflammatory reaction and have a punched-out appearance. Typically the ulcer base is not covered by fibrinous exudate (◘ Fig. 6.4-5a–d).

Treatment. Immunosuppressed patients may be treated with intravenous ganciclovir or oral valganciclovir, depending on the clinical findings.

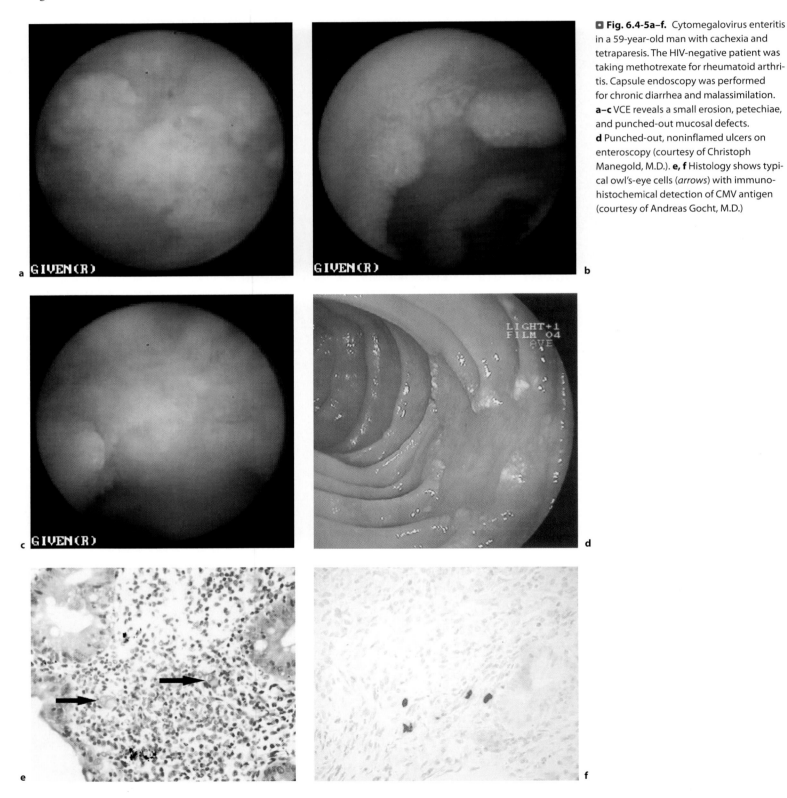

◘ **Fig. 6.4-5a–f.** Cytomegalovirus enteritis in a 59-year-old man with cachexia and tetraparesis. The HIV-negative patient was taking methotrexate for rheumatoid arthritis. Capsule endoscopy was performed for chronic diarrhea and malassimilation. **a–c** VCE reveals a small erosion, petechiae, and punched-out mucosal defects. **d** Punched-out, noninflamed ulcers on enteroscopy (courtesy of Christoph Manegold, M.D.). **e, f** Histology shows typical owl's-eye cells (*arrows*) with immunohistochemical detection of CMV antigen (courtesy of Andreas Gocht, M.D.)

AIDS

AIDS patients can develop enteritis due to a variety of causes. These include mycobacteriosis, histoplasmosis (Gumbs et al. 2000), CMV infection, strongyloidiasis (Overstreet et al. 2003), and cryptosporidiasis (Papp et al. 1996). Histologic and/or microbiologic identification of the causative organism is essential for planning a specific therapy. Malassimilation in AIDS patients may result from enteritis caused by the human immunodeficiency virus (HIV) itself. HIV enteropathy is diagnosed by exclusion (◘ Fig. 6.4-6). These enteropathies have become less common since the widespread use of highly active antiviral therapy (Pollok 2001).

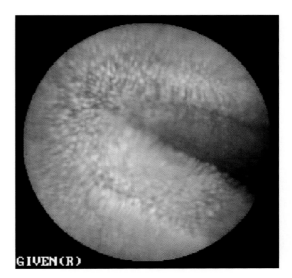

◘ **Fig. 6.4-6.** Diffuse, nonspecific lymphangiectasia in an AIDS patient with malassimilation

Giardiasis

Giardiasis is caused by the protozoon *Giardia lamblia*, which is present worldwide in varying frequency. *G. lamblia* preferably affects the upper gastrointestinal tract.

Clinical Features. The typical manifestation is diarrhea, in some cases causing severe illness. However, most of the infected persons are asymptomatic or have only minor unspecific complaints. The infection may be self-limiting. Treatment is with metronidazole or paromomycin (Lebwohl et al. 2003)

Diagnosis. The first-line diagnostic test is stool examination. The diagnostic yield of an enzyme-linked immunoassay is superior to the previously used microscopic evaluation.

Endoscopy. Endoscopy is usually normal in giardiasis. Rarely, lymphoid hyperplasia of the entire small intestine may be visible (◘ Fig. 6.4-8) or villous atrophy. At endoscopy it is possible to obtain duodenal aspirate for immediate microscopic examination. However, histology from duodenal biopsy is preferable to duodenal aspirate. Histology usually demonstrates normal intestinal architecture and the trophozoites in the overlying mucus (◘ Fig. 6.4-7).

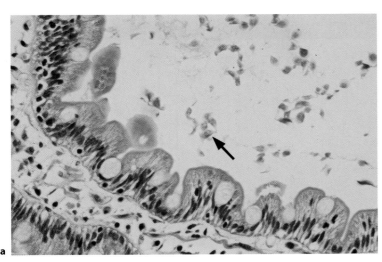

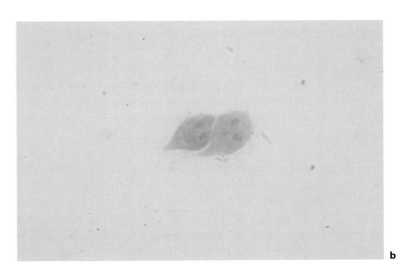

a   b

◘ **Fig. 6.4-7.** Giardiasis. **a** Duodenal biopsy shows trophozoites in the overlying mucus. **b** Trophozoites at higher magnification

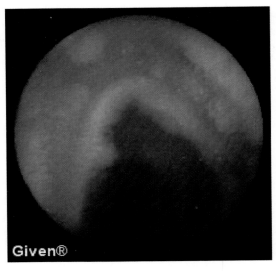

Fig. 6.4-8. Giardiasis. Lymphofollicular hyperplasia throughout the entire small intestine (courtesy of Mark Appleyard, M.D.)

Helminthiases

Epidemiology. Since helminth infections are more prevalent in the tropics and subtropics, it is more common in those regions to find parasitic worms during capsule endoscopy (Sriram et al. 2004). The organisms most commonly found in the small bowel lumen are nematodes (roundworms, threadworms). The largest of these is the roundworm *Ascaris lumbricoides* (Figs. 6.4-9–6.4-11), which may be up to 30 cm long. The smallest are the whipworm *Trichuris trichiura*, the pinworm *Enterobius vermicularis*, and the hookworms *Ankylostoma duodenale* and *Necator americanus* (up to 12 mm) and *Strongyloides stercoralis* (2 mm).

Tapeworms (*Taenia solium* or *Taenia saginata*) may reach a length of up to several meters in the small intestine, causing malnutrition, vitamin deficiency, and even intestinal bleeding (De Simone et al. 2004)

Development. Adult nematodes live in the human intestine, and therefore humans are the definitive host. The infection may be acquired through the oral ingestion of eggs or by larvae penetrating the skin. With strongyloidiasis, autoinfection can occur and may become generalized in immunosuppressed patients.

Endoscopy. Motile worms of varying size may be observed in the bowel lumen (Soares et al. 2003). Ascarids can easily be identified by there large size (Figs. 6.4-9–6.4-11). *Strongyloides* on the other hand is characterized by its tiny dimension, making it hardly visible at all (Fig. 6.4-15). *Enterobius* usually occurs in the cecum, where multiple small worms may be seen (Fig. 6.4-12). *Trichuris* is a long worm, smaller than *Ascaris* with a thin proximal end (Fig. 6.4-14), which is not seen in hookworms (Fig. 6.4-13). The largest helminth is *Taenia*. It consists of multiple proglottides and can reach a length of several meters (Fig. 6.4-16). The outer cuticle of the parasites remains intact, even after the worms have been killed. »Worm-like structures« with irregular outlines in the small bowel are usually food residues.

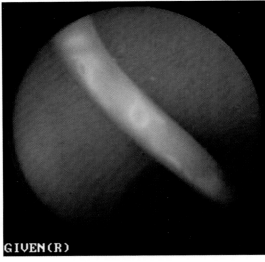

Fig. 6.4-9. *Ascaris* as seen at VCE

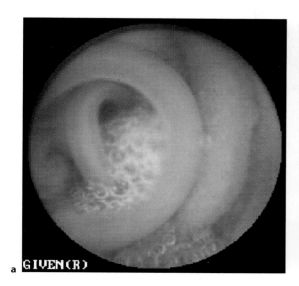

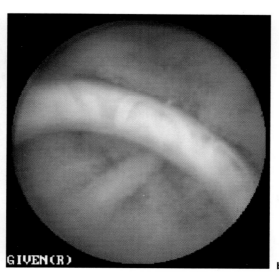

Fig. 6.4-10a, b. Ascarids (reprinted from Soares et al. 2003 with permission from Georg Thieme Verlag)

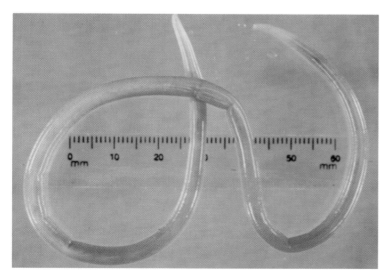

Fig. 6.4-11. Adult *Ascaris*

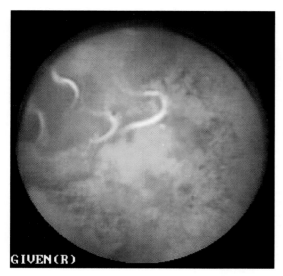

Fig. 6.4-12. Pinworms in the cecum of a child with iron deficiency anemia (courtesy of Ervin Tóth, M.D.)

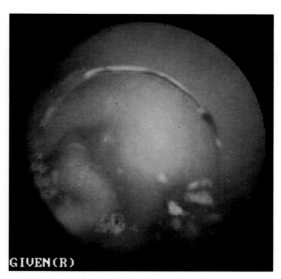

Fig. 6.4-13. Worm in the small intestine, most likely hookworm

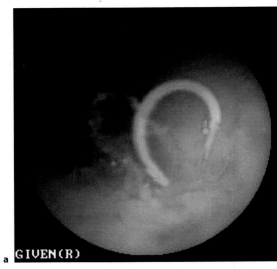
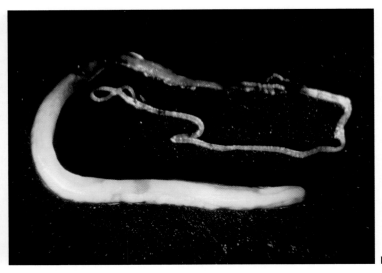

■ **Fig. 6.4-14a, b.** Whipworm. Image from VCE in the small intestine (**a**) (courtesy of Bruno Neu, M.D.). Adult whipworm (**b**)

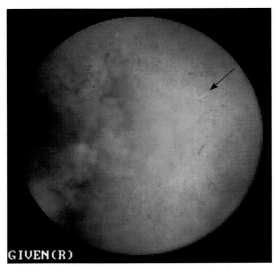

■ **Fig. 6.4-15.** *Strongyloides* (←) (courtesy of Anette Stelzer, M.D.) This small worm is hardly visible on the still image

■ **Fig. 6.4-16a, b.** *Taenia* (courtesy of Michel Delvaux, M.D. and Gerard Gay, M.D.)

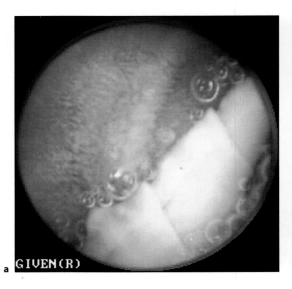
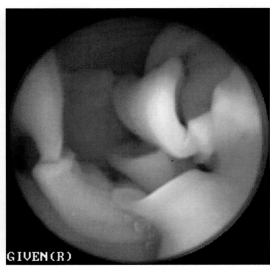

Internet

www.aidsinfo.nih.gov: AIDSinfo (United States Department of Health and Human Services)

www.cdc.gov/ncidod: National Center for Infectious Diseases (USA)

References

Bentley SD, Maiwald M, Murphy LD et al (2003) Sequencing and analysis of the genome of the Whipple's disease bacterium Tropheryma whipplei. Lancet 361:637–644

Chamberlain RS, Atkins S, Saini N, White JC (2000) Ileal perforation caused by cytomegalovirus infection in a critically ill adult. J Clin Gastroenterol 30: 432–435

Collado C, Stirnemann J, Ganne N et al (2005) Gastrointestinal tuberculosis: 17 cases collected in 4 hospitals in the northeastern suburb of Paris. Gastroenterol Clin Biol 29:419–425

De Simone P, Feron P, Loi P et al (2004) Acute intestinal bleeding due to Taenia solium infection (in Italian). Chir Ital 56:151–156

Fenollar F, Raoult D (2003) Whipple's diesease. Curr Gastroenterol Rep 5:379–385

Fritscher-Ravens A, Swain CP, von Herbay A (2004) Refractory Whipple's disease with anaemia: first lessons from capsule endoscopy. Endoscopy 36:659–662

Gay G, Roche JF, Delvaux M (2005) Capsule endoscopy, transit times, and Whipple's disease. Endoscopy 37:272–274

Greinert U, Zabel P (2003) Tuberculosis-current therapeutic principles (in German). Internist 44:1394–1405

Gumbs MA, Girishkumar H, Yousuf A et al (2000) Histoplasmosis of the small bowel in patients with AIDS. Postgrad Med J 76:367–369

Kim SG, Kim JS, Jung HC, Song IS (2003) Is a 9-month treatment sufficient in tuberculous enterocolitis? A prospective, randomized, single-centre study. Aliment Pharmacol Ther 18:85–91

Lebwohl B, Deckelbaum RJ Green PHR (2003) Giardiasis. Gastrointest Endosc 57: 906–913

Overstreet K, Chen J, Rodriguez JW, Wiener G (2003) Endoscopic and histopathologic findings of Strongyloides stercoralis infection in a patient with AIDS. Gastrointest Endosc 58:928–931

Papp JP, DeYoung BR, Fromkes JJ (1996) Endoscopic appearance of cryptosporidial duodenitis. Am J Gastroenterol 91:2235–2236

Pantongrag-Brown L, Krebs TL, Daly BD et al (1998) Frequency of abdominal CT findings in AIDS patients with M. avium complex bacteraemia. Clin Radiol 53: 816–819

Pollok RC (2001) Viruses causing diarrhoea in AIDS. Novartis Found Symp 238: 276–283

Ratnaike RN (2000) Whipple's disease. Postgrad Med J 76:760–766

Reddy DN, Sriram PV, Rao GV, Reddy DB (2003) Capsule endoscopy appearances of small-bowel tuberculosis. Endoscopy 35:99

Soares J, Lopes L, Villas-Boas G, Pinho C (2003) Ascariasis observed by wireless-capsule endoscopy. Endoscopy 35:194

Sriram PV, Rao GV, Reddy DN (2004) Wireless capsule endoscopy: experience in a tropical country. J Gastroenterol Hepatol 19:63–67

6.5 Involvement of the Small Intestine in Systemic Diseases

G. Gay, E. Barth, M. Keuchel

Introduction

Systemic diseases are rare and etiologically diverse. They can affect a variety of organs, and small bowel involvement can occur with varying degrees of frequency (Hagenmüller 1983). The assignment of symptoms, endoscopic and other findings to specific disease entities can be a formidable challenge. A diagnosis cannot be made from endoscopic findings alone.

Amyloidosis

Definition. Amyloidosis is a disorder based on the extracellular deposition of insoluble fibrillary proteins with an antiparallel beta-pleated sheet configuration.

Forms. Both systemic and localized forms occur; they may be acquired or hereditary. The most common systemic form is lambda light-chain amyloidosis (AL) associated with plasmacytoma. Less common is the kappa light-chain form and primary amyloidosis not associated with plasmacytoma. Reactive amyloidosis (AA) caused by serum amyloid A may occur in patients with chronic inflammatory disorders such as Crohn's disease, rheumatoid arthritis, and Still's disease or in the setting of hereditary familial Mediterranean fever or chronic bacterial inflam-

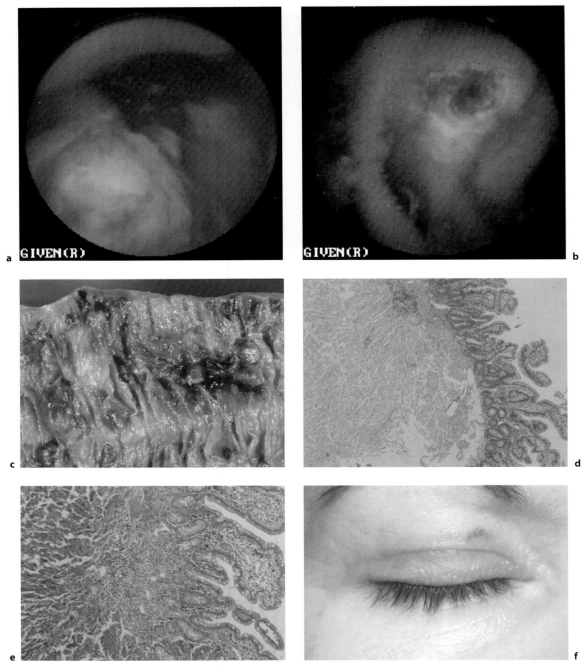

◻ Fig. 6.5-1a–f. Systemic amyloidosis. **a** Multiple bluish-purple masses, some ulcerated (**b**). **c** Diffuse small bowel involvement seen at operation. **d** Histology: massive amyloid infiltration of the small bowel (H&E; courtesy of Michael Amthor, M.D.). **e** Immunohistology: λ-amyloid (courtesy of Wolfgang Saeger, M.D.). The patient presented clinically with recurrent intestinal bleeding and involvement of the skin (**f**) and tongue

mations (e.g., osteomyelitis, tuberculosis, bronchiectasis, etc.). There is also a dialysis-associated amyloidosis ($A\beta_2$-M) caused by β_2-microglobulin, and there are numerous other hereditary forms involving different proteins (Linke et al. 1998; Saeger and Röcken 1998). Small bowel involvement, whether diffuse or localized (Peny et al. 2000), may present with malassimilation (Hayman et al. 2001), bleeding, motility disorders, or perforation (Barzola et al. 1998; Koppelman et al. 2000; Stelzner and Krug 1991).

Endoscopy. Amyloid infiltration of the mucosa may be diffuse, patchy, nodular, or tumorlike (■ Figs. 6.5-1a, b and 6.5-2a, b). The diagnosis is established by histologic examination.

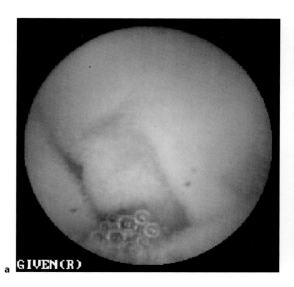
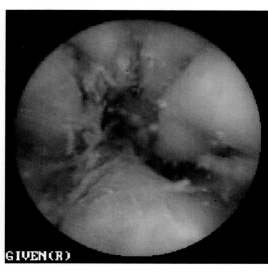

a GIVEN(R)   GIVEN(R) b

■ **Fig. 6.5-2a, b.** Light-chain amyloidosis: κ-amyloid detected in biopsies from the stomach and colon in monoclonal gammopathy. Clinically, the patient had recurring intestinal bleeding. **a** Multiple small red spots in several small bowel segments. **b** Patchy amyloid infiltration in the stomach ·

Abetalipoproteinemia, Hypobetalipoproteinemia

Definition. This condition, known also as Bassen-Kornzweig syndrome, is a very rare, hereditary, autosomal recessive deficiency of β-lipoproteins [very low-density lipoproteins (VLDL) and low-density lipoproteins (LDL)] with no measurable apoprotein B and associated malabsorption with its sequelae.

Etiology. Abetalipoproteinemia is caused by mutations of the gene that encodes larger subunits of the microsomal triglyceride transport protein (MTP). The deficiency of apoprotein B is a secondary phenomenon caused by increased breakdown in the endoplasmic reticulum (Sharp et al. 1993).

Clinical Features. Symptoms are malabsorption with steatorrhea, a fat-soluble vitamin deficiency with its sequelae, retinitis pigmentosa, pro-gressive neurologic symptoms (e.g., ataxia), mental retardation, and massive fatty infiltration of the liver.

Diagnosis. Pathognomonic signs are hypocholesterolemia (<40 mg/dl), hypotriglyceridemia (<10 mg/dl), no detectable VLDL, and the deformation of erythrocytes (acanthocytosis) in blood smears due to membrane lipid abnormalities (■ Fig. 6.5-3c, d).

Endoscopy. Endoscopy shows a grayish-white discoloration of the entire small bowel mucosa (■ Fig. 6.5-3a, b) caused by an accumulation of fat vacuoles (Gay and Delmotte 1998).

Treatment. Treatment consists of triglyceride replacement with medium-chain fatty acids plus the strict avoidance of other fats. High doses of fat-soluble vitamins are also administered.

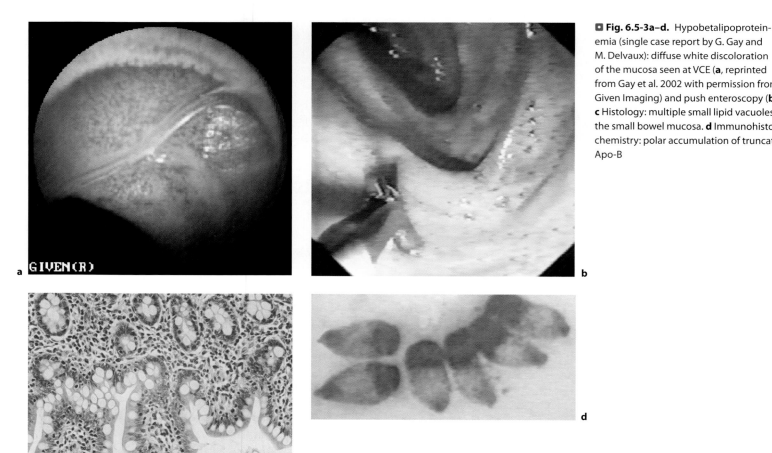

■ **Fig. 6.5-3a–d.** Hypobetalipoprotein-emia (single case report by G. Gay and M. Delvaux): diffuse white discoloration of the mucosa seen at VCE (**a**, reprinted from Gay et al. 2002 with permission from Given Imaging) and push enteroscopy (**b**). **c** Histology: multiple small lipid vacuoles in the small bowel mucosa. **d** Immunohisto-chemistry: polar accumulation of truncated Apo-B

Sarcoidosis

Etiology. Sarcoidosis is a granulomatous systemic disease of unknown cause.

Clinical Features. The chronic form is frequently asymptomatic. Pulmonary involvement is usually predominant, but the disease may also involve the CNS, eyes, myocardium, skin, liver, and kidneys. Small bowel involvement is very rare (Klebl et al. 1999).

Diagnosis. The diagnosis is based on the histologic detection of non-caseating epithelioid cell granulomas, radiologic evidence of bihilar lymphadenopathy, or bronchoalveolar lavage material with a CD4/CD8 ratio greater than 3.5 in the presence of typical clinical manifestations.

Endoscopy. Endoscopy demonstrates nonspecific nodularity and ulcerations of the bowel mucosa (■ Fig. 6.5-4).

Treatment. Steroid therapy may be necessary, depending on the severity of pulmonary lesions and the involvement of extrapulmonary organs. Methotrexate or azathioprine can also be administered to reduce steroid use (Costabel 2003).

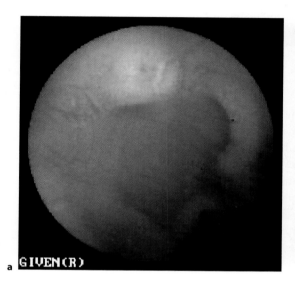
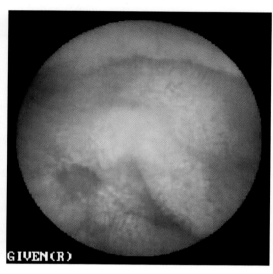

■ **Fig. 6.5-4a, b.** Polypoid mucosal lesion (**a**) and a small ulcer (**b**) in a woman with confirmed pulmonary sarcoidosis (courtesy of Ruprecht Botzler, M.D.)

Vasculitides

Vasculitides may occur as primary entities or may be secondary to other underlying diseases such as infections, tumors, collagen diseases, or drug side effects. The primary vasculitides were defined by the Chapel Hill Consensus Conference (1992) and classified mainly according to the size of the affected blood vessels (large, medium size, and small vessels). Besides clinical and pathologic criteria, immunologic findings are also taken into account, e.g., association with antineutrophil cytoplasmic antibodies (ANCA) in »pauci-immune« vasculitides (no immune complex deposition by histology) or immune complex vasculitides with complement consumption (Jennette et al. 1994).

In simplified terms, the end-organ damage corresponds to the affected type of vessel and ranges from stenosis with hypoxemia and edema to organ infarction or vessel wall destruction with hemorrhage.

Intestinal involvement in vasculitic diseases is relatively common in the following disease entities:

Henoch-Schönlein Purpura. Henoch-Schönlein purpura is an immune complex vasculitis with IgA deposits and involvement of the skin, kidneys, gastrointestinal tract, joints, and rarely the lung. It is characterized by a palpable purpura, abdominal pain, and the biopsy detection of granulocytic infiltrates in the walls of small blood vessels (arterioles and venules). Intestinal involvement occurs in a high percentage of cases (Esaki et al. 2002; Szer 1999). Endoscopic findings include edema, erythema, ulceration, and bleeding (■ Fig. 6.5-5) (Skogestad 2005). Abdominal pain and bloody diarrhea are occasionally the dominant complaints in oligosymptomatic forms and precede renal involvement and purpura. Henoch-Schönlein purpura occurs predominantly in children. Oligosymptomatic forms are more common in adults and can cause problems of differential diagnosis.

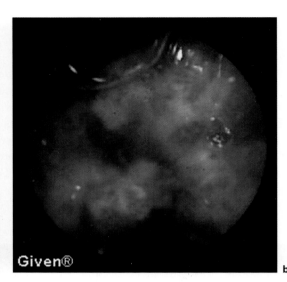

Fig. 6.5-5a, b. Henoch-Schönlein purpura involving the entire small intestine. VCE shows edema, erythema, ulceration, and fibrin exudates (courtesy of Erik Skogestad, M.D.)

Churg-Strauss Syndrome. Churg-Strauss syndrome (formerly called allergic angiitis and granulomatosis) is a necrotizing vasculitis of small and medium size blood vessels characterized by an eosinophilic granulomatous inflammation of the respiratory tract (Churg and Strauss 1951). It is associated clinically with eosinophilia and with a bronchial asthma that often precedes the vasculitis. Particularly serious vasculitic manifestations are myocardial involvement, neuropathies, renal involvement, and alveolitis. Sporadic cases of small bowel ulcers and perforations have been described (Nakamura et al. 2002).

Behçet's Syndrome. Pathologically, Behçet's syndrome usually presents as a vasculitis affecting small arteries and veins. The disease is most common in persons of Turkish descent and is rare in Central Europe. The diagnosis is made clinically; specific serologic markers are unknown. Typical clinical features are oral and genital aphthous ulcers, skin lesions such as eruptions resembling erythema nodosum, joint pain and swelling, and eventually ocular and CNS involvement. Cutaneous hyperreactivity to the pathergy test is observed in Mediterranean Behçet's syndrome but not in the Central European form (Barnes 1999). The intestinal manifestations are similar to those of Crohn's disease (Korman et al. 2003; Pretorius et al. 1996) and include aphthae, ulcerations, fistulae, wall thickening, and pseudopolyps.

Panarteritis Nodosa. By definition, panarteritis nodosa is a necrotizing inflammation of small and medium size arteries. It is classified immunopathologically as an immune complex vasculitis. Researchers have found a serologic association with HBsAg carriers and, increasingly, with antibodies to the hepatitis C virus (Carson et al. 1993). Conventional angiography demonstrates microaneurysms or vascular occlusions, occurring mainly in the mesenteric territory. Additional features are livedo reticularis, myalgias, painful skin nodules, testicular pain, and renal involvement in the form of a vascular nephropathy. Glomerulonephritis is not part of the clinical picture of panarteritis nodosa. The symptoms of intestinal involvement are abdominal pain, nausea, and vomiting. Small bowel involvement is a result of mesenteric ischemia, with lesions ranging from ulceration to mesenteric infarction and subsequent necrosis (Becker et al. 2002).

For historical reasons, panarteritis nodosa requires differentiation from **microscopic polyangiitis (MPA)**, a microvascular vasculitis that chiefly affects the lungs and kidneys causing an alveolitis or glomerulonephritis. MPA is a pauci-immune vasculitis and is associated with the detection of an ANCA directed against myeloperoxidase. Intestinal involvement is rare, but sporadic cases with associated intestinal bleeding have been reported (Ueda et al. 2001).

Wegener's Granulomatosis. Wegener's granulomatosis (WG) is a granulomatous inflammation of the upper respiratory tract that is associated with a necrotizing vasculitis of small blood vessels. All organ systems may be affected during the generalized vasculitic phase, particularly the lung (alveolitis), kidneys, peripheral nervous system, and central nervous system. WG is another pauci-immune vasculitis and is associated with the serologic presence of an ANCA directed against proteinase 3. Small bowel involvement is rare and is manifested by bloody stools, mucoid diarrhea, and abdominal pain resulting from ulcers, active vasculitis, and mucosal inflammation (Storesund et al. 1998).

Collagen Diseases

Collagen diseases is a collective term for inflammatory systemic diseases that manifest common features such as the presence of antinuclear antibodies, elevated serum inflammatory markers, and systemic symptoms such as fever, debilitation, and joint pain. These diseases show considerable variation, however, in their dominant symptoms and prognosis. The named collagen diseases are: systemic lupus erythematosus (SLE), Sjögren's syndrome, systemic sclerosis, CREST (calcinosis, Raynaud's phenomenon, esophageal dysfunction, sclerodactyly, telangiectasia) syndrome, myositis, and dermatomyositis. Additionally, mixed collagen diseases, undifferentiated collagen diseases, and overlap syndromes are also recognized.

SLE is characterized by aphthous lesions of the mucous membranes in the ENT region. Small bowel involvement is generally rare but occurs in the setting of secondary vasculitis, for example. Small bowel involvement may be manifested by aphthae (Fig. 6.5-6), ulcers (Sasamura et al. 1991), perforations (Moriuchi et al. 1989), or intestinal pseudo-obstruction (Nguyen and Khanna 2004).

Systemic sclerosis leads to intestinal motility disturbances, usually beginning in the esophagus, as a result of progressive sclerosis. Affection of the arteries of the hands may lead to Raynaud's phenomenon. Small bowel involvement with hypomotility may be manifested by pseudo-obstruction or malabsorption caused by abnormal bacterial colonization (Marie et al. 1999; Ebert et al. 1997). Abnormal capillaries with distortion and parallel bundles may be observed in the small intestine (Fig. 6.5-7)

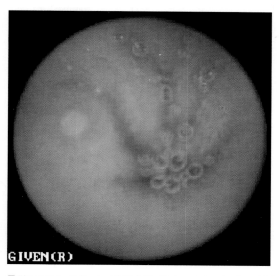

 Fig. 6.5-6. Patient with SLE: Multiple aphthae in the middle third of the small bowel, not clearly distinguishable from Crohn's disease by endoscopy. The patient presented with iron deficiency anemia, albuminuria, arthritis, and positive antinuclear antibodies

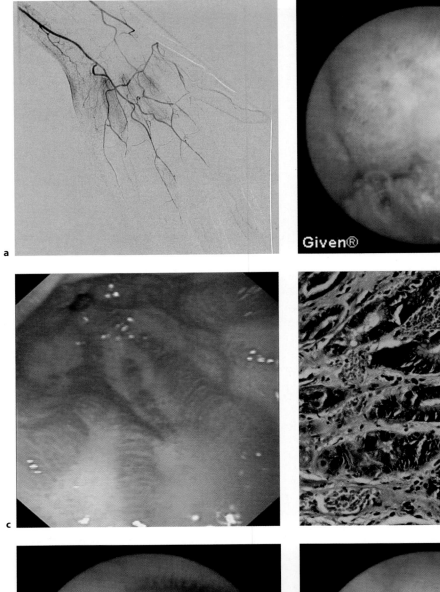

a

b

c

d

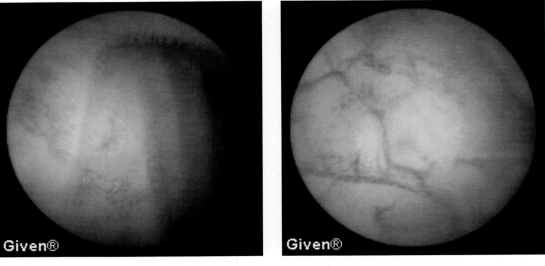

e

f

□ **Fig. 6.5-7a–d.** Affection of multiple blood vessel in a patient with systemic sclerosis. **a** Digital subtraction angiography of the hand shows severe rarefaction of digital arteries (courtesy of Doris Welger, M.D.) Gastric antral venectasia without portal hypertension. **b** VCE. **c** Gastroscopy. **d** Histology (Giemsa stain showing dilated vessel, courtesy of Renate Höhne, M.D.) **e–f** Irregular vessels of the small intestine seen at VCE

Common Variable Immunodeficiency Syndrome (CVID)

This heterogeneous group of congenital or acquired immunodeficiencies is characterized by the inability of B lymphocytes to differentiate to plasma cells, resulting in a panhypogammaglobulinemia. Clinical features include chronic pulmonary infections, lymphadenopathy, fever, diarrhea, and malabsorption. Endoscopy typically reveals diffuse intestinal lymphoid hyperplasia (□ Fig. 6.5-8; Mihaly et al. 2005). Histology shows a wide spectrum of findings such as nodular lymphoid hyperplasia, villous atrophy, granulomas, and lymphocytic infiltration (Washington et al. 1996)

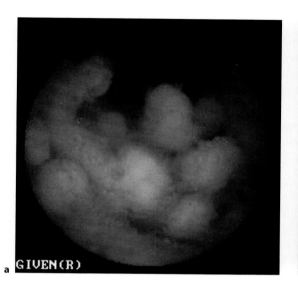
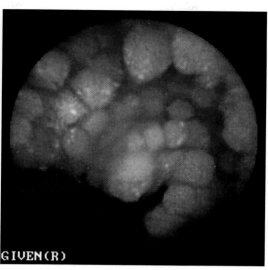

□ Fig. 6.5-8a, b. Common variable immunodeficiency syndrome (CVID). Multiple lymph follicles throughout the small intestine (courtesy of Emese Mihaly, M.D.)

Internet

www.amyloidosis.org: Amyloidosis Support Network
www.eular.org: European League Against Rheumatism
www.lupus.org: Lupus Foundation of America
www.rheumatology.org: American College of Rheumatology

References

Barnes CG (1999) Behçet's syndrome – classification criteria. Ann Med Interne (Paris) 150:477–482

Barzola S, Lespi P, Fuentes R (1998) Intestinal bleeding associated with systemic amyloidosis. Acta Gastroenterol Latinoam 28:257–259

Becker A, Mader R, Elias M et al (2002) Duodenal necrosis as the presenting manifestation of polyarteritis nodosa. Clin Rheumatol 21:314–316

Carson CW, Conn DL, Czaja AJ et al (1993) Frequency and significance of antibodies to hepatitis C virus in polyarteritis nodosa. J Rheumatol 20:304–309

Churg J, Strauss L (1951) Allergic granulomatosis, allergic angiitis, and periarteritis nodosa. Am J Pathol 27:277–301

Costabel U (2003) Sarkoidose. In Paumgartner G, Steinbeck G (eds) Therapie innerer Krankheiten, 10. Aufl. Springer, Berlin Heidelberg New York, pp 414–419

Ebert EC, Ruggiero FM, Seibold JR (1997) Intestinal perforation. A common complication of scleroderma. Dig Dis Sci 42:549–553

Esaki M, Matsumoto T, Nakamura S et al (2002) GI involvement in Henoch-Schönlein purpura. Gastrointest Endosc 56:920–923

Gay G, Delmotte JS (1998) Abeta and hypobetalipoproteinemias. In: Rossini F, Gay G (eds) Atlas of enteroscopy. Springer, Berlin Heidelberg New York, pp 119–120

Gay G, Fassler I, Florent C, Delvaux M (2002) Malabsorption. In: Halpern M, Jacob H (eds): Atlas of capsule endoscopy. Given Imaging, Norcross, GA, USA, pp 83–101

Hagenmüller F (1983) Funktionelle und morphologische Veränderungen des Dünndarms bei systemischen und extraintestinalen Erkrankungen. In: Caspary W (ed) Handbuch der Inneren Medizin. Bd III/3B: Dünndarm. Springer, Berlin Heidelberg New York, pp 611–630

Hayman SR, Lacy MQ, Kyle RA, Gertz MA (2001) Primary systemic amyloidosis: a cause of malabsorption syndrome. Am J Med 111:535–540

Jennette JC, Falk RJ, Andrassy K et al (1994) Nomenclature of systemic vasculitides. Proposal of an international consensus conference. Arthritis Rheum 37: 187–192

Klebl FH, Merger M, Hierlmeier FX et al (1999) Unusual case of disseminated sarcoidosis with prominent gastrointestinal symptoms. Dtsch Med Wochenschr 124:39–44

Koppelman RN, Stollman NH, Baigorri F, Rogers AI (2000) Acute small bowel pseudo-obstruction due to AL amyloidosis: a case report and literature review. Am J Gastroenterol 95:294–296

Korman U, Cantasdemir M, Kurugoglu S et al (2003) Enteroclysis findings of intestinal Behçet disease: a comparative study with Crohn's disease. Abdom Imaging 28:308–312

Linke R, Altland K, Ernst J et al (1998) Praktische Hinweise zur Diagnose und Therapie generalisierter Amyloidosen. Dtsch Ärzteblatt 95:A2626–A2636

Marie I, Levesque H, Ducrotte P, Courtois H (1999) Involvement of the small intestine in systemic scleroderma. Rev Med Interne 20:504–513

Mihaly E, Nemeth A, Zagoni T et al (2005) Gastrointestinal manifestations of common variable immunodeficiency diagnosed by video- and capsule endoscopy. Endoscopy 37:603–604

Moriuchi J, Ichikawa Y, Takaya M et al (1989) Lupus cystitis and perforation of the small bowel in a patient with systemic lupus erythematosus and overlapping syndrome. Clin Exp Rheumatol 7:533–536

Nakamura Y, Sakurai Y, Matsubara T et al (2002) Multiple perforated ulcers of the small intestine associated with allergic granulomatous angiitis: report of a case. Surg Today 32:541–546

Nguyen H, Khanna N (2004) Intestinal pseudo-obstruction as a presenting manifestation of systemic lupus erythematosus: case report and review of the literature. South Med J 97:186–189

Peny MO, Debongnie JC, Haot J, van Gossum A (2000) Localized amyloid tumor in small bowel. Dig Dis Sci 45:1850–1853

Pretorius ES, Hruban RH, Fishman EK (1996) Inflammatory pseudotumor of the terminal ileum mimicking malignancy in a patient with Behçet's disease. CT and pathological findings. Clin Imaging 20:191–193

Saeger W, Röcken C (1998) Amyloid: mikroskopischer Nachweis, Klassifikation und klinischer Bezug. Pathologe 19:345–354

Sasamura H, Nakamoto H, Ryuzaki M et al (1991) Repeated intestinal ulcerations in a patient with systemic lupus erythematosus and high serum antiphospholipid antibody levels. South Med J 84:515–517

Sharp D, Blinderman L, Combs KA et al (1993) Cloning and gene defects in microsomal triglyceride transfer protein associated with abetalipoproteinaemia. Nature 365:65–69

Skogestad E (2005) Capsule endoscopy in Henoch-Schönlein purpura. Endoscopy 37:189

Stelzner M, Krug B (1991) Gastrointestinal amyloidosis: differential diagnosis and indications for surgical therapy. Chirurg 62:493–499

Storesund B, Gran JT, Koldingsnes W (1998) Severe intestinal involvement in Wegener's granulomatosis: report of two cases and review of the literature. Br J Rheumatol 37:387–390

Szer IS (1999) Gastrointestinal and renal involvement in vasculitis: management strategies in Henoch-Schönlein purpura. Cleve Clin J Med 66:312–317

Ueda C, Hirohata Y, Kihara Y et al (2001) Pancreatic cancer complicated by disseminated intravascular coagulation associated with production of tissue factor. J Gastroenterol 36:848–850

Washington K, Stenzel TT, Buckley RH, Gottfried MR (1996) Gastrointestinal pathology in patients with common variable immunodeficiency and X-linked agammaglobulinemia. Am J Surg Pathol 20:1240–1252

6.6   Physical-Chemical Small Intestinal Injury

I. Bjarnason, S.N. Adler, L. Maiden

NSAID-Induced Enteropathy

Etiology. Local damage to enterocytes and the inhibition of both the cyclooxygenases (COX) by nonsteroidal anti-inflammatory drugs (NSAIDs), along with the topical effects of these drugs, can cause injury to the small bowel mucosa (Smale et al. 2001; Bjarnason et al. 1993). The precise pathogenesis is uncertain but it seems likely that there is an initiating local topical effect that involves a NSAID-membrane phospholipid interaction and/or uncoupling of mitochondrial oxidative phosphorylation which compromises intestinal integrity. The consequence of concomitant COX-1 inhibition prevents an increase in microvascular blood flow while COX-2 inhibition may alter inflammatory (immunological) responses to this injury.

Frequency. Enteropathy occurs in up to 70% of patients who take conventional NSAIDs on a short-term basis [defined by measurement of surrogate markers of inflammation in stool (Tibble et al. 1999) or by capsule endoscopy (Maiden et al. 2005; Goldstein et al. 2003)] or on a long-term basis (Graham et al. 2004). It is much less common in patients treated short-term with COX-2 inhibitors (Goldstein et al. 2003). The frequency of the serious outcomes (as described below) is comparable to that seen in the stomach (Laine et al. 2003) with 1–2% of patients encountering problems.

Clinical Features. Many cases of NSAID enteropathy are asymptomatic and only evident if specifically looked for. Potential complications can be classified as

Mild: Occult bleeding and protein loss that may lead to iron deficiency anemia and hypoalbuminemia, respectively.

Serious: Overt bleeding, perforation, and strictures. This bleeding is often only considered after endoscopy and colonoscopy have not disclosed a bleeding site, but the strictures are in particular difficult to diagnose. Some of the patients with strictures present with weight loss, postprandial abdominal pain, and a history of recurrent iron deficiency anemia and hypoalbuminemia. The unique »diaphragmatic«-like strictures are pathognomonic for NSAIDs (Bjarnason et al. 1988), at least when assessed histologically, but macroscopically the smooth concentric strictures are sometimes found in other intestinal diseases.

Treatment. There are no rigorously tested and proven methods for reducing the damage of NSAIDs to the small bowel. A COX-2 selective agent is certainly much safer when given on a short-term basis. Sulfasalazine, misoprostol, and metronidazole have all been shown to be effective in reducing the inflammatory activity and bleeding. The serious complications of the enteropathy demand surgery, but some of these complications may only come to attention at a postmortem examination (Allison et al. 1992).

Endoscopy. After short-term ingestion of NSAIDs there is a range of abnormalities, none of which by themselves are pathognomonic for NSAID-induced damage, and similar pathology may be seen in a number of diseases (Bjarnason et al. 2004). It has been suggested (Maiden et al. 2005) that the damage can be classified as

Endoscopic findings in NSAID enteropathy:
- Reddened folds (■ Fig. 6.6-1)
- Denuded areas (■ Fig. 6.6-2)
- Petechia/red spots (■ Fig. 6.6-3)
- Mucosal breaks that encompass lesions resembling erosions (■ Fig. 6.6-4) and
- Ulcers (■ Fig. 6.6-5); sometimes with luminal blood (■ Fig. 6.6-6).

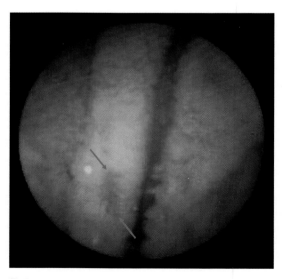

■ **Fig. 6.6-1.** Patchy mucosal reddened folds with a suspicion of villous blunting

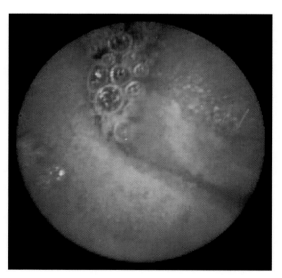

■ **Fig. 6.6-2.** Denuded area with clear loss of villi, but lacking the central pallor of erosions-ulcers

The precise temporal relationship between these lesions is at present uncertain, but it is likely that NSAIDs denude the mucosa (via a topical effect) with loss of villi and that this then progresses to erosions and ulcers (because of COX-1 and/or COX-2 inhibition). The petechia/red spot (not seen in normal volunteers) may represent microvascular damage (a COX-1 mediated effect).

The long-term endoscopic damage is similar as demonstrated by patchy redness (◘ Fig. 6.6-7), erosions (◘ Fig. 6.6-8), and ulcers (◘ Fig. 6.6-9) that cannot be distinguished easily from the acute damage. However, the web-like diaphragm strictures (◘ Fig. 6.6-10) are highly suggestive of long-term NSAID-induced damage (Chutkan and Toubia 2004; Morris 1999; Bjarnason et al. 1988). A representative macroscopic appearance of NSAID-induced small bowel stricture(s) is shown in ◘ Fig. 6.6-11.

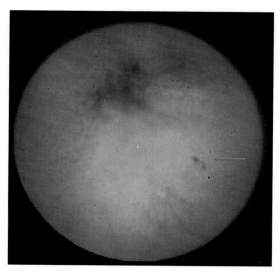

◘ **Fig. 6.6-3.** Localized mucosal petechia or red spot without any other mucosal abnormality

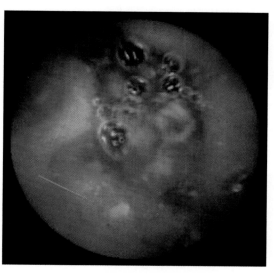

◘ **Fig. 6.6-4.** Mucosal break resembling an erosion with central pallor and surrounding erythema

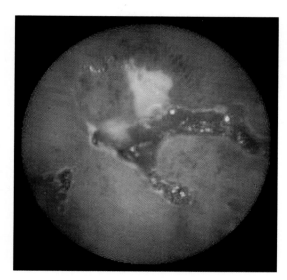

◘ **Fig. 6.6-5.** Mucosal break resembling an ulcer. However, as neither this figure nor ◘ Fig. 6.6-4 clearly demonstrates depth, these two lesions are categorized together. Furthermore, these lesions cannot be positively distinguished from Crohn's disease by endoscopy

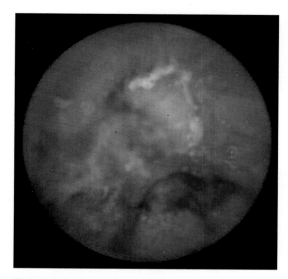

◘ **Fig. 6.6-6.** Mucosal break with luminal blood

6

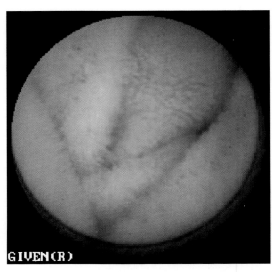

Fig. 6.6-7. Patchy mucosal redness and petechia in a patient on long-term NSAID

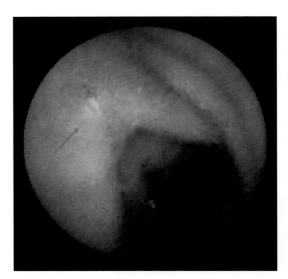

Fig. 6.6-8. Mucosal break resembling an erosion in a patient on long-term NSAID

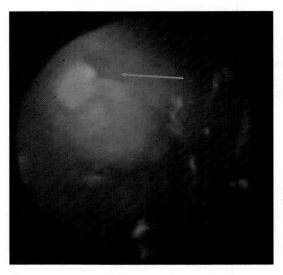

Fig. 6.6-9. Mucosal break resembling an ulcer in a patient on long-term NSAID

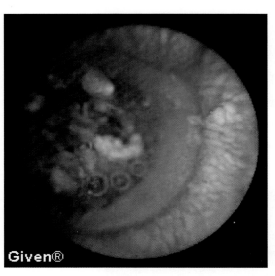

Fig. 6.6-10. A smooth diaphragm-like stricture with the leading edge of the diaphragm showing evidence of ulceration

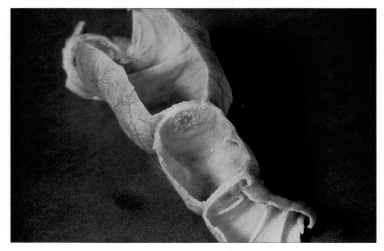

Fig. 6.6-11. A small bowel resection specimen from a patient with NSAID-induced diaphragm-like strictures. There is prestenotic dilatation and the diaphragm (2–3 mm thick) can be seen to close the lumen down to a pinhole (reprinted from Bjarnason et al 1988 with permission from the American Gastroenterological Association)

Chronic Radiation Enteritis

Occurrence. Chronic radiation enteritis can occur within 1 year or up to many years after radiotherapy to the small bowel, especially if the bowel is fixed due to adhesion or other lesions. The disease is caused by a progressive endarteritis which leads to a state of chronic ischemia.

Clinical Features. Symptoms include diarrhea, maldigestion-malabsorption (Cosnes et al. 1988), vomiting, and in particular abdominal pain (Cosnes et al. 1983). Potential complications are perforation, bleeding, and stenosis, but these are very rare indeed.

Diagnosis. The diagnosis of chronic radiation enteritis is often difficult and relies currently on ileoscopy, enteroclysis, and computed tomography (CT) scans (Chen et al. 2003) which will identify only very advanced cases. The present experience with capsule endoscopy supports the notion that radiation-induced enteritis will be diagnosed earlier with greater ease and certainty (Lee et al. 2004; Martinez et al. 2004), provided that the Patency Capsule is used first.

Treatment. Treatment is often targeted towards possible small bowel overgrowth, bile acid malabsorption etc., and symptomatic treatment (dietary management with antidiarrheal agents and antispasmodics) is the norm. Surgical treatment for adhesions and strictures is associated with a high complication rate (Frede and Bories-Azeau 1990; Wobbes et al. 1984).

Endoscopy. It is advisable to exclude significant stenosis by the ingestion of a Patency Capsule prior to carrying out a capsule study in patients who have been subjected to abdominal radiation, especially those with postprandial pain, nausea, and vomiting (Chap. 1.5).

By the nature of the problem many patients undergoing chemotherapy and abdominal radiation have significant abdominal symptoms during active treatment and it is often these symptoms that limit the amount of cytotoxic drugs administered. However, the symptoms are expected and accepted by those caring for these patients so that they are not investigated for these symptoms. Many patients find their way to gastroenterologists 5 years or more after treatment. The early events in the small bowel damage of radiation enteritis are, at present, not known but it is suggested that the damage may be similar to that seen following conventional NSAIDs (Bjarnason et al. 2004).

A range of lesions is evident with the long-term damage.

A very common feature of radiation enteritis is the clubbing of villi with lymphangectasia. These can be subtle such as radiation of 1 year's duration (◘ Fig. 6.6-12) or immediately obvious in severe cases of 25 year's duration (◘ Fig. 6.6-13), with denuded mucosa (◘ Fig. 6.6-14), red spots (neovascularization) (◘ Fig. 6.6-15), and reddened folds (◘ Fig. 6.6-16) similar to that seen in NSAID enteropathy or indeed this may be a common final mechanism of damage seen in a number of diseases (Bjarnason et al. 2004).

> **Endoscopic findings in radiation enteritis:**
> — Lymphangiectasia
> — Denuded mucosa
> — Neovascularization
> — Reddened folds

◘ Figure 6.6-17 shows a characteristic radiation stricture of the small bowel. It resembles NSAID-induced strictures, but there is more nodularity and the inflammatory activity is not on the leading edge of the diaphragm.

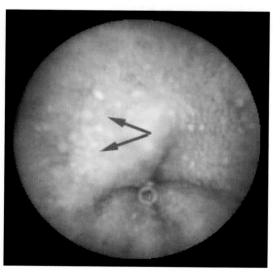

◘ **Fig. 6.6-12.** Subtle villous clubbing with lymphangiectasia suggestive of radiation damage

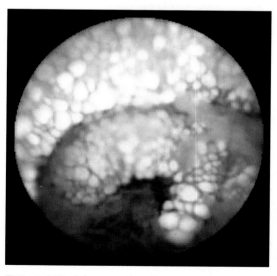

◘ **Fig. 6.6-13.** Pronounced lymphangiectasia with clubbing of villi characteristic of severe radiation damage

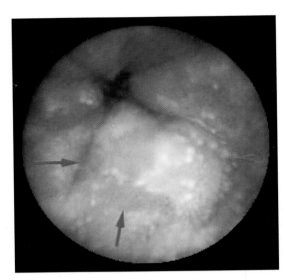

■ **Fig. 6.6-14.** Denuded mucosa outlined by the *long arrows* while the *arrowhead* points to the villous clubbing

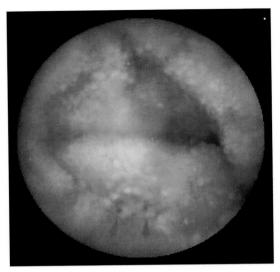

■ **Fig. 6.6-15.** Mild clubbing with lymphangiectasia and redness. The *arrows* point to red spots that may represent neovascularization

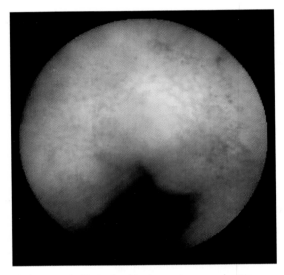

■ **Fig. 6.6-16.** Marked reddening and some red spots

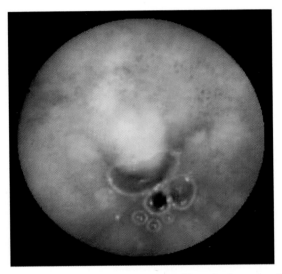

■ **Fig. 6.6-17.** Radiation-induced small bowel stricture (confirmed at surgery)

References

Allison MC, Howatson AG, Torrance CJ, Lee FD, Russell RI (1992) Gastrointestinal damage associate d with the use of nonsteroidal anti-inflammatory drugs. N Engl J Med 327:749–754

Bjarnason I, Price AB, Zanelli G, Smethurst P, Burke M, Gumpel JM, Levi AJ (1988) Clinicopathological features of nonsteroidal antiinflammatory drug-induced small intestinal strictures. Gastroenterology 94:1070–1074

Bjarnason I, Hayllar J, Macpherson AJ, Russell AS (1993) Side effects of nonsteroidal anti-inflammatory drugs on the small and large intestine in humans. Gastroenterology 104:1832–1847

Bjarnason I, Takeuchi K, Bjarnason A, Adler SN, Teahon K (2004) The G.U.T. of gut. Scand J Gastroenterol 39:807–815

Chen S, Harisinghani MG, Wittenberg J (2003) Small bowel CT fat density target sign in chronic radiation enteritis. Australas Radiol 47:450–452

Chutkan R, Toubia N (2004) Effect of nonsteroidal anti-inflammatory drugs on the gastrointestinal tract: diagnosis by wireless capsule endoscopy. Gastrointest Endosc Clin N Am 14:67–85

Cosnes J, Gendre JP, Le Quintrec Y (1983) Chronic radiation enteritis. II. General consequences and prognostic factors. Gastroenterol Clin Biol 7:671–676

Cosnes J, Laurent-Puig P, Baumer P et al (1988) Malnutrition in chronic radiation enteritis. Study of 100 patients. Ann Gastroenterol Hepatol (Paris) 24:7–12

Frede KE, Bories-Azeau A (1990) Strahlenfolgen am Darm. In: Siewert J, Harder F, Allgöwer M et al (eds) Chirurgische Gastroenterololgie. Springer, Berlin Heidelberg New York, pp 1008–1015

Goldstein JL, Eisen G, Lewis B et al (2003) Celecoxib is associated with fewer small bowel lesions than naproxen + omeprazole in healthy subjects as determined by capsule endoscopy. Gut 52:A16–A17

Graham DY, Qureshi WA, Willingham F et al (2004) Visible small-intestinal mucosal injury in chronic NSAID. Clin Gastroenterol Hepatol 3:55–59

Laine L, Connors LG, Reicin A, Hawkey CJ, Burgos-Vargas R, Schnitzer TJ, Yu Q, Bombardier C (2003) Serious lower gastrointestinal clinical events with nonselective NSAID or coxib use. Gastroenterology 124:288–292

Lee DW, Poon AO, Chan AC (2004) Diagnosis of small bowel radiation enteritis by capsule endoscopy. Hong Kong Med J 10:419–421

Maiden L, Thjodleifsson B, Theodors A, Gonzalez J, Bjarnason I (2005) A quantitative analysis of NSAID-induced small bowel pathology by capsule enteroscopy. Gastroenterology 128:1172–1178

Martinez AD, Gonzalez CB, Souto RJ, Vazquez Millan MA, Estevez PE, Alonso AP, Vazquez Iglesias JL (2004) Obscure gastrointestinal bleeding: a complication of radiation enteritis diagnosed by wireless capsule endoscopy. Rev Esp Enferm Dig 96:132–137

Morris AJ (1999) Nonsteroidal anti-inflammatory drug enteropathy. Gastrointest Endosc Clin N Am 9:125–133

Smale S, Tibble J, Sigthorsson G, Bjarnason I (2001) Epidemiology and differential diagnosis of NSAID-induced injury to the mucosa of the small intestine. Best Pract Res Clin Gastroenterol 15:723–738

Tibble JA, Foster R, Sigthorsson G, Scott D, Roseth A, Bjarnason I (1999) Faecal calprotectin: a simple method for the diagnosis of NSAID-induced enteropathy. Gut 45:362–366

Wobbes T, Verschueren RC, Lubbers EJ et al (1984) Surgical aspects of radiation enteritis of the small bowel. Dis Colon Rectum 27:89–92

6.7 Acute Gastrointestinal Graft-Versus-Host Disease After Bone Marrow Transplantation

S.N. Adler, V. Maunoury

Definition

Acute graft-versus-host disease (GVHD) is a major complication following allogeneic stem cell transplantation (allo-SCT) and carries a high morbidity and mortality rate (Ferrara and Deeg 1991). This disease may affect skin, liver, and the gastrointestinal tract (acute GI GVHD). Mismatched histocompatibility antigens cause graft T cells to attack the host's tissues in acute GI GVHD. Histologic findings in the intestine include crypt epithelial cell apoptosis, crypt destruction, and variable lymphocytic infiltration of the epithelium and lamina propria. Severe GVHD (☐ Table 6.7-1) affects the small bowel causing extensive damage with a large spectrum of endoscopic findings (Adler et al. 2004). Patients with acute GI GVHD have a higher mortality than patients without acute GI GVHD (Cruz-Correa et al. 2002). Treatment of acute GI GVHD requires aggressive immunosuppressive therapy which is associated with infectious complications.

Chronic GVHD occurs months later after stem cell transplantation and primarily involves the skin. It may involve the GI tract affecting the esophagus or leading to intestinal strictures.

Diagnosis

The diagnosis of acute GI GVHD may be challenging. Whereas diarrhea is the most common symptom in acute GI GVHD it is by far not specific. Diarrhea may be treatment related or caused by GI infections such as cytomegalovirus (CMV), other viruses, *Clostridium difficile* toxin, toxoplasmosis, fungi, and other pathogens (Einsele et al. 1994). Diagnosis of acute GI GVHD usually requires upper or lower GI endoscopy with biopsies. Stage 3 and 4 GVHD patients are very ill and only with difficulty can they tolerate an upper GI endoscopy which examines merely the very proximal part of the small bowel. The diagnostic accuracy of endoscopy when compared to histologic findings is high (Cruz-Correa et al. 2002). The precise diagnosis of acute GI GVHD is important since therapy for GVHD-associated diarrhea necessitates the increase of immunosuppressive therapy whereas diarrhea associated with infectious pathogens requires specific antiviral or antibacterial agents. The addition of immunosuppression in the latter group will have grave consequences in these already severely compromised patients.

Video Capsule Endoscopy in Acute GI GVHD

The authors used VCE in acute GI GVHD patients to evaluate feasibility and diagnostic yield of this method. A total of 28 patients who had received allo-SCT were examined: 25 patients with acute GI GVHD and 3 patients with chronic GVHD. All patients had undergone intensive investigations in the evaluation of diarrhea, which included stool cultures, testing for *C. difficile* toxin, serum polymerase chain reaction (PCR), and serology for Epstein-Barr virus (EBV) and adenovirus, viral cultures of throat, stool, and urine, and an assay for CMV pp65 antigen in blood.

☐ **Table 6.7-1.** Stages of acute GI GVHD affecting the digestive tract

	Endoscopic classification	Diarrhea
Stage 1	Focal mild erythema and edematous mucosa	>30 ml/kg or >500 ml/24 h
Stage 2	Rough, reddish, and atrophic mucosa	>60 ml/kg or >1000 ml/24 h
Stage 3	Erosive changing and oozing	>90 ml/kg or >1500 ml/24 h
Stage 4	Ulceration with extensive exudates	>90 ml/kg or >2000 ml/24 h or severe abdominal pain with or without ileus

VCE was performed in all patients. One patient had difficulties swallowing the capsule and in one patient the video capsule remained lodged in the esophagus for the entire study. No untoward side effects to the patients were noted in any of the 28 patients. VCE was performed safely in even the severest cases of acute GI GVHD and was far better tolerated than invasive endoscopic procedures.

A normal video capsule study (☐ Fig. 6.7-1) essentially rules out acute GI GVHD. The normal findings at capsule endoscopy in some patients led to the reduction of immunosuppression(Yakoub-Agha et al. 2004). In patients with **chronic** GVHD the capsule endoscopy findings of the small bowel are normal even if they suffer from diarrhea (Adler et al. 2004). However, all patients with grade 2 to 4 acute GI GVHD have abnormal findings on capsule endoscopy of the small bowel. The extent and severity of the lesions parallel the stage of the disease. VCE was at least as sensitive as upper GI endoscopy and histology in diagnosing acute GI GVHD (Yakoub-Agha et al. 2004). In two cases, despite invasive tests it was only VCE that made the diagnosis of acute GI GVHD (Shapira et al. 2005). Finally VCE findings have a direct impact on clinical management in these critically ill patients.

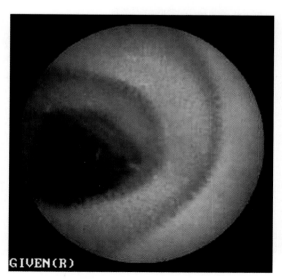

GIVEN(R)

☐ **Fig. 6.7-1.** Normal mucosa in a patient with suspected acute GI GVHD

Findings at Capsule Endoscopy in Acute GI GVHD

VCE findings characteristic of the mucosal damage include the following:

- Destruction of the mucosa (◘ Fig. 6.7-3)
- Diffuse superficial mucosal disease, mucosal breaks
- Loss of villous formation, scalloped folds
- Erythema (◘ Fig. 6.7-2)
- Ulcerations, aphthous lesions
- Mucosal erosive changes and inflammatory exudates (◘ Fig. 6.7-5)
- Vascular malformation
- Mucosal hemorrhages, fresh bleeding (◘ Fig. 6.7-4)
- Strictures (◘ Fig. 6.7-6)

Capsule endoscopy also revealed new findings previously not described in patients with acute GI GVHD such as strictures (◘ Fig. 6.7-6). The anemia of some patients is worsened by spontaneous bleeding of friable mucosa (◘ Fig. 6.7-4).

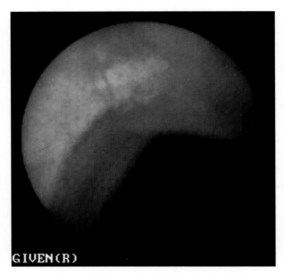

◘ **Fig. 6.7-2.** Grade 1 acute GI GVHD with focal mild erythema

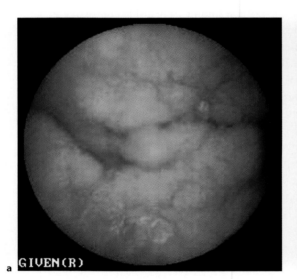

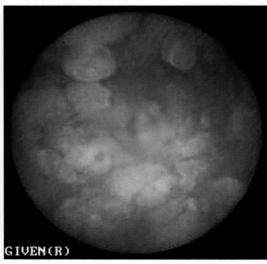

◘ **Fig. 6.7-3a–c.** Grade 2 acute GI GVHD with rough, reddish atrophic mucosa and erosive changes

a

b

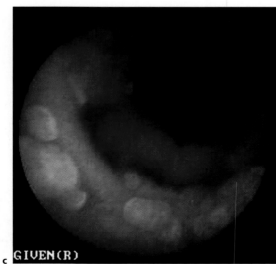

c

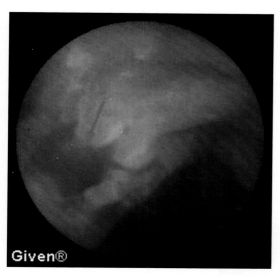

■ **Fig. 6.7-4.** Grade 3 acute GI GVHD. Spontaneous mucosal bleeding in a patient with acute GVHD

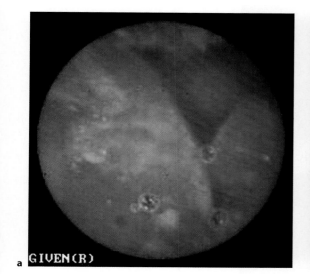

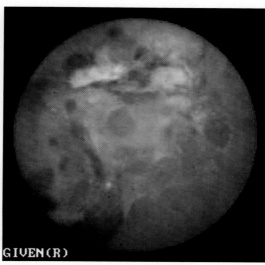

■ **Fig. 6.7-5a, b.** Grade 3 acute GI GVHD: erosive changes and inflammatory exudates

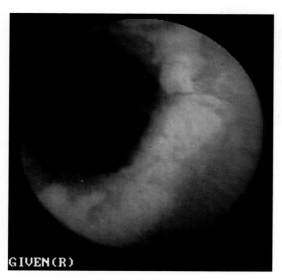

■ **Fig. 6.7-6.** Inflammatory stricture in a patient with acute GVHD

Transit Times in Acute GI GVHD

Gastric emptying of the video capsule was delayed, especially in grades 3 and 4 acute GI GVHD. This fact has to be taken into account when performing capsule endoscopy in patients with severe acute GI GVHD. These patients may require prokinetic agents and should be kept in the right lateral position for an extended period of time to facilitate passage into the small bowel (Sachdev et al. 2004).

Small bowel transit time characteristically is prolonged either due to segments of small bowel with no propagated contractions or because of the presence of inflammatory strictures (◘ Fig. 6.7-6).

Differential Diagnosis

Yakoub-Agha et al. 2004 and Adler et al. 2004 describe two patients with deep ulcers and sharply demarcated borders (◘ Figs. 6.7-7a, b and 6.7-8). Both patients were demonstrated to have CMV infections and were successfully treated with ganciclovir.

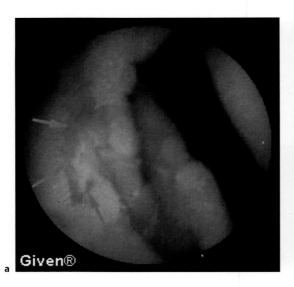
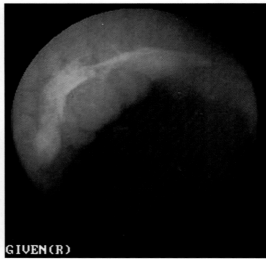

◘ **Fig. 6.7-7a, b.** Sharply demarcated deep ulcer in a patient with acute GVHD and CMV infection

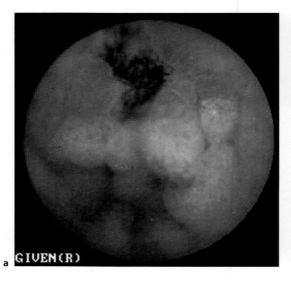
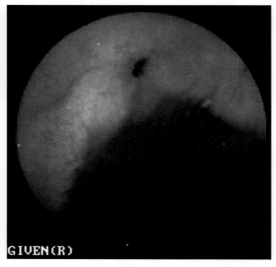

◘ **Fig. 6-7-8a, b.** Necrotic ulcerations related to CMV in a patient with acute GVHD

Internet

www.marrow.org/MEDICAL/graft_vs_host_disease.html: National Marrow Donor Program

References

Adler SN, Jacob H, Shapira MY, Or R, Rosenmann E (2004) Capsule endoscopy of the small intestine in graft versus host disease. Gastrointest Endosc 59:AB174

Cruz-Correa M, Poonawala A, Abraham SC, Wu TT, Zahurak M, Vogelsang G, Kalloo AN, Lee LA (2002) Endoscopic findings predict the histologic diagnosis in gastrointestinal graft-versus-host disease. Endoscopy 34:808–813

Einsele H, Ehninger G, Hebart H et al (1994) Incidence of local CMV infection and acute intestinal GVHD in marrow transplants recipients with severe diarrhoea. Bone Marrow Transplant 14:955–963

Ferrara JL, Deeg HJ (1991) Graft-versus-host disease. N Engl J Med 324:667–674

Sachdev R, Hibberd P, Mammen A, Cave DR (2004) Reduction of gastric transit time of video capsule endoscopy by right lateral positioning. Gastrointest Endosc 59:AB176

Shapira MY, Adler SN, Jacob H, Resnick IB, Slavin S, Or R (2005) New insights into the pathophysiology of gastrointestinal graft-versus-host disease using capsule endoscopy. Haematologica 90:1003-1004

Yakoub-Agha I, Maunoury V, Wacrenier S et al (2004) Impact of small bowel exploration using video-capsule endoscopy in the management of acute gastrointestinal graft-versus-host disease. Transplantation 78:1697–1701

Tumors of the Small Intestine

7.1   **Benign Tumors**

M. Keuchel, W.A. Selby, E.Tóth

Definition. Benign tumors of the small intestine consist of various entities such as tumorlike inflammatory or hyperplastic lesions, hamartomas (organoid malformations), ectopic tissues, and true neoplasms of epithelial or mesenchymal origin.

Benign small bowel tumors

Inflammatory lesions
- Inflammatory polyps
- Suture granulomas

Hyperplasias
- Hyperplastic polyps (☐ Fig. 2.3-5)
- Brunneromas

Hamartomas
- Hamartomatous polyps (Peutz-Jeghers polyps)
- Juvenile polyps (☐ Fig. 7.3-1)

Ectopic tissues
- Ectopic pancreatic tissue
- Ectopic gastric mucosa
- Endometriosis

Epithelial tumors
- Adenomas

Mesenchymal tumors
- Hemangiomas
- Lymphangiomas
- Leiomyomas
- Lipomas
- Neurofibromas

Clinical Features. Benign tumors of the small intestine often remain asymptomatic for years. They may be manifested clinically by bleeding, iron deficiency anemia, or abdominal pain. Possible complications are obstruction, intussusception, and perforation.

Endoscopy. Hyperplasias, hamartomas, ectopic gastric mucosa, foci of endometriosis, and adenomas may appear as flat or raised lesions on the mucosal surface. Ectopic pancreatic tissue and mesenchymal tumors are usually located beneath normal mucosa, have smooth margins, and are raised. The surface may show a generally circumscribed ulceration that can cause bleeding. Vascular tumors often have a reddish or bluish appearance.

❶ Benign and malignant small intestinal tumors cannot be reliably differentiated by endoscopic examination.

Inflammatory Lesions

Suture Granuloma

Granulomas may develop as an inflammatory reaction caused by suture material. These granulomas rarely cause symptoms, but may be confused with neoplastic lesions.

Endoscopy. Polypoid lesions can be visible at an anastomosis; the suture itself may be hidden by the granuloma (☐ Fig. 7.1-1).

Inflammatory Polyps

Inflammatory fibroid polyps are a rare finding in the gastrointestinal tract, occasionally involving the small intestine. Histologically, they show a fibroblast proliferation and eosinophilia (Santos et al. 2004). They can cause intussusception or bleeding.

Endoscopy. Sessile or pedunculated polyps (☐ Fig. 7.1-2) may be seen, sometimes with ulceration, hemorrhage, or hematoma.

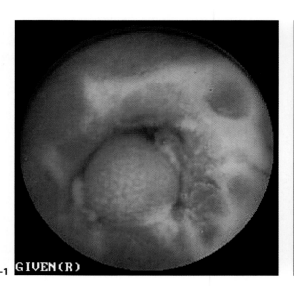

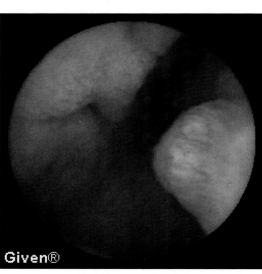

☐ **Fig. 7.1-1.** Tumorlike suture granuloma and ulcerated stricture in the ileum in a patient with previously resected small bowel Crohn's disease.

☐ **Fig. 7.1-2.** Pyloric inflammatory fibroid polyp seen at VCE.

7.1-1   GIVEN(R)

Given®   7.1-2

Ectopic Tissues

Definition. Ectopic tissues are structurally normal but occur at an abnormal location in the body.

Ectopic Pancreatic Tissue

Occurrence. Ectopic pancreatic tissue is rare, but it is the most common tumorlike lesion in the jejunum and ileum (Matsuo et al. 1994).

Endoscopy. Endoscopy demonstrates a submucosal mass (◘ Figs. 7.1-3 and 7.1-4). Histologic examination establishes the diagnosis.

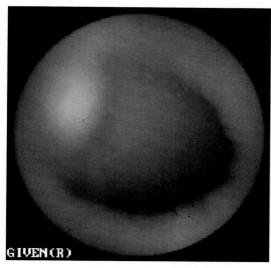

a

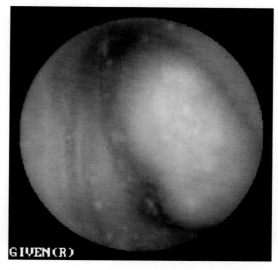

◘ **Fig. 7.1-4.** Ectopic pancreatic tissue in the terminal ileum (courtesy of Ingo Franke, M.D.). The patient presented with intermittent bowel obstruction.

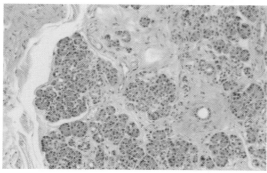

b

◘ **Fig. 7.1-3a, b.** Small, submucosal tumor in the jejunum **(a)**. Histology of the resected specimen **(b)** shows normal pancreatic tissue with glands and excretory ducts (H&E, courtesy of Jürgen Schmoll, M.D.). The patient presented with obscure gastrointestinal bleeding years after undergoing a small intestine resection for carcinoid.

Ectopic Gastric Mucosa

Occurrence. Though relatively rare, ectopic gastric mucosa is the most common polyp in the duodenal bulb besides inflammatory polyps (each comprise 35%) (Stolte and Lux 1983). Ectopic gastric mucosa is a common finding in Meckel's diverticula.

Endoscopy. A typical raised, brightly colored mosaic pattern of gastric mucosa with no villi is seen at endoscopy. Sometimes the tissue is found to be in contact with the distal, duodenal aspect of the pylorus (◘ Fig. 7.1-5).

Endometriosis

Ectopic endometrial tissue is rarely found in the small intestine. In women of childbearing age, these lesions may cause obstructive symptoms caused by subserosal, rather than by transmural involvement (Ridha and Cassaro 2003).

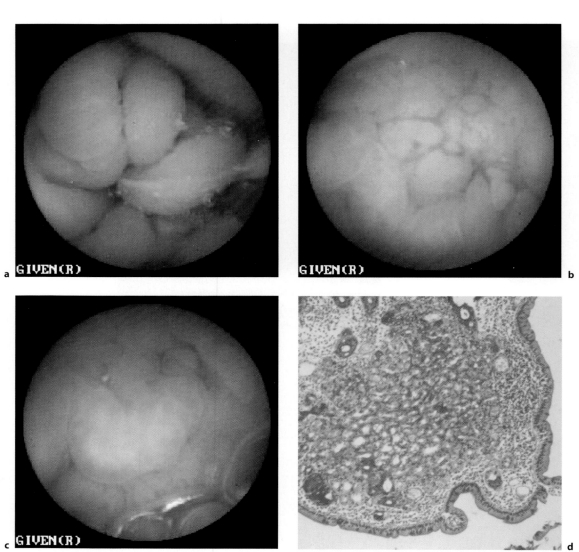

◘ **Fig. 7.1-5.** **a** Typical gastric mucosa extends through the pylorus into the duodenal bulb (capsule in the duodenum). **b, c** Raised, pseudopolypous gastric mucosa with irregular marginal extensions, appearing on normal small intestine mucosa with villi. **d** Histology: corpus-type gastric mucosa (PAS, courtesy of Martin Bergmann, M.D.).

Hyperplasias

Brunneroma

Definition. A brunneroma is a mass formed by hyperplasia of the mucus-forming Brunner's glands in the duodenum. It often has an inflammatory etiology (Merine et al. 1991).

Prevalence. Brunneromas account for 7% of all tumorlike lesions in the duodenum (Stolte and Lux 1983).

Clinical Features. Brunneromas are usually asymptomatic. Rarely, they can be large, known as Brunner's gland adenoma, and can result in bleeding or obstruction.

Endoscopy. Endoscopy reveals a polypoid bulge of mucosa in the duodenal bulb with normal-appearing villi (☐ Fig. 7.1-6). Large lesions are usually found on the posterior wall at the junction of the first and second parts of the duodenum (☐ Fig. 7.1-7) and can be removed endoscopically (Gao et al. 2004).

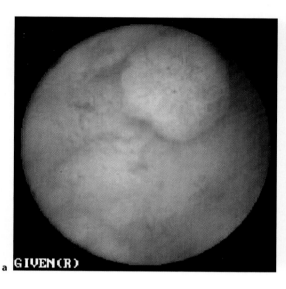
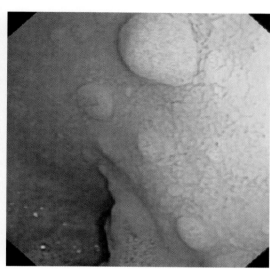

☐ **Fig. 7.1-6a, b.** Biopsy-confirmed hyperplasia of Brunner's glands in the duodenal bulb with superficial villi. **a** VCE, **b** side-viewing duodenoscopy.

a GIVEN(R)   b

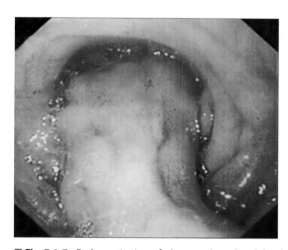

☐ **Fig. 7.1-7.** Endoscopic view of a large pedunculated duodenal Brunner's gland adenoma.

Hyperplastic Polyps

Hyperplastic polyps are rare in the small intestine (■ Fig. 2.3-5); they are mostly found in the duodenum (Matsuura et al. 1990).

Lymphoid Hyperplasia

Some degree of hyperplasia of lymphoid tissue in the terminal ileum is not uncommon, especially in children (Chap. 11).

Endoscopy. Nodular or polypoid lesions, sometimes aggregated, are typically found in the terminal ileum (■ Fig. 7.1-8).

■ Fig. 7.1-8 a, b. Lymphoid hyperplasia in the terminal ileum. **a** VCE, **b** ileoscopic view.

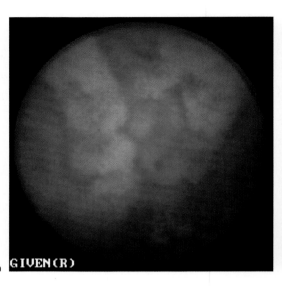

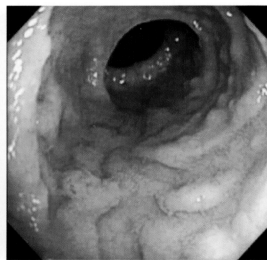

a GIVEN(R)   b

Hamartomas

Definition. Hamartomas are tumorlike developmental anomalies in which different tissue components are abnormally combined.

Juvenile Polyps

Occurrence. Juvenile polyps occur predominantly in the colon and less commonly in the stomach and small intestine (◘ Fig. 7.3-1). They may be a manifestation of familial juvenile polyposis (see Chap. 7.3).

Histology. The term »juvenile« refers to the histologic type with inflammatory infiltrate and mucus-filled glands of the lamina propria.

Endoscopy. Endoscopy sometimes shows inflammatory surface changes in the polyps.

Hamartomatous Polyps

Clinical Features. Hamartomatous polyps may occur as sporadic or multiple manifestations in patients with Peutz-Jeghers syndrome (► Chap. 7.3). Polyps of sufficient size may produce symptoms of intestinal obstruction or may bleed (◘ Fig. 7.1-9).

Histology. The lesions have a characteristic histologic appearance marked by an arborizing pattern of the muscular layer of the polyps (◘ Fig. 7.1-10c).

Endoscopy. Endoscopy demonstrates reddish polyps, often pedunculated, that may completely occupy the intestine lumen (◘ Figs. 7.1-10 and 7.3-2–7.3-4).

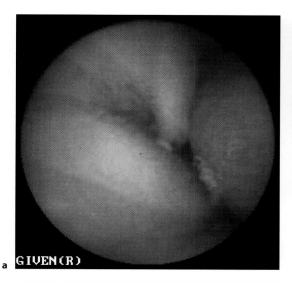

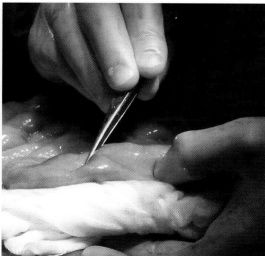

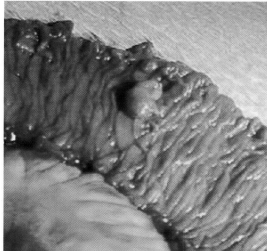

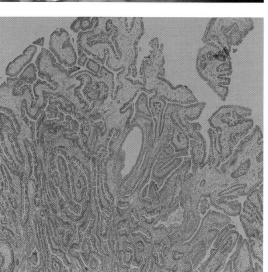

◘ **Fig. 7.1-9a–d.** Hamartomatous polyp (15×15 mm in size) in the proximal jejunum. **a** VCE finding, **b** intraoperative view, **c** resected surgical specimen, **d** histology of benign hamartomatous polyp (courtesy of Otto Ljungberg, M.D.). Patient with a 1-year history of persistent iron deficiency anemia (lowest hemoglobin level 60 g/l). Normal preoperative enteroclysis. After 2 years of follow-up the patient is symptom-free, with normal laboratory tests.

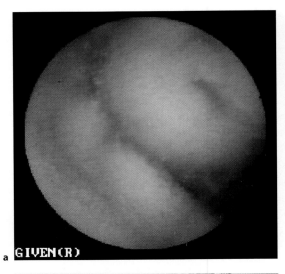

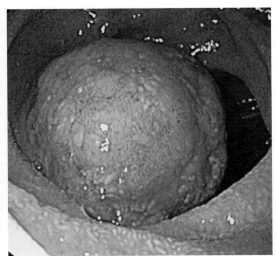

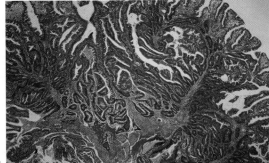

Fig. 7.1-10. a Peutz-Jeghers polyp of the small intestine, **b** push enteroscopy, **c** histology showed arborization of the muscle layer (courtesy of Renate Höhne, M.D.).

Epithelial Neoplasms

Adenomas

Definition. An adenoma is a benign neoplasm that arises from the crypt epithelium.

Occurrence. Adenomas occur sporadically in rare cases. Their incidence is increased in patients with polyposis syndromes (▶ Chap. 7.3).

Location. Adenomas occur predominantly in the duodenum, often in the peripapillary region.

Endoscopy. Adenomas in the duodenum often appear as flat lesions with a typical whitish surface (■ Fig. 7.1-11). Adenomatous polyps of the small intestine occur in all sizes and may be sessile, broad-based, or pedunculated (■ Fig. 7.3-6 and 7.3-7).

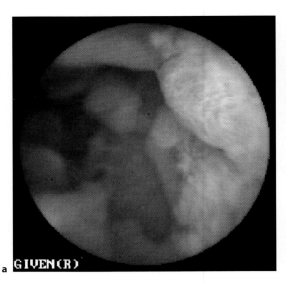

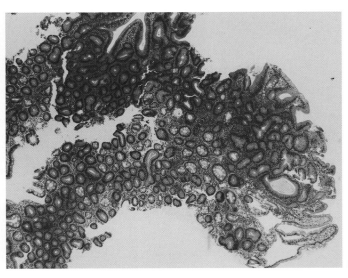

Fig. 7.1-11. a Flat, multifocal duodenal adenomas. **b** Histology showed tubular adenomas with moderate dysplasia (courtesy of Wilhelm-Wolfgang Höpker, M.D.). Familial adenomatous polyposis in a patient who had previously undergone colectomy.

Mesenchymal Tumors

Definition. Mesenchymal tumors are benign neoplasms that arise from various mesodermal cells. They are classified according to the underlying cell type, which often can be characterized only with the help of additional immunohistochemical methods.

Hemangioma

Occurrence. Hemangiomas of the small intestine are rare. There are capillary (Kim at al. 2004) (■ Fig. 7.1-12), cavernous (Khurana et al. 2004) (■ Fig. 7.1-13), and mixed types. Hemangiomas may occur as singular lesions or may be multiple, for instance, in blue rubber bleb nevus syndrome (Fish et al. 2004; Maunoury et al. 1990), which also comprises cutaneous lesions (■ Figs. 7.1-14 and 5.1-7, and 5.1-8) .

Clinical Features. The main symptoms are episodes of bleeding.

Endoscopy. Hemangiomas appear as soft, bluish vascular tumors, sometimes reaching giant dimensions (■ Fig. 7.1-13). Occasionally, active bleeding is observed during VCE (■ Fig. 7.1-12).

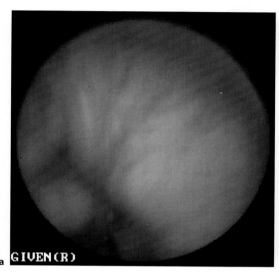

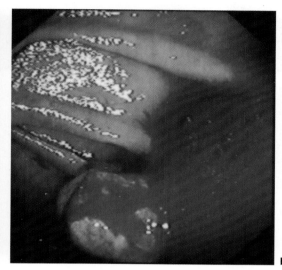

a GIVEN(R)

b

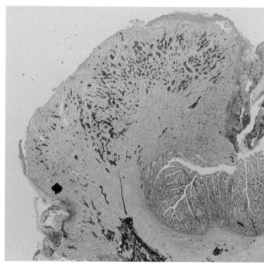

c

■ Fig. 7.1-12a–c. Bleeding capillary hemangioma. **a** Ongoing bleeding and narrow lumen in the proximal jejunum (VCE), **b** 1-cm large polypoid, bleeding tumor (push enteroscopy), **c** histology of the surgically resected tumor showed a benign capillary hemangioma with dilated submucosal blood vessels (courtesy of Otto Ljungberg, M.D.). An 82-year-old lady presented with a 6-week history of obscure GI bleeding requiring transfusion. After 2 years of follow-up the patient is symptom free, without further bleeding.

a b c d

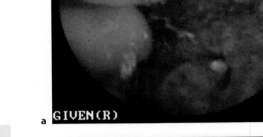

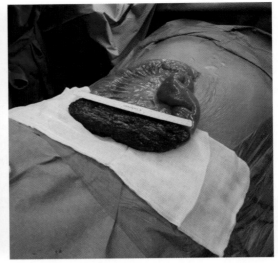

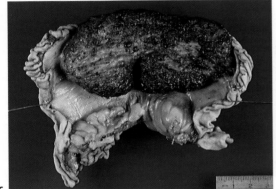

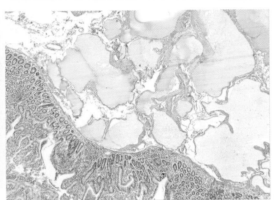

Fig. 7.1-13a–d. Giant hemangioma (case courtesy of André Van Gossum, M.D.) **a** VCE shows a vascular polypoid lesion, **b** laparotomy reveals the presence of a giant intestinal hemangioma, **c** surgical specimen, **d** histology showing dilated vessels.

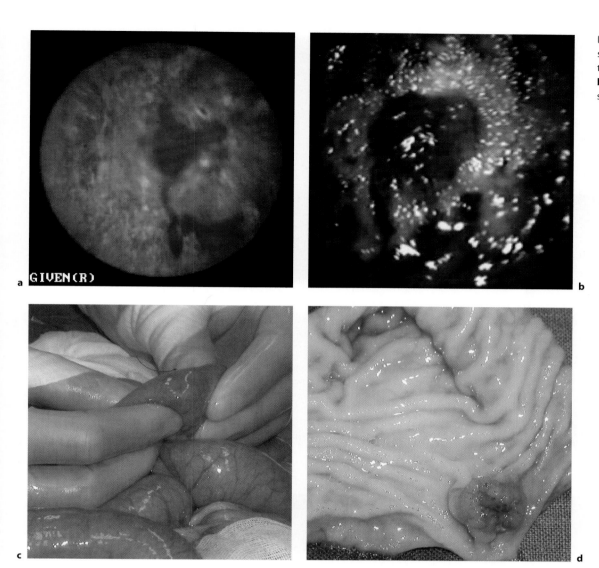

Fig. 7.1-14a–d. Blue rubber bleb nevus syndrome. **a** VCE showing polypoid bluish tumor with bleeding in the distal ileum, **b** preoperative ileoscopy, **c** intraoperative situs, **d** surgical specimen.

Lymphangioma, Cystic Lymphangiectasia

Occurrence. Cystic lymphangiectasia is a frequent associated finding in video capsule endoscopy of the small intestine. It was found in up to 20% of cases in an older autopsy series (Shilkin et al. 1968).

Clinical Features. The lesion itself apparently has no clinical significance. An extremely large lesion (◘ Fig. 7.1-18) can lead to intestinal obstruction, and erosion can cause bleeding.

Endoscopy. A submucosal, yellowish-white mass is observed at endoscopy (◘ Figs. 7.1-16 and 7.1-17). In some cases the villi over the cyst are white and thickened (◘ Fig. 7.1-15). The submucosal vessels are often clearly visible in lesions with normal mucosa and normal villi.

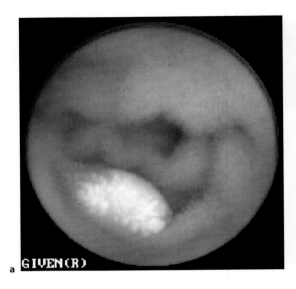

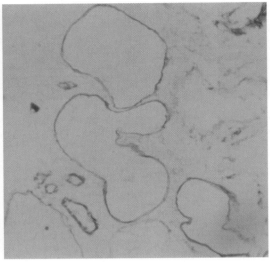

a   GIVEN(R)   b

◘ **Fig. 7.1-15a, b.** Microcystic lymphangiectasia: **a** white, thickened villi over a submucosal bulge. **b** Immunohistology: submucosal-like dilatation of lymphatic vessels (endothelial marker CD34, courtesy of Jörg Caselitz, M.D.).

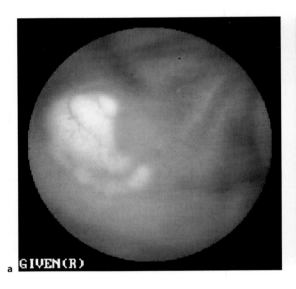

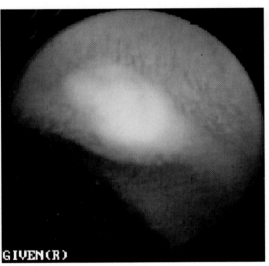

a   GIVEN(R)   GIVEN(R)   b

◘ **Fig. 7.1-16a, b.** Cystic lymphangiectasias: **a** en face view with a visible vascular pattern. **b** Tangential view with a pseudotumor appearance, normal mucosa.

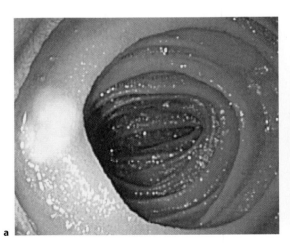

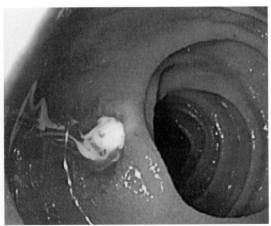

a   b

◘ **Fig. 7.1-17a, b.** Cystic lymphangiectasias: **a** push enteroscopy, **b** white lymph exudes from an endoscopic biopsy site.

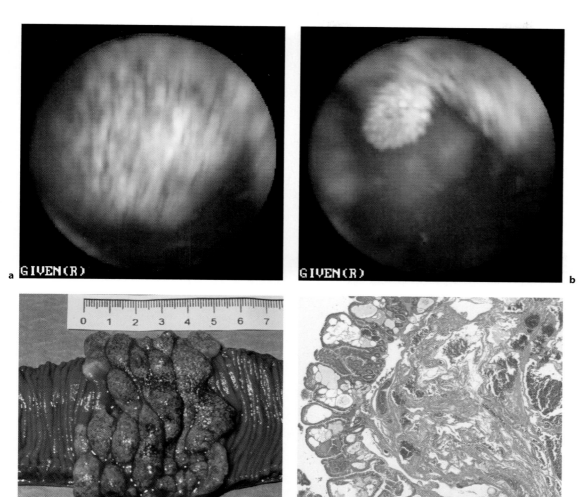

Fig. 7.1-18a–d. Large, segmental lymphangiectasia completely filling the intestine lumen (**a, b**). Motion unsharpness due to swift capsule passage through the stenotic small intestine segment. **c** Resected specimen. **d** Histology: marked cystic dilatation of the lymph vessels (case courtesy of Siegbert Faiss, M.D.) (**□** Figs. 7.1a–d).

Leiomyoma

Definition. Leiomyoma is a benign mesenchymal tumor of smooth muscle cells. It can be distinguished immunohistologically from gastrointestinal stromal tumors (GIST) (Miettinen et al. 2000).

Clinical Features. Leiomyomas are frequently asymptomatic. Anemia is sometimes present (Rice et al. 2001).

Endoscopy. Endoscopy demonstrates a submucosal tumor (**□** Fig. 7.1-19) of highly variable size, occasionally with ulceration of the otherwise normal-appearing mucosa. Endoscopic biopsies are often unrewarding due to the submucosal tumor location, since only the normal mucosa overlying the submucosal tumor is evaluated.

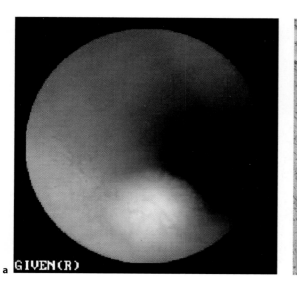

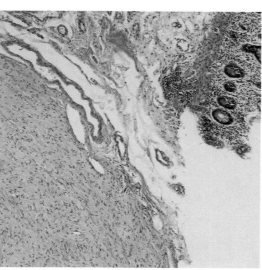

Fig. 7.1-19a, b. Small leiomyoma of the ileum: **a** submucosal tumor at VCE. **b** Histologically, the tumor is composed of smooth muscle cells (PAS, courtesy of Renate Höhne, M.D.). Note the normal mucosa over the tumor.

Lipoma

Clinical Features. Although small intestinal lipomas are mainly asymptomatic, they can cause intestinal bleeding or obstruction, requiring surgery (Zissin 2004) (◻ Fig. 7.1-24).

Endoscopy. Endoscopy reveals a soft, yellowish-whitish, mobile, sometimes pedunculated tumor (◻ Fig. 7.1-20) that is often located near the ileocecal valve (◻ Figs. 7.1-21 and 7.1-23).

Rarely, multiple lipomas present as intestinal lipomatosis (◻ Fig. 7.1-22). Fibrolipomas are characterized by additional fibrosis of the stroma, changing the endoscopic appearance to a more consistent, reddish tumor with a somewhat irregular surface (◻ Fig. 7.1-24).

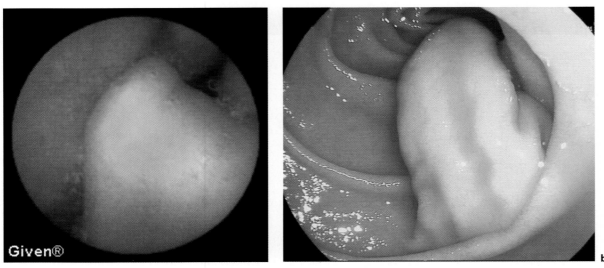

◻ **Fig. 7.1-20a, b.** Lipoma. **a** VCE: submucosal, pedunculated tumor. **b** Push enteroscopy: submucosal tumor with soft impressible content. Superficial biopsy showed normal mucosa.

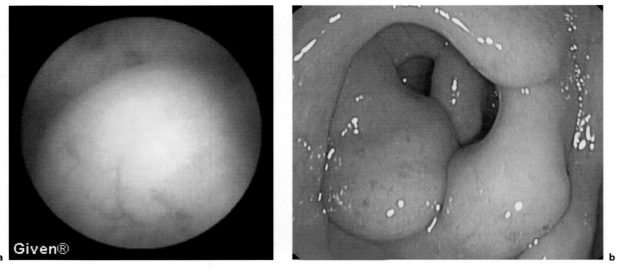

◻ **Fig. 7.1-21.** **a** Lipomatous thickening of the ileocecal valve at VCE, **b** corresponding colonoscopic view.

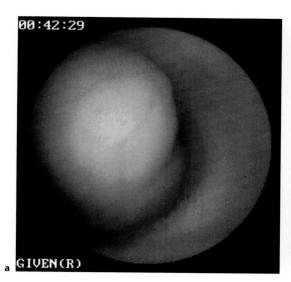

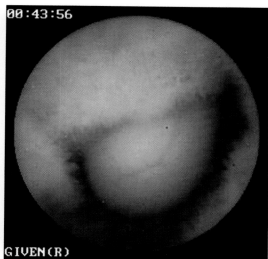

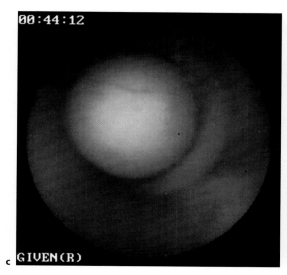

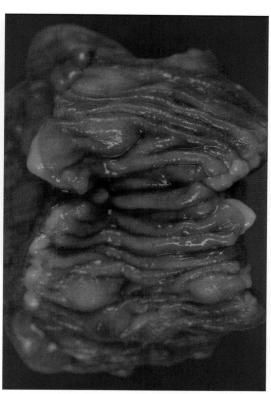

■ **Fig. 7.1-22a–d.** Intestinal lipomatosis. **a–c** Multiple bulging submucosol yellowish tumors of the jejunum. **d** Resected specimen with multiple lipomas. 48-year old patient wih postprandial abdominal pain and weight loss of 20 kg. After resection of 110 cm of small intestine complete resolution of pain (courtesy of Frank Stenschke, M.D. and Henryk Dancygier, M.D.).

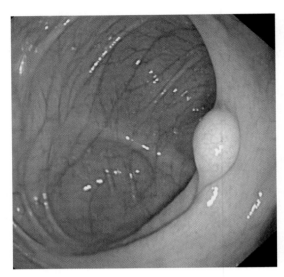

◘ Fig. 7.1-23. Colonoscopic view of a lipoma on the ileocecal valve.

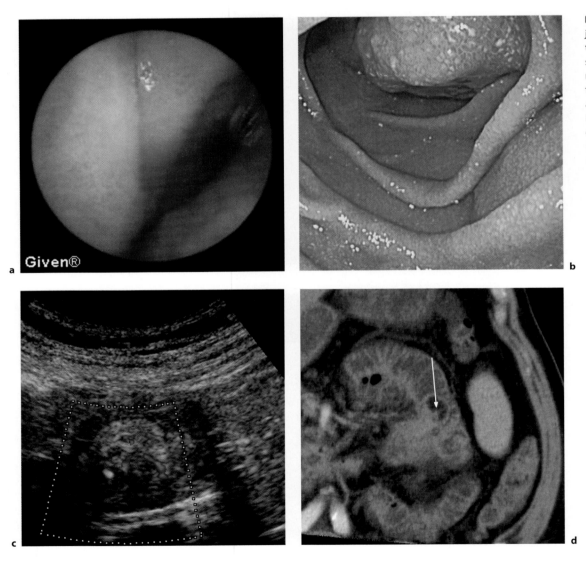

◘ Fig. 7.1-24a–d. Fibrolipoma of the jejunum. **a** VCE demonstrates a submucosal tumor. **b** Push enteroscopy. **c** Sonography shows a tumor with hyperechogenic inhomogeneous pattern and hypervascularization in power Doppler mode. **d** CT reveals an intraluminal, inhomogeneous tumor of low density, typical of fat (*arrow*) (courtesy of Ernst Malzfeldt, M.D.). The patient was referred because of relapsing severe intestinal hemorrhage.

Neurofibroma

Definition. Neurofibromas are benign tumors with neural and connective tissue differentiation.

Occurrence. Neurofibromas occur rarely in the setting of neurofibromatosis type I (Recklinghausen's disease) due to a mutation of the NF-1 gene on chromosome 17. Other small intestinal tumors, including malignant lesions, may also occur (Behranwala et al. 2004). Sporadic neurofibroma of the small intestine is a rarity (Watanuki et al. 1995).

Endoscopy. Neurofibromas have nonspecific endoscopic features, appearing as firm, submucosal tumors on the mesenteric side of the intestine. They are occasionally ulcerated (◻ Fig. 7.1-25).

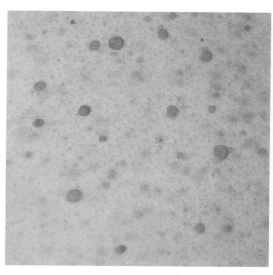
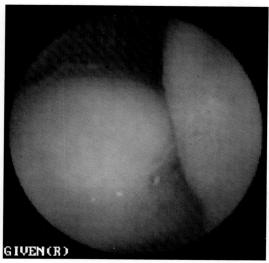

◻ **Fig. 7.1-25a–e.** Neurofibromas: **a** Cutaneous lesions. **b, c** Firm, white submucosal tumors at VCE, partly ulcerated. **d** Resected fibrotic tumor. **e** Histology: neurofibroma covered by normal small bowel mucosa (H&E, courtesy of Jörg Caselitz, M.D.).

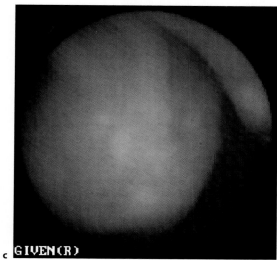
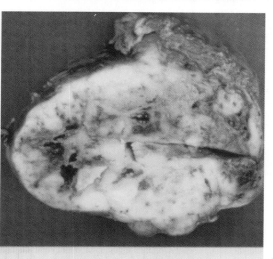
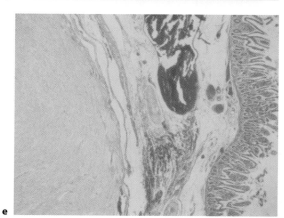

Intussusception

Occasionally a (benign) small intestinal tumor can lead to intussusception. This condition appears as an intraluminal duplication of the mucosa when observed by VCE (■ Fig. 7.1-26).

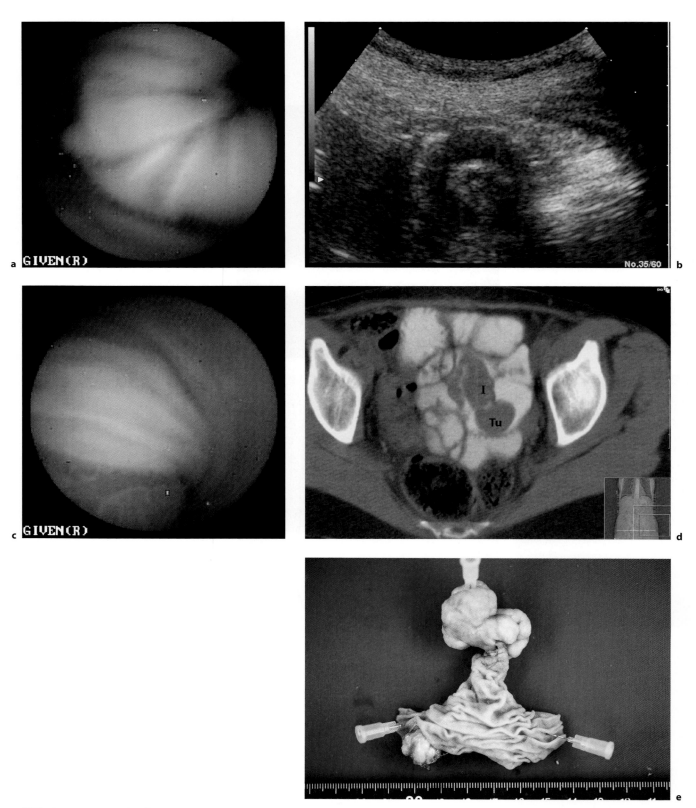

■ **Fig. 7.1-26a–e. a, c** Small intestine intussusception caused by a tumor. **b** Target sign in a transverse ultrasound scan of the small intestine. **d** The tumor *(Tu)* and intussusceptum *(I)* produce an intraluminal filling defect on CT (courtesy of Ernst Malzfeldt, M.D.). **e** Resected specimen (courtesy of Renate Höhne, M.D.). Histology revealed adenoma

Internet

http://ghr.nlm.nih.gov Genetics Home reference (U.S. National Library of Medicine)
http://www.nf.org National Neurofibromatosis Foundation
www.geneclinics.org/profiles Gene reviews NIH/University of Washington, Seattle
http://www.rarediseases.org National Organization for Rare Disorders

References

Behranwala KA, Spalding DR, Wotherspoon A et al (2004) Small bowel gastrointestinal stromal tumours and ampullary cancer in type 1 neurofibromatosis. World J Surg Oncol 2:1–4

Fish L, Fireman Z, Kopelman Y, Sternberg A (2004) Blue rubber bleb nevus syndrome: small-bowel lesions diagnosed by capsule endoscopy. Endoscopy 36:836

Gao Y-P, Zhu J-S, Zheng W-J (2004) Brunner's gland adenoma of duodenum: a case report and literature review. World J Gastroenterol 10:2616–2617

Khurana V, Dala R, Barkin JS (2004) Small bowel cavernous hemangioma. Gastrointest Endosc 60:96

Kim YS, Chun HJ, Jeen YT, Um SH, Kim CD, Hyun JH (2004) Small bowel capillary hemangioma. Gastrointest Endosc 60:599

Matsuo S, Eto T, Tsunoda T, Kanematsu T, Shinozaki T (1994) Small bowel tumors: an analysis of tumor-like lesions, benign and malignant neoplasms. Eur J Surg Oncol 20:47–51

Matsuura H, Kuwano H, Kanematsu T, Sugimachi K, Haraguchi Y (1990) Clinicopathological features of elevated lesions of the duodenal bulb. J Surg Oncol 45:79–84

Maunoury V, Turck D, Brunetaud JM et al (1990) Blue rubber bleb nevus syndrome. 3 cases treated with a Nd:YAG laser and bipolar electrocoagulation (in French). Gastroenterol Clin Biol 14:593–595

Merine D, Jones B, Ghahremani GG et al (1991) Hyperplasia of Brunner glands: the spectrum of its radiographic manifestations. Gastrointest Radiol 16:104–108

Miettinen M, Sobin LH, Sarlomo-Rikala M (2000) Immunohistochemical spectrum of GISTs at different sites and their differential diagnosis with a reference to CD117 (KIT). Mod Pathol 13:1134–1142

Ridha JR, Cassaro S (2003) Acute small bowel obstruction secondary to ileal endometriosis: report of a case. Surg Today 33:944–947

Rice DC, Bakaeen F, Farley DR et al (2001) Surgical management of duodenal leiomyomas. World J Surg 25:562–566

Santos G, Alves AF, Wakamatsu A, Zucoloto S (2004) Inflammatory fibroid polyp. An immunohistochemical study. Arq Gastroenterol 41:104–107

Shilkin KB, Zerman JB, Blackwell JB (1968) Lymphangiectatic cysts of the small bowel. Pathol Bacteriol 96:353–358

Stolte M, Lux G (1983) Duodenum und Papilla Vateri: Tumoren und tumorähnliche Läsionen – ein klinisch pathologisches Gespräch. Leber Magen Darm 13: 227–241

Watanuki F, Ohwada S, Hosomura Y et al (1995) Small ileal neurofibroma causing intussusception in a non-neurofibromatosis patient. J Gastroenterol 30:113–116

Zissin R (2004) Enteroenteric intussusception secondary to a lipoma: CT diagnosis. Emerg Radiol 11:107–109

7.2 Malignant Tumors

B. Lewis, M. Keuchel, J. Caselitz

Prevalence. Tumors of the small bowel account for 5% of all gastro-intestinal tract tumors and 2% of the cancers. Prior to the advent of capsule endoscopy, the methods for examining the small bowel proved inadequate, so the accuracy of the above statement is unknown. The diagnosis of small bowel tumors is often delayed, contributing to the poor prognosis in patients with malignant tumors. In 1995, 4600 new cases of small intestinal cancer were reported along with 1120 deaths (Conn 1997). Tumors are typically missed by most radiographic tests and thus prior to small intestinal endoscopy, tumors of the small bowel generally carried a dismal prognosis. In 1980, Herbsman et al. (1980) reported that survival of more than 6 months for adenocarcinoma of the small bowel was rare. More recently in the era of earlier detection due to small bowel endoscopic techniques, the overall 5-year survival is reported to be 57% and the median survival is 52 months (North and Pack 2000).

Malignant small bowel tumors:

- ▬ Primary small bowel malignancies
  - – Adenocarcinomas (47%)
  - – Neuroendocrine tumors (28%)
  - – Sarcomas (12%)
  - – Lymphomas (12%)
- ▬ Metastases
- ▬ Small bowel infiltration by extraintestinal malignancies

Clinical Features. Malignant tumors of the small bowel are asymptomatic in their early stages. Later the complaints are often uncharacteristic, causing a delay in diagnosis. An important warning sign is gastrointestinal bleeding or iron deficiency anemia of unknown cause. Abdominal pain, weight loss, (partial) bowel obstruction, or perforation are seen with advanced tumors (Rossini et al. 1999).

Endoscopy. The endoscopic appearance of a small bowel mass can be deceiving to the endoscopist. The variety of pathologies seen within the small bowel cannot be matched by the colon or the stomach. Thus the well-trained endoscopist may still be only able to say that a tumor was present and not know the true pathology. Many small bowel tumors are submucosal also adding to the difficulty of visual diagnosis and even diagnosis by endoscopic biopsy. Submucosal tumors include leiomyomas, carcinoids, lipomas, and metastatic disease. With the small space of the small bowel and the large nature of a tumor, the typical changes suggestive of a submucosal process may be missed. Typically the endoscopist looks for visible mucosa and a vascular pattern across the tumor to confirm its submucosal nature. Bridging folds may also help in this regard. In the small bowel, the mucosa may be pulled so tightly over the mass that it becomes transparent, masking the standard changes. Leiomyomas can vary in size and the endoscopic appearance does not judge the size of the extramucosal component. Occasionally central ulceration or umbilication may be seen. Lymphomas can have several different appearances. A classification of these appearances has been created and includes a nodular pattern, an infiltrative pattern, and an ulcerating pattern (Barakat 1982). Halphen et al. (1986), in a review of 120 patients with primary small bowel lymphoma, found the infiltrative pattern, in which the mucosa is firm and motionless, to be most indicative of lymphoma. The other patterns may be mimicked by celiac disease and radiation enteritis among others. Adenocarcinoma is circumferential and often quite exophytic appearing like the endoscopic appearance of colon cancer. Metastatic melanoma can often be suspected by its pigmented nature. Carcinoid often appears as multiple submucosal nodules. Most small bowel tumors diagnosed by VCE have been detected in patients evaluated for intestinal bleeding (Mascarenhas-Saraiva and da Silva Araujo Lopes 2003; Cobrin et al. 2004; Keuchel et al. 2004). VCE is more sensitive than imaging procedures in detecting these lesions. False-negative VCE findings have been described in cases where the viewing axis of the capsule was deflected by a tumor-related stricture (Madisch et al. 2003) or vision was obscured due to tumor bleeding (Knop et al. 2003) or inadequate preparation (Hara et al. 2004).

Treatment. Complete surgical removal of the tumor is the treatment of choice (Brucher et al. 1998). Other adjuvant or alternative treatment modalities may be considered, depending on the tumor entity and stage.

Adenocarcinoma

Location. From 41 to 76% of adenocarcinomas are located in the duodenum, and approximately 38% can be reached by esophagogastroduodenoscopy (Abrahams et al. 2002).

Risk Factors. Risk factors for small bowel adenocarcinoma are several polyposis syndromes, sprue, Crohn's disease, and previous radiotherapy.

Endoscopy. Endoscopy may reveal an infiltrating lesion (◪ Fig. 7.2-1) or exophytic tumor (◪ Figs. 7.2-2–7.2-4), which may show ulceration, stricturing, and/or bleeding.

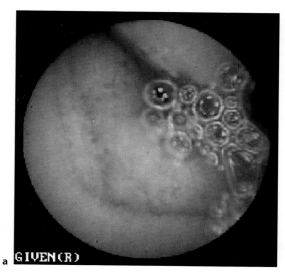

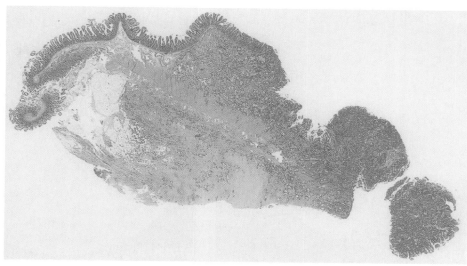

■ Fig. 7.2-1a, b. Adenocarcinoma. **a** Semicircumferential, infiltrating tumor partially obstructing the small bowel lumen. The capsule did not pass spontaneously through the stricture. **b** Histology shows infiltration of all wall layers (T3 lesion, courtesy of Brigitte Mahn, M.D.). The patient presented with bleeding requiring transfusion and recurrent partial bowel obstruction; enteroclysis was negative

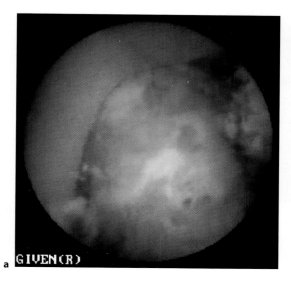

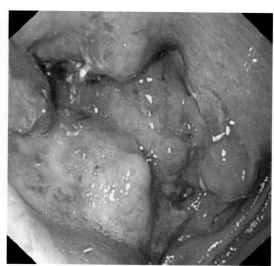

■ Fig. 7.2-2a, b. Adenocarcinoma of the jejunum (courtesy of Michel Delvaux, M.D. and Gerard Gay, M.D.): large exophytic, ulcerated tumor at VCE **(a)** and push enteroscopy **(b)**. Intrinsic malignant stricture did not obstruct capsule passage

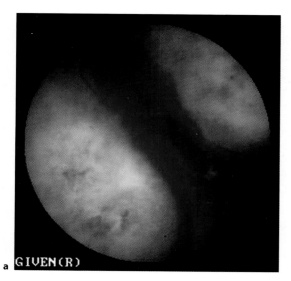

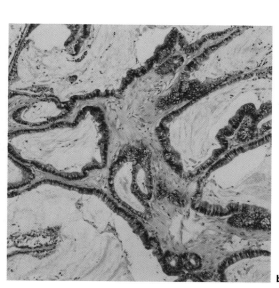

■ Fig. 7.2-3a, b. Stenosing and bleeding adenocarcinoma. **a** VCE. **b** Histology reveals a mucinous adenocarcinoma of the small bowel

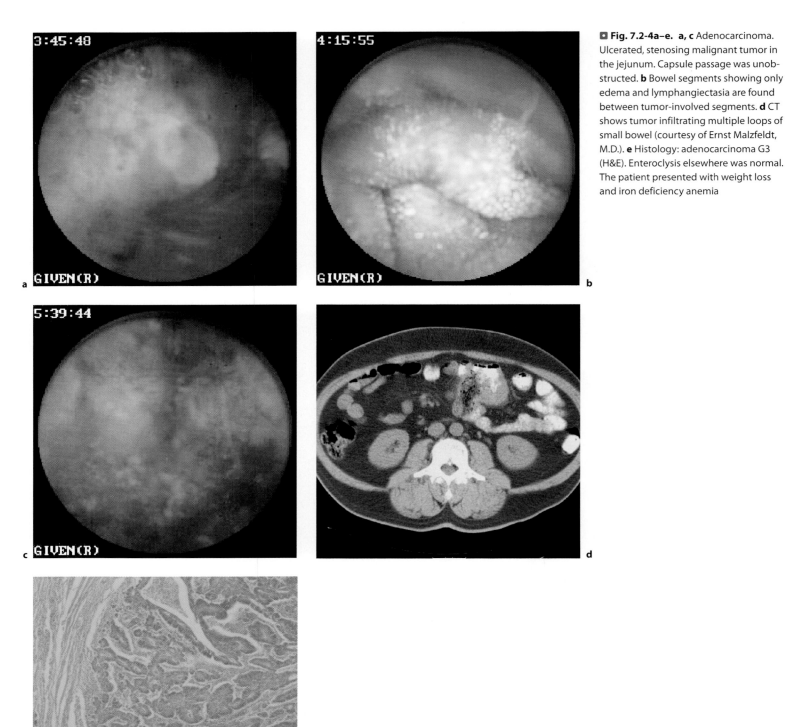

Fig. 7.2-4a–e. a, c Adenocarcinoma. Ulcerated, stenosing malignant tumor in the jejunum. Capsule passage was unobstructed. **b** Bowel segments showing only edema and lymphangiectasia are found between tumor-involved segments. **d** CT shows tumor infiltrating multiple loops of small bowel (courtesy of Ernst Malzfeldt, M.D.). **e** Histology: adenocarcinoma G3 (H&E). Enteroclysis elsewhere was normal. The patient presented with weight loss and iron deficiency anemia

Neuroendocrine Tumors (Carcinoids)

Definition. These tumors originate from neuroendocrine cells, are often hormone producing, and are of varying biologic behavior.

Nomenclature. Neuroendocrine tumors of the gastroenteropancreatic system are subdivided into well-differentiated neuroendocrine tumors with a benign pattern of behavior (e.g., carcinoid) and well- or poorly differentiated neuroendocrine carcinomas (e.g., malignant carcinoid; Klöppel et al. 2004).

Location. Most carcinoids occur in the small intestine (Modlin et al. 2003).

Clinical Features. Localized carcinoids of the small bowel are frequently asymptomatic (Hemminki and Li 2001). Pain, bleeding, and bowel obstruction may occur, and symptoms of carcinoid syndrome can occur with hepatic metastases.

Diagnosis. Special tests include the serum determination of chromogranin A, specific hormone determinations [e.g., gastrin, insulin, glucagon, vasoactive intestinal peptide (VIP)], the determination of breakdown products (urinary 5-hydroxyinsolacetic acid with carcinoids), and somatostatin receptor scintigraphy (⬛ Figs. 7.2-6b and 7.2-8b) as a localizing study (Horton et al. 2004).

Endoscopy. Endoscopy usually shows submucosal (☐ Figs. 7.2-5–7.2-7) or infiltrating tumors (☐ Figs. 7.2-8 and 7.2-9) of varying size. They can be classified only by histologic examination.

Treatment. Hormone-related symptoms in advanced cases may respond to treatment with somatostatin (Oberg et al. 2004). Other options are interferon, chemotherapy if necessary, and experimental radiation therapy (Buscombe et al. 2003).

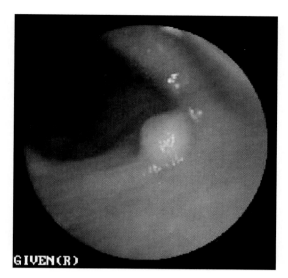

☐ **Fig. 7.2-5.** Small carcinoid tumor in the ileum: submucosal tumor (courtesy of Wilfred Landry, M.D.)

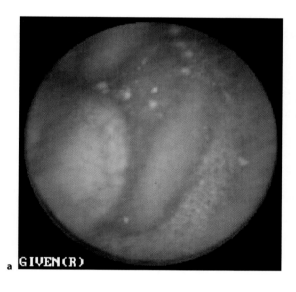

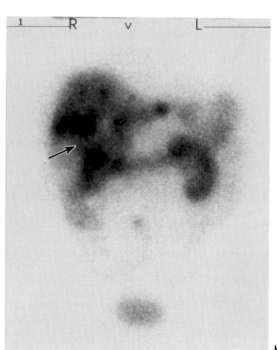

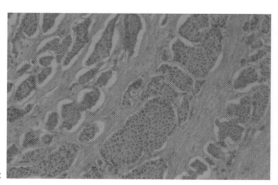

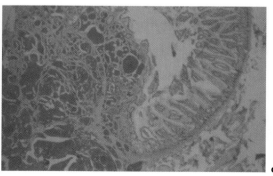

☐ **Fig. 7.2-6a–d.** Well-differentiated neuroendocrine carcinoma (malignant carcinoid). **a** Small, infiltrating tumor of the jejunum. **b** Somatostatin-receptor scintigraphy shows large hepatic metastases (*arrow*) and slightly increased uptake in the midabdomen (courtesy of Bernhard Leisner, M.D.). **c, d** Histology: small cell tumor with marked connective tissue reaction and presence of somatostatin receptors (courtesy of Wilhelm-Wolfgang Höpker, M.D.). The small bowel tumor noted at scintigraphy could not be demonstrated by laparoscopy or CT. The VCE findings were confirmed by open laparotomy

7

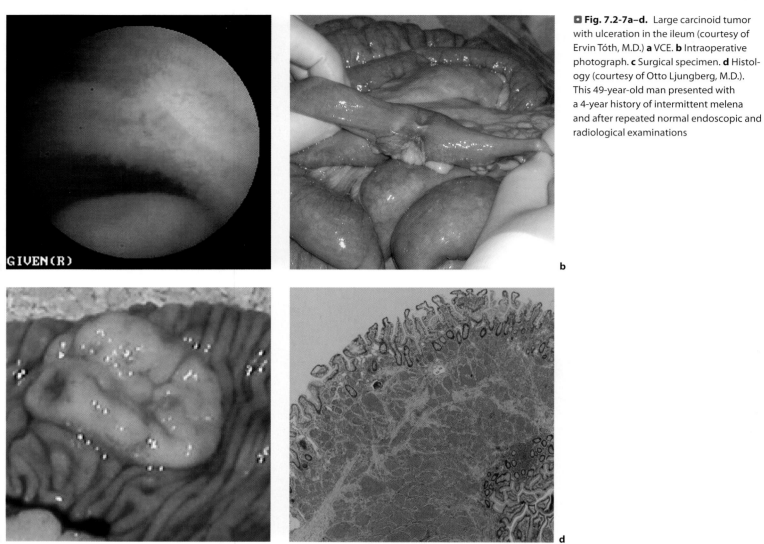

◻ **Fig. 7.2-7a–d.** Large carcinoid tumor with ulceration in the ileum (courtesy of Ervin Tóth, M.D.) **a** VCE. **b** Intraoperative photograph. **c** Surgical specimen. **d** Histology (courtesy of Otto Ljungberg, M.D.). This 49-year-old man presented with a 4-year history of intermittent melena and after repeated normal endoscopic and radiological examinations

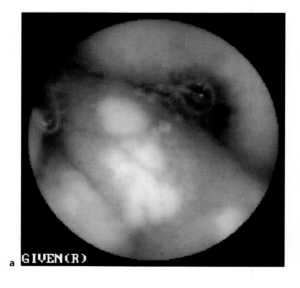

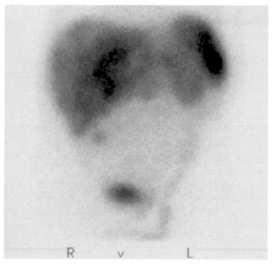

◻ **Fig. 7.2-8a, b.** Well-differentiated neuroendocrine carcinoid tumor of the ileum. **a** Infiltrating tumor causing subtotal stenosis, confirmed at operation. The capsule passed spontaneously. **b** Somatostatin-receptor scintigraphy shows hepatic metastases and a tumor of the terminal ileum (courtesy of Bernhard Leisner, M.D.). The patient presented with flush symptoms and increased 5-hydroxyindolacetic acid excretion

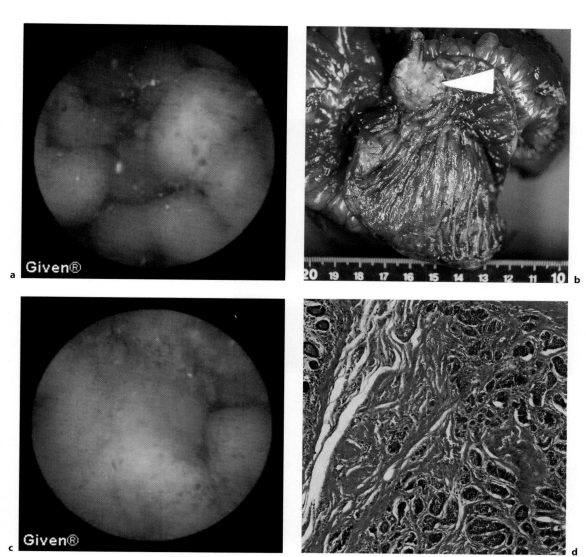

◘ Fig. 7.2-9a–d. Infiltrating carcinoid tumor of the ileum. **a**, **c** VCE shows thickened folds with multiple red spots, capsule did not pass. **b** Resected tumor, infiltrating the small bowel and mesentery. **d** Histology

Melanoma of the Small Intestine

Melanoma is the most common metastatic tumor to the small bowel
(■ Figs. 7.2-25 and 7.2-26). Primary small bowel melanoma (■ Fig. 7.2-10)
is a rarity (Khosrowshahi and Horvath 2002).

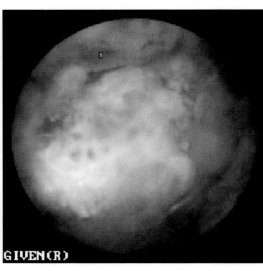

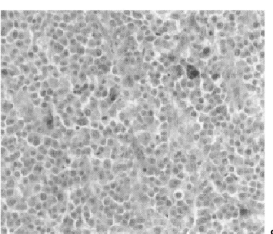

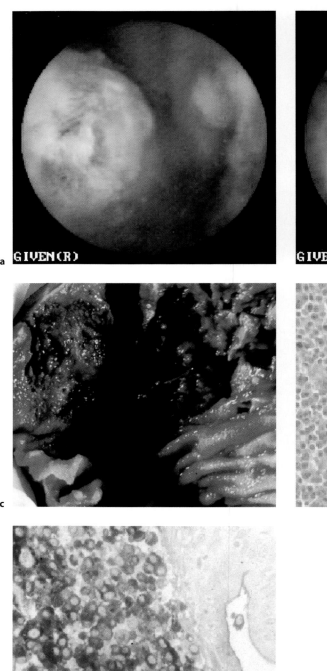

■ **Fig. 7.2-10a–e.** Primary melanoma of the small bowel. **a, b** Exophytic ulcerated tumor of the ileum causing partial stenosis, with active bleeding. **c** Surgical specimen. **d** Histology: small cell tumor with melanin pigment (H&E). **e** Strongly positive expression of the melanoma marker HMB 45 (**c–e**, courtesy of Stefan Krüger, M.D.). The patient presented with intestinal bleeding and normal enteroclysis with no additional foci of melanoma

Gastrointestinal Stromal Tumors

Definition. Gastrointestinal stromal tumors (malignant GISTs) are mesenchymal tumors that express the CD117 marker. They presumably have a similar origin to intestinal pacemaker cells (Logrono et al. 2004). Their biologic behavior is variable. In the absence of metastasis and local invasion, their prognosis can be assessed (favorable/intermediate/unfavorable) based on criteria such as tumor size, histologic type, and rate of mitosis.

Prevalence. GISTs are rare, with an incidence of 1 or 2 cases per 100,000 population per year, but they are the most common mesenchymal tumor of the small bowel.

Location. GISTs are generally more common in the stomach than in the small bowel, but the malignant form tends to be located in the small bowel (Burkill et al. 2003). The malignant potential of the tumor correlates with its size and intestinal location (Tazawa et al. 1999).

Endoscopy. Endoscopy often shows a firm, submucosal tumor that may be smooth (◘ Fig. 7.2-12) or cauliflower-like (◘ Fig. 7.2-11). An extraintestinal tumor site may produce visible mucosal infiltration (◘ Fig. 7.2-13), but this is a nonspecific sign.

Treatment. An option for advanced tumor stages is treatment with the specific tyrosine kinase inhibitor imatinib.

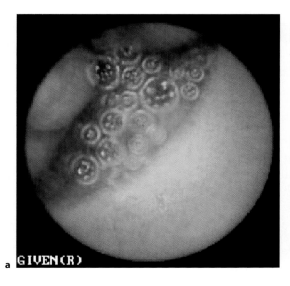

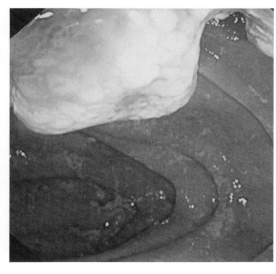

◘ Fig. 7.2-11a, b. Malignant GIST: exophytic tumor of the jejunum at VCE **(a)** and push enteroscopy **(b)**. The patient presented with bleeding that required a transfusion (courtesy of Ingo Franke, M.D.)

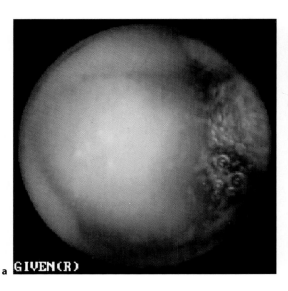

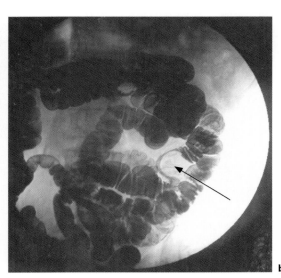

◘ Fig. 7.2-12a, b. GIST with a favorable prognosis. **a** Large submucosal tumor causing partial stenosis, slightly constricted at the base; smooth mucosa (VCE). **b** Smooth-bordered tumor producing an intraluminal filling defect at enteroclysis (courtesy of Christian Müller, M.D.). The patient presented with gastrointestinal bleeding. Histology showed a low mitotic rate

7

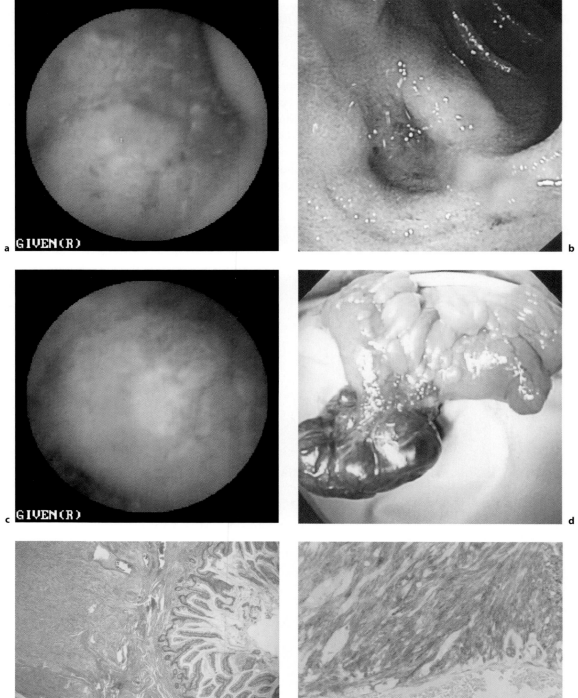

■ **Fig. 7.2-13a–f.** Extraluminal growth of GIST. **a, c** Tumor with dilated vessels embedded in the ileum. **b** Surgical specimen, intraluminal aspect with excavation. **d** Tumor attached externally to the small bowel, also a small Meckel's diverticulum (**b** and **d**, courtesy of Johannes Krüger, M.D.). **e, f** Histology: GIST with increased mitotic rate, CD117-positive (courtesy of Joachim Gottschalk, M.D.). The patient presented clinically with recurrent intestinal bleeding

Hemangiosarcoma

This very rare malignant tumor deriving from endothelial cells can cause intestinal perforation or bleeding (Knop et al. 2003).

Endoscopy. Endoscopy may show reddish black polypoid tumors (◻ Fig. 7.2-14). Rarely, multiple nodules may be distributed throughout the small intestine (◻ Fig. 7.2-15).

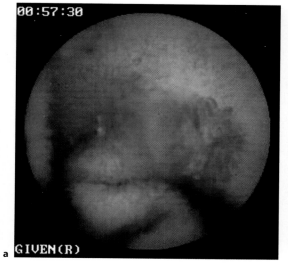

◻ **Fig. 7.2-14.** Hemangiosarcoma. Polypoid, vascular tumor with irregular surface (courtesy of Filip Knop, M.D., reprinted from Knop et al. 2003 with permission from Georg Thieme Verlag, Stuttgart)

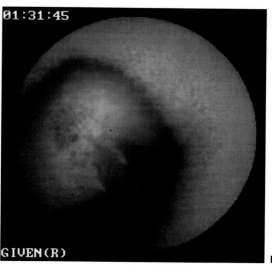
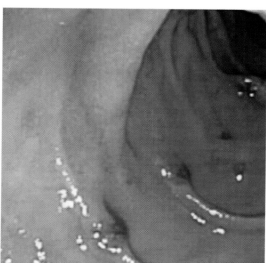
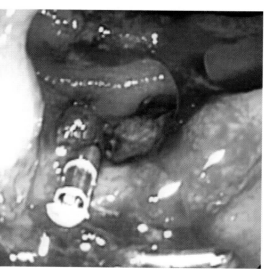

◻ **Fig. 7.2-15a–d.** Diffuse intestinal epitheloid angiosarcoma in a patient under immunosuppressive therapy after liver transplantation. VCE shows flat (**a**) and polypoid (**b**) small reddish tumors with central ulceration throughout the entire small intestine. Multiple small tumors seen at push enteroscopy in the jejunum (**c**), some of them bleeding, requiring hemostasis by clipping (**d**) (case courtesy of Virender Sharma, M.D.)

Kaposi's Sarcoma

Definition. Kaposi's sarcoma is a malignant angiosarcoma that is associated with human herpesvirus 8.

Clinical Features. The most common lesion is the cutaneous Kaposi's sarcoma observed in acquired immunodeficiency syndrome (AIDS) patients. The involvement of internal organs, including the small bowel, can occur. Small bowel involvement is usually asymptomatic, but some patients present with bleeding (Neville et al. 1996), intussusception, or exudative enteropathy.

Endoscopy. Typical endoscopic findings consist of bluish-red nodules or tumors (◘ Fig. 7.2-16).

Treatment. Treatment for the AIDS-associated form consists of antiretroviral therapy. Other options are chemotherapy and radiation. Resection is advised only in emergency situations due to the high risk of recurrence.

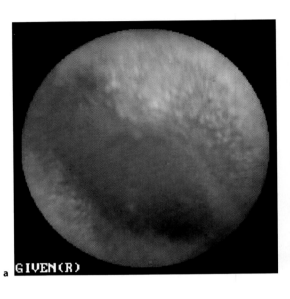 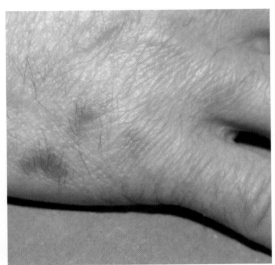

◘ **Fig. 7.2-16. a** Bluish-red polypoid lesions in the jejunum. **b** AIDS patient with recurrent intestinal bleeding and cutaneous Kaposi's sarcoma

Intestinal Lymphomas

Gastrointestinal lymphomas are the most common extranodal manifestation of non-Hodgkin's lymphoma (Feller and Diebold 2004). Ninety percent originate from B lymphocytes and 10% from T lymphocytes, and most are highly malignant. The most common site of occurrence is the stomach, followed by the small bowel and colon. Celiac disease and IPSID (immunoproliferative disease of the small intestine) are considered predisposing factors.

Endoscopy. Endoscopy shows a variegated pattern of nodular polypoid tumors, ulcerations, infiltrative growth, thickened folds, and focal atrophy (Flieger et al. 2004; Hartmann et al. 2003).

Treatment. Whenever possible, treatment should be provided within the framework of studies based on histology- and stage-oriented concepts with consideration of all modalities: chemotherapy (CHOP regimen/high-dose), radiotherapy, and surgical resection (Fischbach 2004).

Intestinal lymphomas:

B-cell lymphomas
- High-grade malignancies
  - Diffuse large-cell B-cell lymphomas (centroblastic, immunoblastic; ◘ Figs. 7.2-17 and 7.2-18)
  - Burkitt's lymphoma (mainly in the terminal ileum, more prevalent in developing countries)
- Low-grade malignancies
  - Extranodal marginal zone lymphoma of the MALT type (Western-type lymphoma; ◘ Fig. 7.2-19)
  - Mantle cell lymphoma (◘ Fig. 7.2-20)
  - Alpha heavy-chain disease (Mediterranean-type lymphoma; ◘ Fig. 7.2-21)
  - Follicular lymphoma (rare as primary intestinal tumor; ◘ Fig. 7.2-22)

T-cell lymphomas
- Enteropathy-associated T-cell lymphoma (EATL; ◘ Figs. 7.2-23 and 6.2-10)

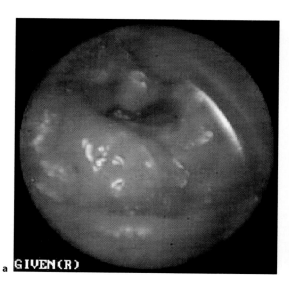

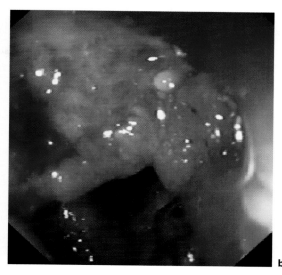

Fig. 7.2-17a, b. Large cell centroblastic lymphoma of the jejunum: polypoid tumor at VCE (**a**) and push enteroscopy (**b**). The patient presented with intestinal bleeding and had a prior history of renal transplantation (courtesy of Winfried Voderholzer, M.D.)

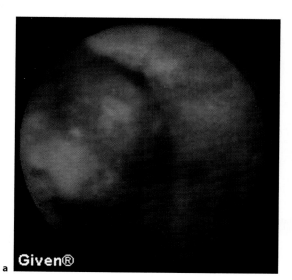

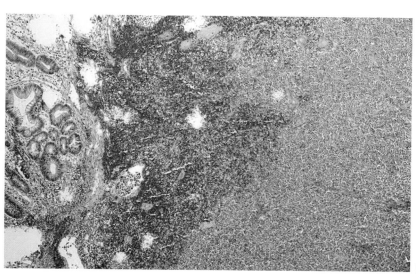

Fig. 7.2-18. a Large-cell B lymphoma, centroblastic variant. Stenosing tumor of the ileum (courtesy of Axel de Rossi, M.D.) **b** Histology (courtesy of Hans-Michael Schneider, M.D.)

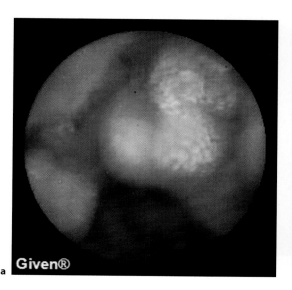

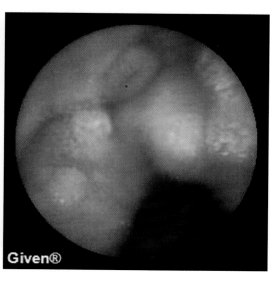

Fig. 7.2-19a, b. MALT lymphoma. Infiltrating, polypoid tumor (courtesy of Markus Oeyen, M.D.)

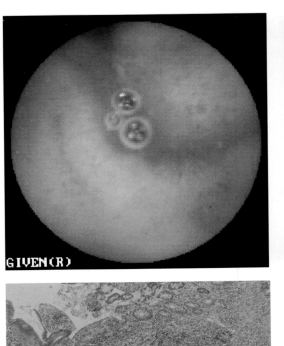

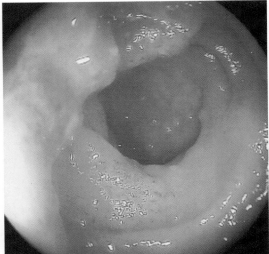

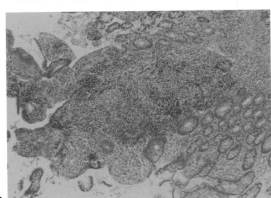

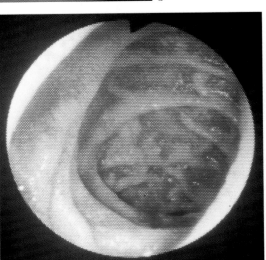

Fig. 7.2-20a–c. Mantle cell lymphoma: polypoid tumor in the terminal ileum at VCE (**a**) and deep ileoscopy (**b**). Histology: diffuse lymphomatous infiltration of the small bowel (**c**). The patient presented with diarrhea and previously had only nodal manifestations

Fig. 7.2-21. Alpha heavy-chain disease with diffuse, white infiltration of the mucosa at fiberoptic endoscopy of the duodenum

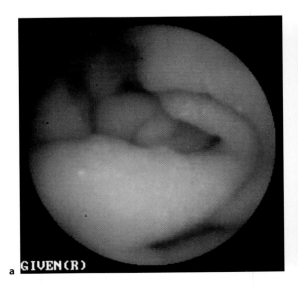

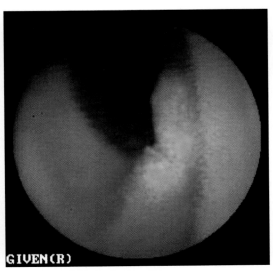

Fig. 7.2-22a, b. Follicular centroblastic/centrocytic lymphoma: circumscribed thickening of folds in the jejunum (**a**) with an eroded surface (**b**) (courtesy of Jann Erdmann, M.D.). The patient presented with intestinal bleeding. Intraoperative endoscopy showed a circumscribed recurrence 4 years after initially successful chemotherapy

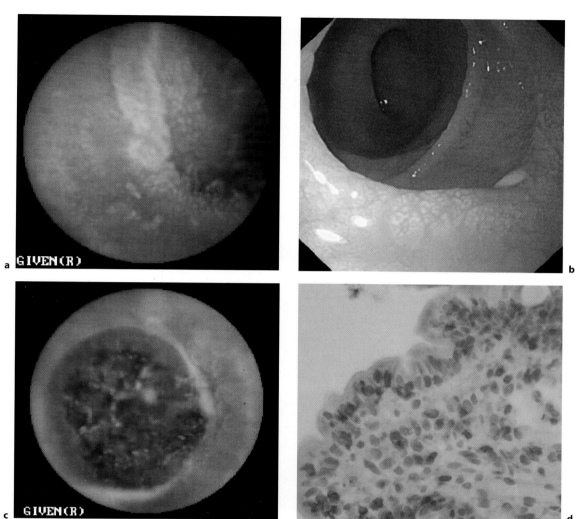

⬛ **Fig. 7.2-23a–d.** Refractory villous atrophy, T-cell lymphoma (case courtesy of Michel Delvaux, M.D. and Gerard Gay, M.D.). **a** VCE. **b** Push enteroscopy. **c** Ulcerative jejunoileitis is also present. **d** Lymphocytic T-cell infiltrate. Molecular biology: monoclonal T-cell receptor

Metastases

Metastases in the small bowel are very rare. They usually originate from melanomas (■ Figs. 7.2-25 and 7.2-26) and less commonly from carcinomas of the ovaries, bladder, breast, bronchi (■ Fig. 7.2-24), and pancreas (Washington and McDonagh 1995).

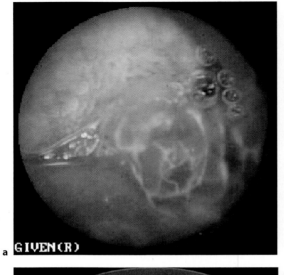

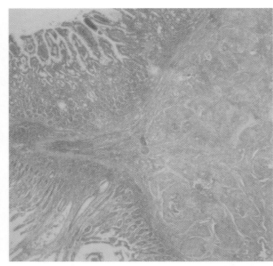

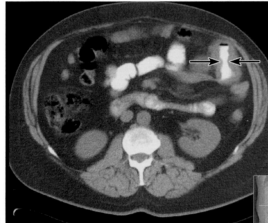

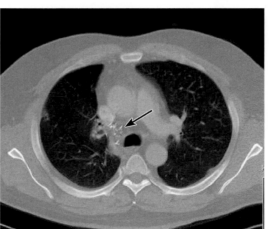

■ **Fig. 7.2-24a–d.** Small bowel metastasis from a large-cell bronchial carcinoma. **a** Tumor infiltrating and stenosing the jejunum (VCE). **b** Histology: tumor composed of atypical large cells (H&E). **c** CT (*arrows*). **d** Thoracic CT shows clips (*arrows*) after right upper lobectomy (**c**, **d**, courtesy of Ernst Malzfeldt, M.D.). The patient presented with intestinal bleeding requiring transfusion

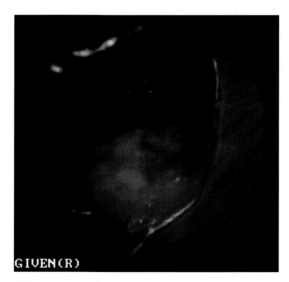

■ **Fig. 7.2-25.** Melanoma metastasis to the small intestine. Ulcerated, polypoid tumor

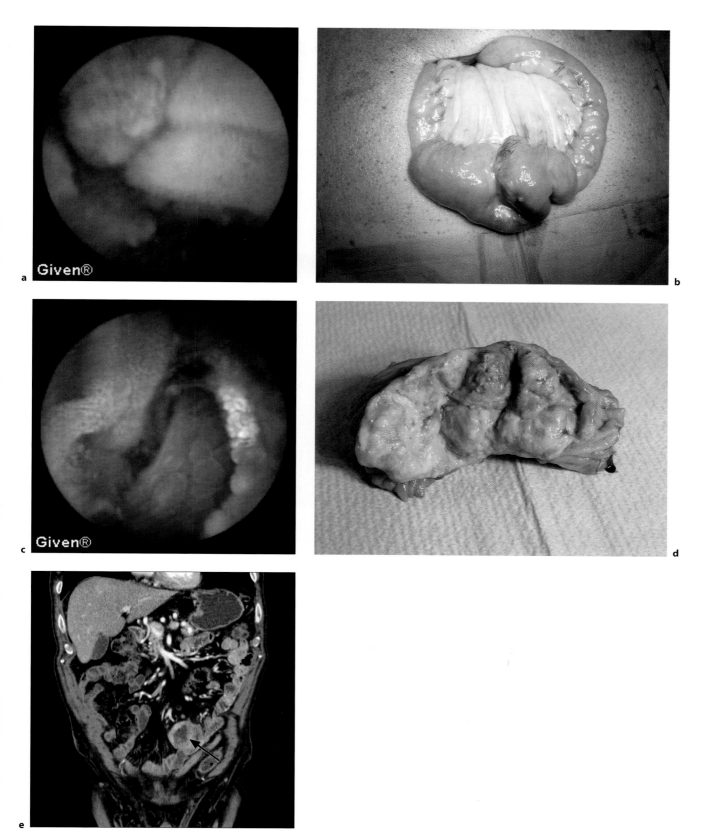

□ Fig. 7.2-26a–e. Melanoma metastasis to the jejunum. **a**, **c** Diffusely infiltrating tumor with circumscript lymphangiectasia seen at VCE. Infiltrated and locally enlarged jejunal loop at CT (**e**) (courtesy of Ernst Malzfeldt, M.D.) and at laparoscopically assisted mini-laparotomy (**b**) (**b**, **d**, courtesy of Christopher Pohland, M.D.). Surgical specimen reveals an infiltrating, stenosing tumor; the capsule was temporarily retained, but passed spontaneously before surgery. A 75-year-old man with cutaneous malignant melanoma and relapsing intestinal bleeding

Contiguous Invasion of the Small Intestine

When VCE findings in the small bowel are equivocal, the examiner should also consider the rare possibility of small bowel invasion by the contiguous spread of malignant tumors from neighboring organs. Ultrasound, endosonography, computed tomography/magnetic resonance imaging, and laparoscopy can accomplish the diagnosis in these cases.

Peritoneal Mesothelioma

This tumor, which arises from the peritoneal mesothelium, is much rarer than pleural mesothelioma (Neumann et al. 2004).

Endoscopy. Nonspecific superficial mucosal defects or patchy red areas may be seen (◻ Fig. 7.2-27). The diagnosis is established by laparoscopy or laparotomy.

Treatment. A complete resection is not feasible in most cases. (Hyperthermal) intraperitoneal chemotherapy has been proposed (Loggie 2001). It is reasonable to expect that the multidirectional folic acid antagonist pemetrexed will one day be used as successfully for this lesion as it has for pleural mesothelioma (Adjei 2003).

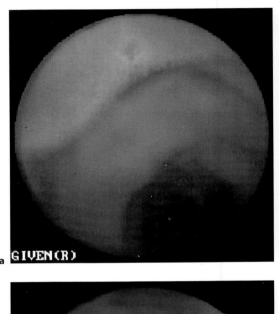

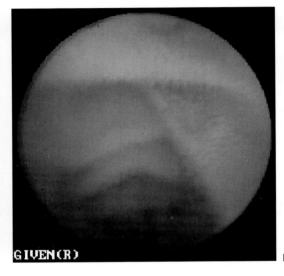

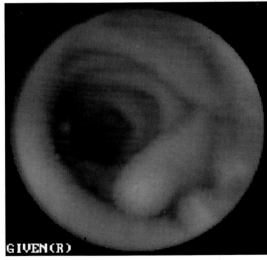

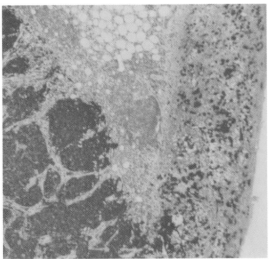

◻ **Fig. 7.2-27a–d.** Peritoneal mesothelioma. **a** Circumscribed villous denudation. **b** Faint red patch. **c** Small pedunculated polyp. **d** Open resection of a tumor infiltrating the greater omentum: papillary proliferative epithelioid tumor (calretinin-positive; courtesy of Wilhelm-Wolfgang Höpker, M.D.)

Pancreatic Head Carcinoma

Since the video capsule tends to pass swiftly through the proximal duodenum, the region of the pancreatic head and papilla often cannot be adequately evaluated. Relevant findings are occasionally noted when the video capsule is favorably positioned (◘ Fig. 7.2-28).

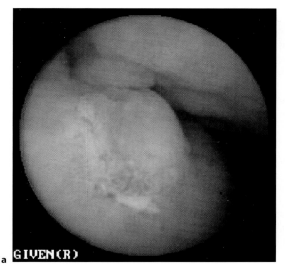

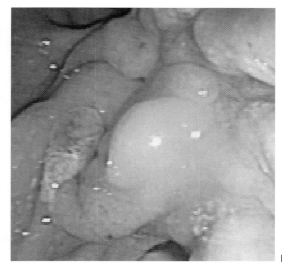

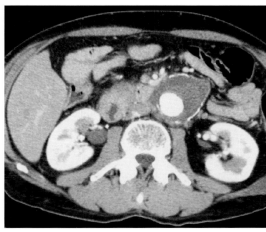

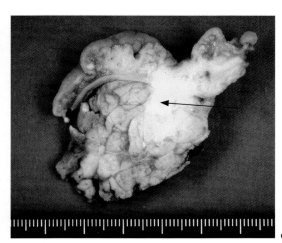

◘ Fig. 7.2-28a–d. Duodenal infiltration. VCE was performed to investigate chronic diarrhea and a 15-kg weight loss: **a** duodenal infiltration, **b** confirmed with a side-viewing duodenoscope. Several prior esophagogastroduodenoscopic examinations showed nonspecific duodenitis. Magnetic resonance cholangiopancreatography was normal. **c** CT demonstrates a pancreatic head tumor (with an aortic aneurysm as an incidental finding, courtesy of Ernst Malzfeldt, M.D.). **d** Tumor resected by a pancreaticoduodenectomy (Whipple's operation): pancreatic head carcinoma (*arrow*)

Internet

www.cancer.org: American Cancer Organization

www.carcinoid.org: The Carcinoid Cancer Foundation

www.eortc.be: European Organisation for Research and Treatment of Cancer

www.liferaftgroup.org: Support Organization for patients with GIST

www.lymphoma.org: Lymphoma Research Foundation

References

Abrahams NA, Halverson A, Fazio VW et al (2002) Adenocarcinoma of the small bowel: a study of 37 cases with emphasis on histologic prognostic factors. Dis Colon Rectum 45:1496–1502

Adjei AA (2003) Pemetrexed (Alimta): a novel multitargeted antifolate agent. Expert Rev Anticancer Ther 3:145–156

Barakat M (1982) Endoscopic features of primary small bowel lymphoma: a proposed endoscopic classification. Gut: 23:36–41

Brucher BL, Roder JD, Fink U et al (1998) Prognostic factors in resected primary small bowel tumors. Dig Surg 15:42–51

Burkill GJ, Badran M, Al Muderis O et al (2003) Malignant gastrointestinal stromal tumor: distribution, imaging features, and pattern of metastatic spread. Radiology 226:527–532

Buscombe JR, Caplin ME, Hilson AJ (2003) Long-term efficacy of high-activity 111 in-pentetreotide therapy in patients with disseminated neuroendocrine tumors. J Nucl Med 44:1–6

Cobrin GM, Pittman RH, Lewis BS (2004) Diagnosing small bowel tumors with capsule endoscopy. Gastroenterology 126 [Suppl 2]:A194–A195

Conn M (1997) Tumors of the small intestine. In: DiMarino A, Benjamin S (eds) Gastrointestinal disease: an endoscopic approach. Blackwell Science, Malden, MA, pp 551–566

Feller AC, Diebold J (2004) Histopathology of nodal and extranodal non-Hodgkin's lymphomas, 3rd edn. Springer, Berlin Heidelberg New York

Fischbach W (2004) Gastrointestinal lymphomas (in German). Z Gastroenterol 42:1067–1072

Flieger D, Keller R, Fischbach W (2004) Capsule endoscopy in gastric MALT lymphoma and other gastrointestinal lymphomas. Gastroenterology 126 [Suppl 2]: A621

Halphen M, Najjar T, Jaafoura H et al (1986) Diagnostic value of upper intestinal fiber endoscopy in primary small intestinal lymphoma. Cancer 58:2140–2145

Hara AK, Leighton JA, Sharma VK, Fleischer DE (2004) Small bowel: preliminary comparison of capsule endoscopy with barium study and CT. Radiology 230:260–265

Hartmann D, Schilling D, Rebel M et al (2003) Diagnosis of a high-grade B-cell lymphoma of the small bowel by means of wireless capsule endoscopy. Z Gastroenterol 41:171–174

Hemminki K, Li X (2001) Incidence trends and risk factors of carcinoid tumors: a nationwide epidemiologic study from Sweden. Cancer 92:2204–2210

Herbsman H, Wetstein L, Rosen Y et al (1980) Tumors of the small intestine. Curr Probl Surg 17:121

Horton KM, Kamel I, Hofmann L, Fishman EK (2004) Carcinoid tumors of the small bowel: a multitechnique imaging approach. AJR Am J Roentgenol 182:559–567

Keuchel M, Thaler C, Caselitz J, Hagenmüller F (2004) Diagnosis of small bowel tumors with video capsule endoscopy – report of 16 cases. Gastroenterology 126 [Suppl 2]:A347

Khosrowshahi E, Horvath W (2002) Primary malignant melanoma of the small intestine – a case report. Röntgenpraxis 54:220–223

Klöppel G, Perren A, Heitz PU (2004) The gastroenteropancreatic neuroendocrine cell system and its tumors: the WHO classification. Ann N Y Acad Sci 1014:13–27

Knop FK, Hansen MB, Meisner S (2003) Small-bowel hemangiosarcoma and capsule endoscopy. Endoscopy 35:637

Loggie BW (2001) Malignant peritoneal mesothelioma. Curr Treat Options Oncol 2:395–399

Logrono R, Jones DV, Faruqi S, Bhutani MS (2004) Recent advances in cell biology, diagnosis, and therapy of gastrointestinal stromal tumor (GIST). Cancer Biol Ther 3:251–258

Madisch A, Schimming W, Kinzel F et al (2003) Locally advanced small-bowel adenocarcinoma missed primarily by capsule endoscopy but diagnosed by push enteroscopy. Endoscopy 35:861–864

Mascarenhas-Saraiva MN, da Silva Araujo Lopes LM (2003) Small-bowel tumors diagnosed by wireless capsule endoscopy: report of five cases. Endoscopy 35:865–868

Modlin IM, Lye KD, Kidd M (2003) A 5-decade analysis of 13,715 carcinoid tumors. Cancer 97:934–959

Neumann V, Rutten A, Scharmach M et al (2004) Factors influencing long-term survival in mesothelioma patients—results of the German mesothelioma register. Int Arch Occup Environ Health 77:191–199

Neville CR, Peddada AV, Smith D et al (1996) Massive gastrointestinal hemorrhage from AIDS-related Kaposi's sarcoma confined to the small bowel managed with radiation. Med Pediatr Oncol 26:135–138

North JH, Pack MS (2000) Malignant tumors of the small intestine: a review of 144 cases. Am Surg 66:46–51

Oberg K, Kvols L, Caplin M et al (2004) Consensus report on the use of somatostatin analogs for the management of neuroendocrine tumors of the gastroenteropancreatic system. Ann Oncol 15:966–973

Rossini FP, Risio M, Pennazio M (1999) Small bowel tumors and polyposis syndromes. Gastrointest Endosc Clin N Am 9:93–114

Tazawa K, Tsukada K, Makuuchi H, Tsutsumi Y (1999) An immunohistochemical and clinicopathological study of gastrointestinal stromal tumors. Pathol Int 49:786–798

Washington K, McDonagh D (1995) Secondary tumors of the gastrointestinal tract: surgical pathologic findings and comparison with autopsy survey. Mod Pathol 8:427–433

7.3 Polyposis Syndromes

K. Schulmann, C. Burke, W. Schmiegel

Small bowel polyps are very rare in the general population. However, in patients with hereditary colon cancer syndromes, polyps occur not only in the colon and rectum but also in the stomach and small bowel with varying frequency. The risk for intestinal and extraintestinal malignancies is significantly increased in these syndromes (Giardiello et al. 2001).

Patients with Lynch syndrome, also called **hereditary nonpolyposis colon cancer** (HNPCC), have a 1–4% lifetime risk of developing small bowel cancer; 50% of these cancers are located in the duodenum (Schulmann et al. 2005b). Duodenal carcinoma after colectomy is the leading cause of cancer death in **familial adenomatous polyposis** (FAP) (Galle et al. 1999). Duodenal adenomas (■ Table 7.3-1) are predominantly diagnosed in the duodenum (Saurin et al. 1999) (■ Fig. 7.3-6). Additional small bowel polyps are detectable in FAP patients depending on the severity of duodenal polyposis (Schulmann et al. 2005a; Burke et al.

2005) (■ Fig. 7.3-7). The small bowel is the most common site of polyp occurrence in **Peutz-Jeghers syndrome** (PJS) seen in 78% of patients (Pennazio and Rossini 2000; Schulmann et al. 2005a; Burke et al. 2005) (■ Figs. 7.3-2–7.3-4). Perioral pigmentation is a common clinical sign in PJS (■ Fig. 7.3-5). Small bowel polyps are occasionally found in patients with **familial juvenile polyposis** (FJP) (■ Fig. 7.3-1).

■ **Table 7.3-1.** Spigelman score for staging duodenal adenomas. Zero points = stage 0, 1–4 points = stage I, 5–6 points = stage II, 7–8 points = stage III, 9–12 points = stage IV (Spigelman et al. 1989)

Points	1	2	3
Number of adenomas	1–4	5–20	>20
Size	1–4 mm	5–10 mm	>10 mm
Histology	Tubular	Tubulovillous	Villous
Dysplasia	Mild	Moderate	Severe

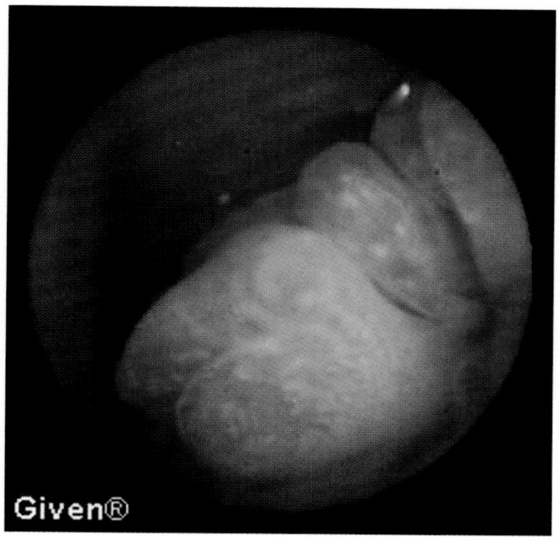

■ **Fig. 7.3-1.** Juvenile polyp of the duodenum

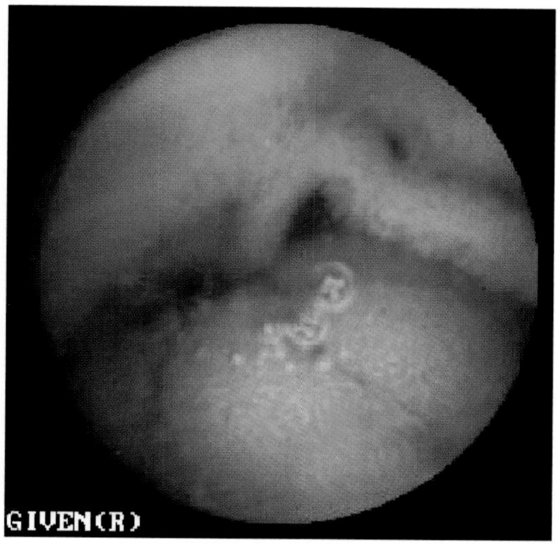

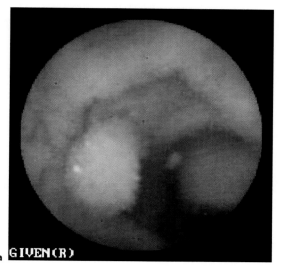

■ **Fig. 7.3-2.** Large Peutz-Jeghers polyp (courtesy of Ullrich Wahnschaffe, M.D.)

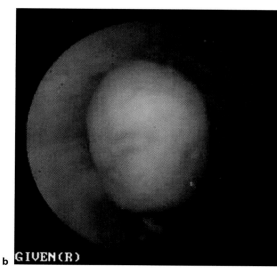

■ **Fig. 7.3-3a, b.** Peutz-Jeghers polyp of the small intestine: **a** small and **b** medium size

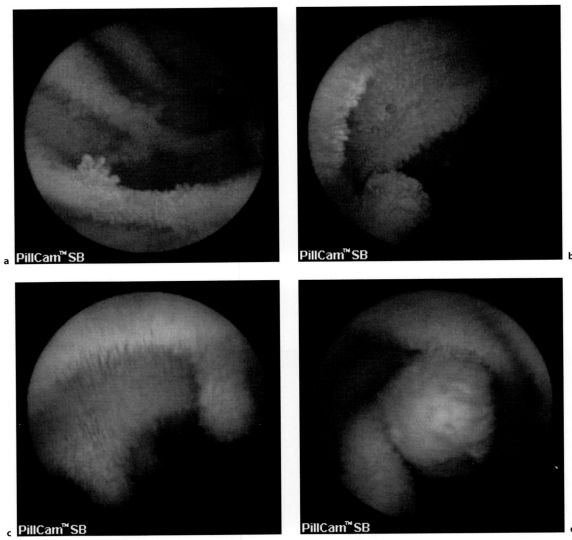

Fig. 7.3-4a–d. Peutz-Jeghers polyps in the jejunum and ileum; varying sizes illustrate their development

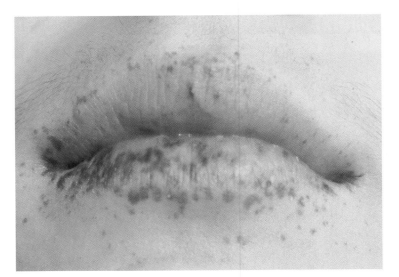

Fig. 7.3-5. Typical perioral pigmentation in a patient with Peutz-Jeghers syndrome

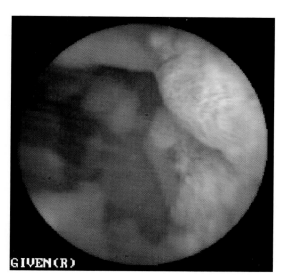

◘ **Fig. 7.3-6.** Flat, multifocal duodenal adenoma. Familial adenomatous polyposis in a patient who had previously undergone colectomy

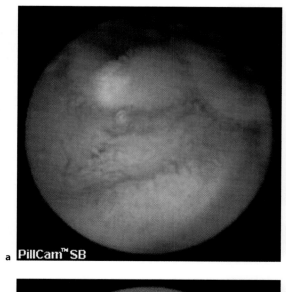

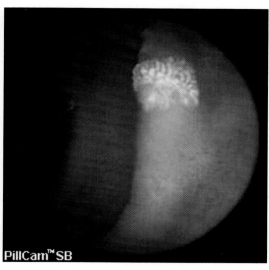

◘ **Fig. 7.3-7a–d.** Jejunal polyps in familial adenomatous polyposis

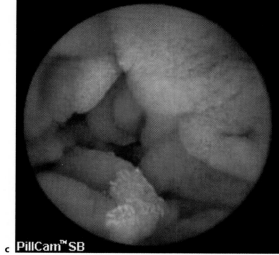

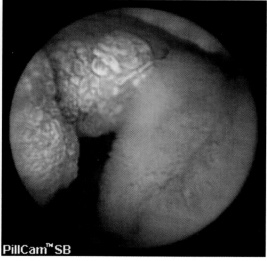

Given the rarity of these diseases and incomplete understanding of the prevalence and clinical significance of polyps beyond the duodenum in FAP and FJP, there is limited evidence to establish definitive guidelines for jejunal and ileal surveillance in HNPCC, FAP, and FJP (Dunlop 2002). Forward and side viewing endoscopy with biopsy of the papilla (even if normal) is recommended in FAP (Schmiegel et al. 2004; Burke et al. 1999), and esophagogastroduodenoscopy is recommended in HNPCC patients with a positive family history of gastric carcinoma (Schmiegel et al. 2004). Biennial upper endoscopy and small bowel radiography are recommended in PJS. However, capsule endoscopy has been recently recommended as a radiation-free and preferred method of jejunal and ileal surveillance in patients with PJS (Burke et al 2005; Caspari et al. 2004; Parsi and Burke 2004; Schulmann and Schmiegel 2004; Schulmann et al. 2005a; Soares 2004).

The risk of capsule impaction may be theoretically increased in patients with large polyps or prior intestinal surgery (◻ Fig. 10-15). However, four series did not observe capsule retention in a total of 100 patients.

Cowden syndrome is a rare autosomal dominant syndrome with hamartomatous polyps of the gastrointestinal tract (◻ Fig. 7.3-8) and a high risk of thyroid and breast cancer (Bencheqroun et al. 2005; Pilarski and Eng 2004). To date there is no convincing evidence for an increased risk of developing gastrointestinal cancer.

Cronkhite-Canada syndrome, a rare, noninherited syndrome of unknown origin, consists of ectodermal abnormalities such as discoloration and dystrophy of nails, alopecia areata, and polyposis (Blonski et al. 2005). These polyps can occur throughout the gastrointestinal tract and show a pseudopolypoid-inflammatory appearance with cystic dilatation at histology (Kim et al. 2004)

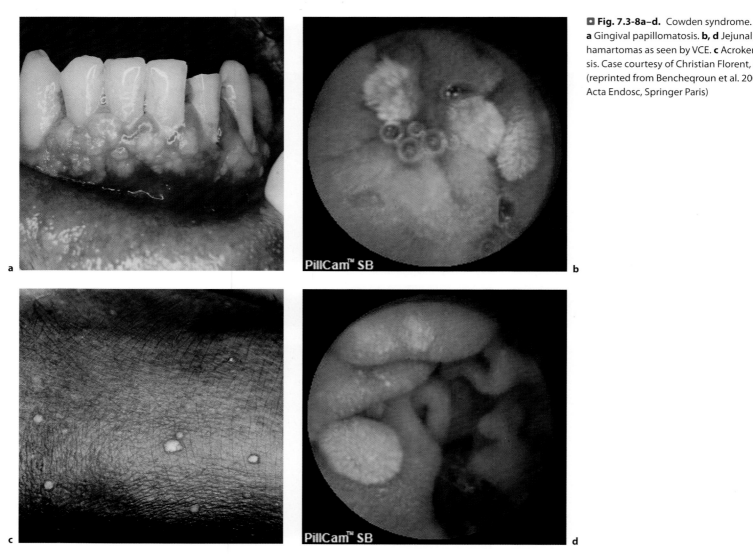

◻ **Fig. 7.3-8a–d.** Cowden syndrome. **a** Gingival papillomatosis. **b, d** Jejunal hamartomas as seen by VCE. **c** Acrokeratosis. Case courtesy of Christian Florent, M.D. (reprinted from Bencheqroun et al. 2005, Acta Endosc, Springer Paris)

References

Bencheqroun R, Meary N, Laroche L et al (2005) Cowden syndrome, first case investigated using electronic video capsule. Acta Endosc 35:227–232

Blonski WC, Furth EE, Kinosian BP et al (2005) A case of Cronkhite-Canada syndrome with taste disturbance as a leading complaint. Digestion 71:201–205

Burke CA, Beck GJ, Church JM, van Stolk RU (1999) The natural history of untreated duodenal and ampullary adenomas in patients with familial adenomatous polyposis followed in an endoscopic surveillance program. Gastrointest Endosc 49:358–364

Burke CA, Santisi J, Church J, Levinthal G (2005) The utility of capsule endoscopy small bowel surveillance in patients with polyposis. Am J Gastroenterol 100:1498–1502

Caspari R, von Falkenhausen M, Krautmacher C et al (2004) Comparison of capsule endoscopy and magnetic resonance imaging for the detection of polyps of the small intestine in patients with familial adenomatous polyposis or with Peutz-Jeghers' syndrome. Endoscopy 36:1054–1059

Dunlop MG (2002) Guidance on gastrointestinal surveillance for hereditary non-polyposis colorectal cancer, familial adenomatous polyposis, juvenile polyposis and Peutz-Jeghers syndrome. Gut 51:21–27

Galle TS, Juel K, Bulow S (1999) Causes of death in familial adenomatous polyposis. Scand J Gastroenterol 34:808–812

Giardiello FM, Brensinger JD, Petersen GM (2001) AGA technical review on hereditary colorectal cancer and genetic testing. Gastroenterology 121:198–213

Kim YS, Chun HJ, Jeen YT et al. (2004) Cronkhite-Canada syndrome. Gastrointest Endosc 60:432–433

Parsi M, Burke CA (2004) Utility of capsule endoscopy in Peutz-Jeghers syndrome. Gastrointest Endosc Clin N Am 14:159–167

Pennazio M, Rossini FP (2000) Small bowel polyps in Peutz-Jeghers syndrome: management by combined push enteroscopy and intraoperative enteroscopy. Gastrointest Endosc 51:304–308

Pilarski R, Eng C (2004) Will the real Cowden syndrome please stand up (again)? Expanding mutational and clinical spectra of the PTEN hamartoma tumour syndrome. J Med Genet 41:323–326

Saurin JC, Chayvialle JA, Ponchon T (1999) Management of duodenal adenomas in familial adenomatous polyposis. Endoscopy 31:472–478

Schmiegel W, Pox C, Adler G et al (2004) Deutsche Gesellschaft fur Verdauungs- und Stoffwechselkrankheiten. S3-Guidelines Conference »Colorectal Carcinoma« 2004. Z Gastroenterol 42:1129–1177

Spigelman AD, Williams CB, Talbot IC (1989) Upper gastrointestinal cancer in patients with familial adenomatous polyposis. Lancet 2:783–785

Schulmann K, Schmiegel W (2004) Capsule endoscopy for small bowel surveillance in hereditary intestinal polyposis and non-polyposis syndromes. Gastrointest Endosc Clin N Am 14:149–158

Schulmann K, Hollerbach S, Kraus K et al (2005a) Feasibility and diagnostic utility of video capsule endoscopy for the detection of small bowel polyps in patients with hereditary polyposis syndromes. Am J Gastroenterol 100:27–37

Schulmann K, Brasch F, Kunstmann E et al (2005b) HNPCC-associated small bowel cancer: clinical and genetic characteristics. Gastroenterology 128:590–599

Soares J, Lopes L, Vilas Boas G, Pinho C (2004) Wireless capsule endoscopy for evaluation of phenotypic expression of small-bowel polyps in patients with Peutz-Jeghers syndrome and in symptomatic first-degree relatives. Endoscopy 36:1060–1066

Findings Outside the Small Intestine

8.1   Mouth, Pharynx, and Esophagus

V.K. Sharma, M. Keuchel, T. Rösch

Mouth and Pharynx

Figures 8.1-1–8.1-5 illustrate images recorded from the oral cavity and pharynx.

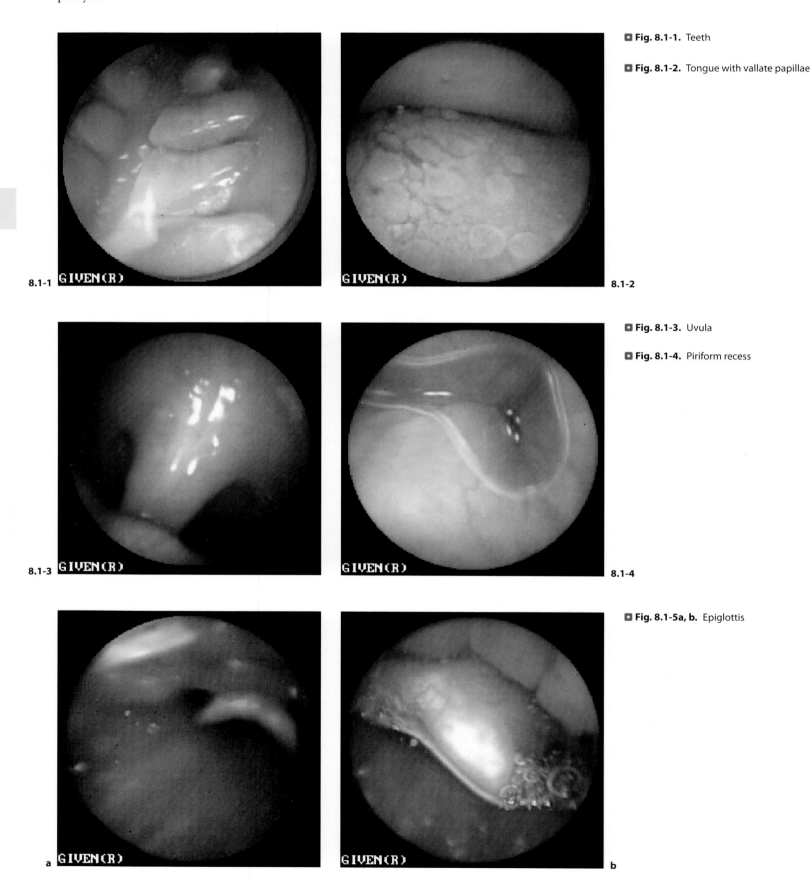

Fig. 8.1-1. Teeth

Fig. 8.1-2. Tongue with vallate papillae

Fig. 8.1-3. Uvula

Fig. 8.1-4. Piriform recess

Fig. 8.1-5a, b. Epiglottis

Esophagus

VCE for the esophagus often supplies only a few recognizable images of the esophagus (■ Fig. 8.1-6). The entire esophagus cannot be reliably evaluated due to the exceptionally swift passage of the capsule (Neu et al. 2003). Pathologic findings are occasionally seen, most commonly at the cardioesophageal junction (■ Figs. 8.1-7–8.1-16). Resolution in these cases is equal to that achieved with modern flexible video endoscopes.

A possible solution is a new capsule with two cameras and faster recording specially designed for the esophagus (Eliakim et al. 2004). Findings with this special esophageal capsule are not addressed in this chapter. A detailed description of the procedure and findings is given in Chap. 13.

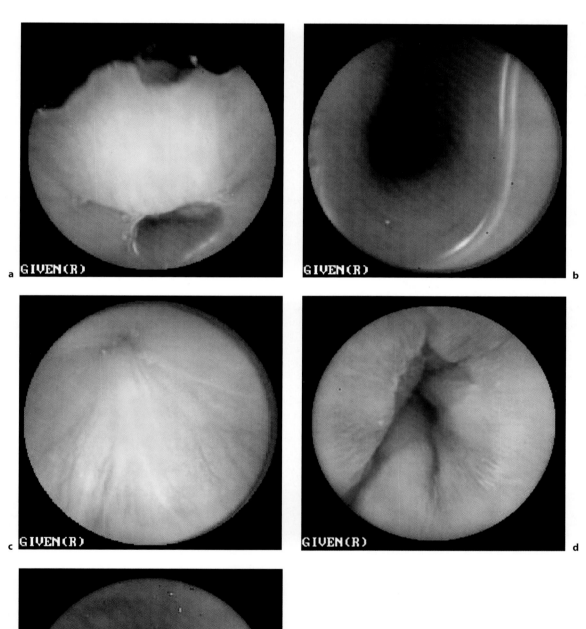

■ **Fig. 8.1-6a–e. a** Upper esophageal sphincter. **b** Tubular esophagus – view through an air bubble. **c** Distal esophagus with longitudinal vessels. **d** Normal Z line. **e** Glycogen acanthosis

8

Sliding Hiatal Hernia

The Z line is not visualized with the standard capsule in most cases (Enns et al. 2003). A Z line that is clearly visible at VCE may signify a sliding hiatal hernia (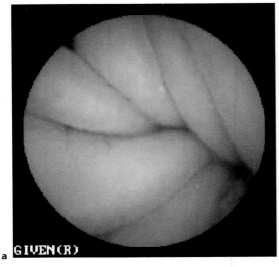 Fig. 8.1-8). A characteristic feature of a hiatal hernia is the presence of longitudinal gastric folds above the hiatal constriction. The hernia cannot be examined from within the stomach by capsule endoscopy (as it can with a retroflexed endoscope). The capsule may become trapped in a very large hernia for some time (◻ Fig. 8.1-7).

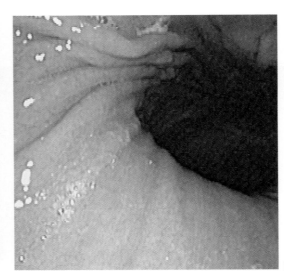

◻ **Fig. 8.1-7a–c.** Large sliding hiatal hernia with gastric folds above the hiatal constriction. **a** VCE. **b** Flexible endoscopy. **c** Retroflexion view. After more than a 3-h delay, the capsule had to be retrieved endoscopically from the hernia

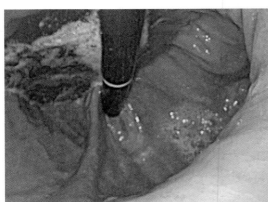

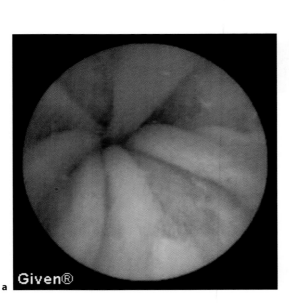

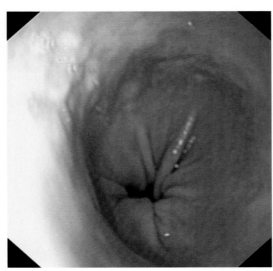

◻ **Fig. 8.1-8. a** Small sliding hiatal hernia: Z line and hiatus are visible in one image at VCE. **b** Corresponding image of flexible endoscopy

Reflux Esophagitis

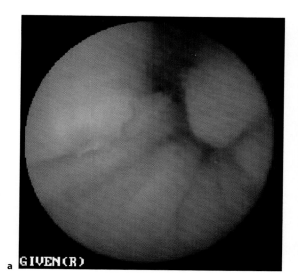

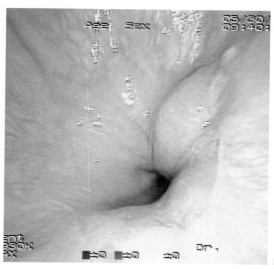

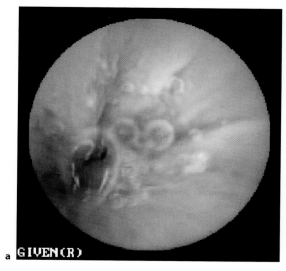

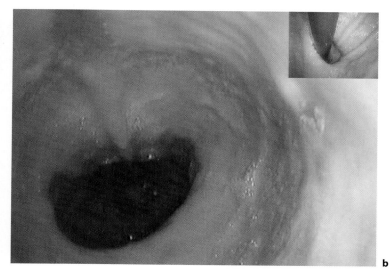

◻ **Fig. 8.1-9a, b.** Inflammatory pseudo-polyp resulting from reflux esophagitis (»sentinel polyp«) and patchy inflammation. **a** VCE. **b** Esophagoscopy

◻ **Fig. 8.1-10a, b.** Streaky areas of inflammation. **a** VCE. **b** Esophagoscopy also demonstrates a hiatal hernia

Barrett's Esophagus

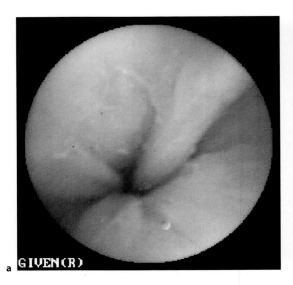

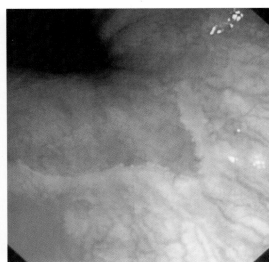

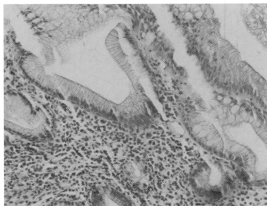

◻ **Fig. 8.1-11a–c.** Cardiac intestinal metaplasia (ultra-short segment Barrett's esophagus). **a** Peaked Z line at VCE. **b** Esophagoscopy. **c** Histology: intestinal metaplasia (PAS stain; courtesy of Jörg Caselitz, M.D.)

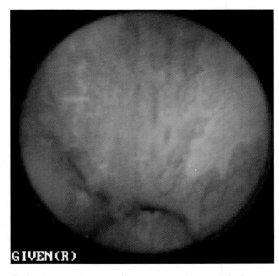

◻ **Fig. 8.1-12.** Tongue of Barrett's esophagus with characteristic longitudinal vessels in the distal esophagus

Esophageal Varices

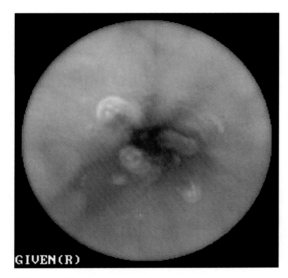

Fig. 8.1-13. Small venectasia

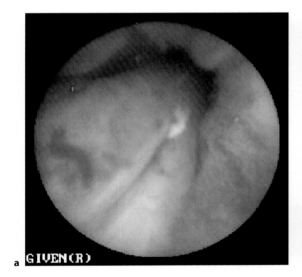

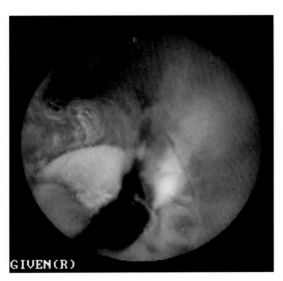

Fig. 8.1-15. Ligated esophageal varix

Fig. 8.1-14a, b. Grade II esophageal varices with vasa vasorum. **a** VCE. **b** Esophagoscopy

Esophageal Diverticulum

Both Zenker's diverticula and epiphrenic diverticula (■ Fig. 8.1-16) can lead to capsule retention.

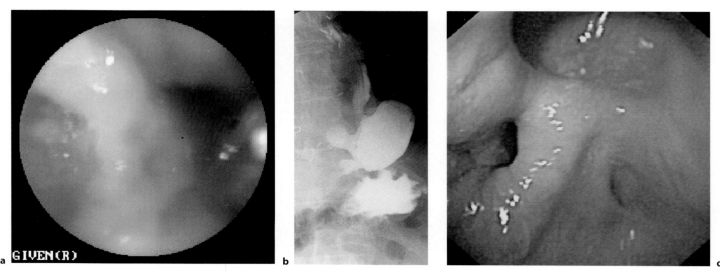

a **GIVEN(R)**   b   c

■ **Fig. 8.1-16a–c.** Epiphrenic diverticulum in a hiatal hernia. **a** Two lumina and a septum in the distal esophagus (VCE). **b** Contrast radiograph (courtesy of Uwe Paul Eggers, M.D.). **c** Esophagoscopy (■ Fig. 10-4)

Motility Disorders

Ingesting the standard capsule while lying down can significantly delay passage of the capsule through the esophagus but does not guarantee a complete survey (Neu et al. 2003). Even when the capsule is ingested in an upright position, motility disorders can greatly delay its passage through the esophagus (■ Figs. 8.1-17–8.1-19).

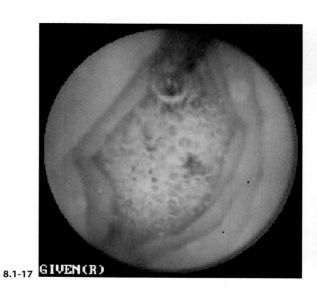

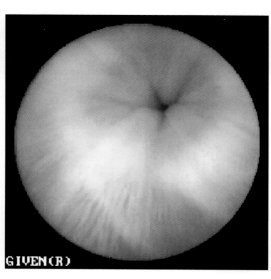

■ **Fig. 8.1-17.** Synchronous contractions

■ **Fig. 8.1-18.** Powerful closure of the distal esophageal sphincter. Brief discomfort was reported during capsule passage

8.1-17 **GIVEN(R)**

GIVEN(R)   8.1-18

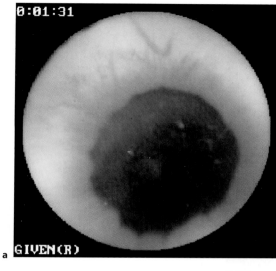

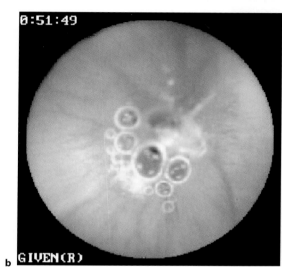

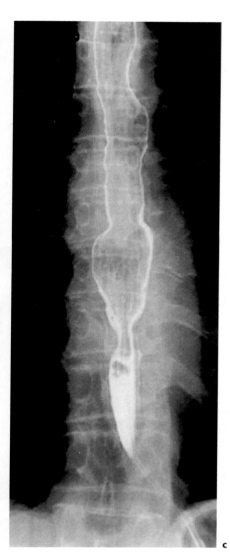

Fig. 8.1-19a–c. Fluid-filled esophageal lumen (**a**) with forceful contractions (**b**), esophageal transit time 2 h 25 min. **c** Hypermotility of the esophagus with radiographically nonpropulsive peristalsis (courtesy of Sybille Othmar, M.D.). The patient complained of occasional retrosternal discomfort

References

Enns R, Mergener K, Yamamoto K (2003) Capsule endoscopy for the assessment of the gastroesophageal junction. Gastrointest Endosc 57:AB169

Neu B, Wettschureck E, Rösch T (2003) Is esophageal capsule endoscopy feasible? Results of a pilot study. Endoscopy 35:957–961

Eliakim R, Yassin K, Shlomi I, Suissa A, Eisen GM (2004) A novel diagnostic tool for detecting oesophageal pathology: the PillCam oesophageal video capsule. Aliment Pharmacol Ther 20:1083–1089

8.2   Stomach

M. Keuchel, M. Delvaux, F. Hagenmüller

The distal body and antrum of the stomach are often clearly visualized by VCE, while the proximal portions are not. Changing the patient's position after capsule ingestion may be able to increase the diagnostic yield in the stomach (Adler and Fireman 2003), but even so the stomach cannot be reliably evaluated with VCE. Nevertheless, attention should be given to any gastric pathology that may be observable at VCE as bleeding lesions in the stomach may be missed at prior gastroscopy (Van Gossum et al. 2003; Delvaux et al. 2004).

Normal Anatomy

Normal findings are illustrated in ◻ Fig. 8.2-1. After the capsule has entered the stomach, it usually passes quickly to the antrum and displays the pylorus. When the camera is pointing at the pylorus, the pressure of the capsule against the pylorus can sometimes be clearly recognized (◻ Fig. 8.2-2). Occasionally the duodenal mucosa with its villi can be seen before the capsule falls back into the stomach. The time of definitive passage into the duodenum is noted for the determination of transit time.

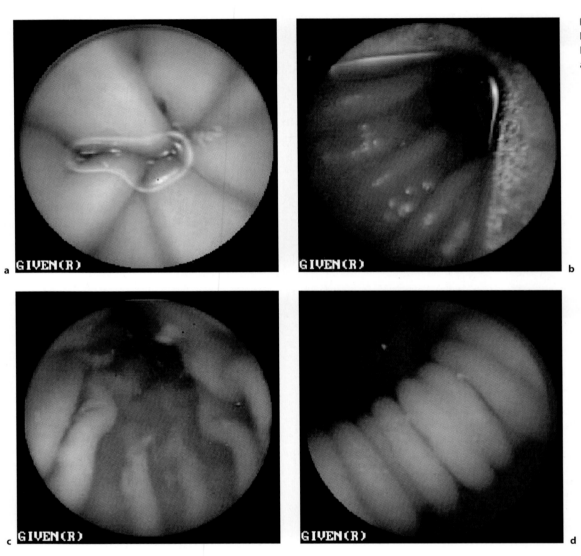

◻ **Fig. 8.2-1a–d.** Gastric folds in a collapsed (**a**), air-filled (**b**), and fluid-filled lumen (**c**). En face view of the gastric angulus (**d**)

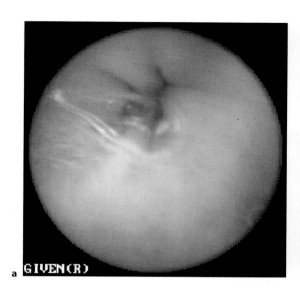

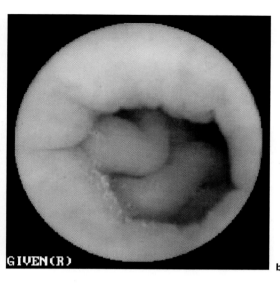

Fig. 8.2-2a, b. Pylorus: **a** closed; **b** partially open

Diverticula

Gastric diverticula are rare. As video capsule endoscopy does not provide a reliable localization in the stomach, they may be difficult to differentiate from the pylorus (■ Fig. 8.2-3).

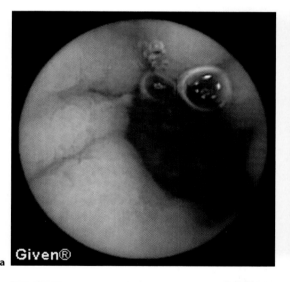

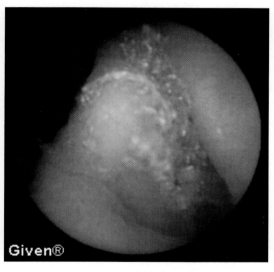

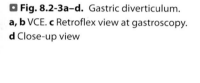
Fig. 8.2-3a–d. Gastric diverticulum. **a, b** VCE. **c** Retroflex view at gastroscopy. **d** Close-up view

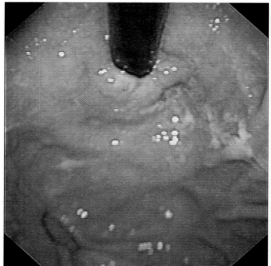

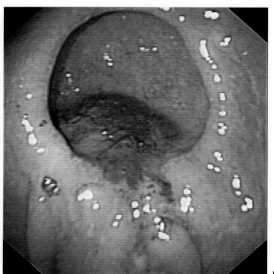

8

Vascular Lesions

Angiectasias present as sharply circumscribed red areas in the stomach (■ Fig. 8.2-4), while the gastric antral vascular ectasia (GAVE) syndrome leads to the typical picture of watermelon stomach (■ Fig. 8.2-5) (Mascarenhas-Saraiva et al. 2003). The vascular ectasia as the origin of these red areas becomes evident if the pressure of the capsule against the mucosa leads to emptying of the vessels (■ Fig. 8.2-6) and refilling is observed as the pressure is relieved (Raju et al. 2003).

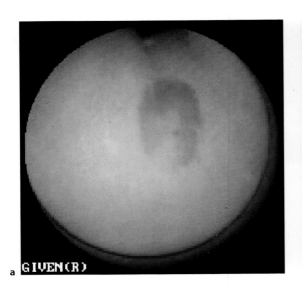
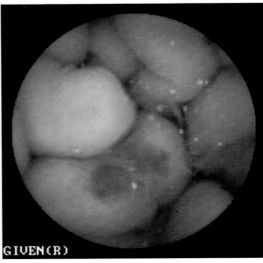

■ **Fig. 8.2-4a, b.** Angiectasias in the antrum (**a**) and corpus (**b**)

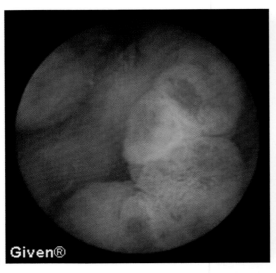
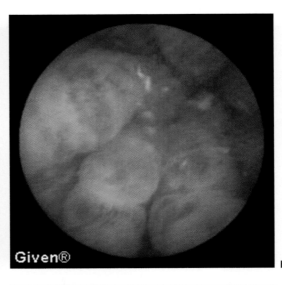

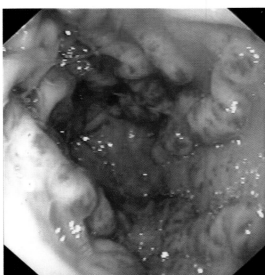
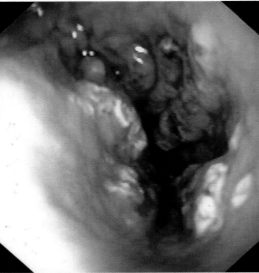

■ **Fig. 8.2-5a-d.** Gastric antral vascular ectasia (GAVE syndrome) in a patient with end-stage renal disease. Image of watermelon stomach seen at VCE (**a**, **b**) and at repeated gastroscopy. **d** Image after treatment with argon plasma coagulation (**c**, **d** courtesy of Thomas Thomsen, M.D.). Lesions had not been described at initial gastroscopy performed elsewhere

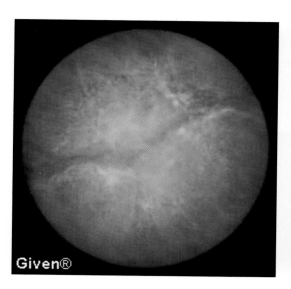

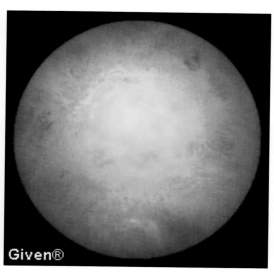

◻ **Fig. 8.2-6a, b.** Gastric antral vascular ectasia (GAVE syndrome). Pressure of the capsule against the mucosa empties the ectatic vessels

Inflammatory and Infiltrative Lesions

Amyloidosis

The stomach can be involved in systemic amyloidosis. Endoscopy shows irregular red spots or larger red infiltrated areas (◻ Fig. 8.2-7) that can be confused with angiectasias, GAVE, or peptic erosions. Biopsy gives a diagnostic clue.

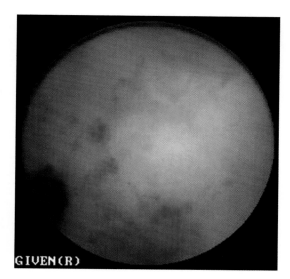

◻ **Fig. 8.2-7.** Gastric amyloidosis

Gastritis

Because the absence of air insufflation and mucosal distention in VCE presents the examiner with an unaccustomed view (■ Figs. 8.2-8, 8.2-9, and 8.2-10a), it is difficult to interpret the images in the same way as in conventional gastroscopy (■ Fig. 8.2-10b).

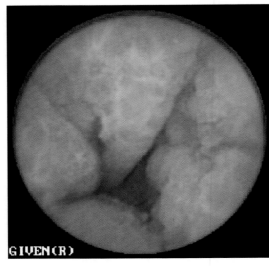

■ **Fig. 8.2-8.** Edema of the gastric mucosa, histologically confirmed

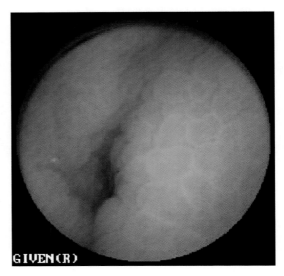

■ **Fig. 8.2-9.** Stomach of a patient with histologically confirmed chronic *Helicobacter*-positive gastritis with inflammatory activity

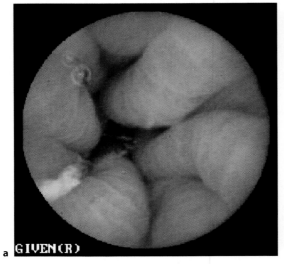

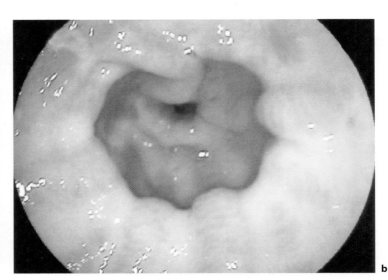

■ **Fig. 8.2-10a, b.** Markedly red, edematous longitudinal folds radiating to the pylorus. **a** VCE. **b** Gastroscopy with air insufflation shows red streaks in the prepyloric antrum. Biopsy: type C gastritis

Erosions

Erosions at VCE appear as flat or raised mucosal defects, with or without fibrin, that are most clearly appreciated in the gastric antrum (■ Fig. 8.2-11a, b). Accompanying hematin traces visible in the stomach (■ Fig. 8.2-12) or even fresh blood may reinforce the impression of these erosions as a potential source of bleeding. The examiner should be aware of any previous biopsies (■ Fig. 8.2-13) due to their similar appearance.

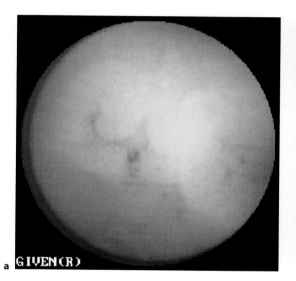

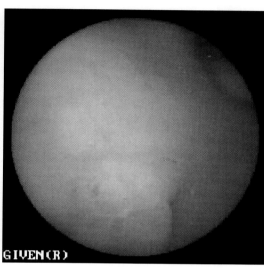

■ Fig. 8.2-11a, b. Flat (**a**) and raised erosions (**b**)

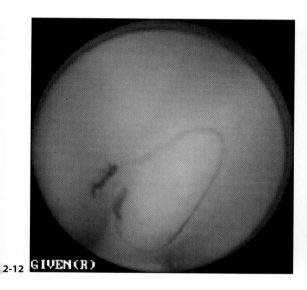

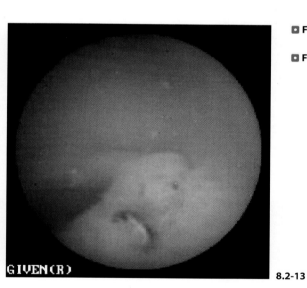

■ Fig. 8.2-12. Hematin trace

■ Fig. 8.2-13. Biopsy site after 1 day

Ulcers

Fibrin-coated ulcers (■ Fig. 8.2-14) are routinely detected at preceding esophagogastroduodenoscopy (EGD). Dieulafoy's ulcers, however, may easily be missed, if they are not actually bleeding. If intermittent bleeding occurs during VCE recording, they can become evident (■ Fig. 8.2-15)

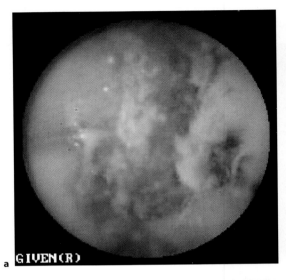

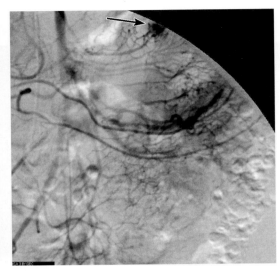

■ **Fig. 8.2-14a–c.** Fibrin-coated gastric ulcer, diabetic gastric emptying disorder. **a** VCE. **b** Angiography shows a small mass of tangled vessels in the gastric wall (courtesy of Andreas Wandler, M.D.). Initial gastroscopy was normal. The ulcer was endoscopically confirmed and clipped (**c**), and the bleeding did not recur

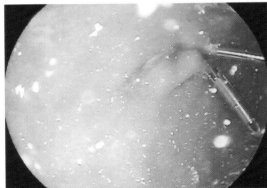

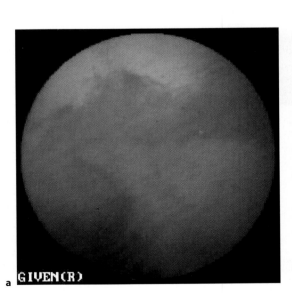

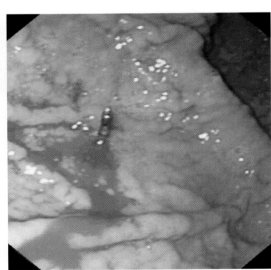

■ **Fig. 8.2-15a, b.** Dieulafoy's ulcer of the stomach. **a** Active bleeding at VCE. **b** Punctate bleeding source at gastroscopy, clipped

Tumors

Polyps, adenomas, and glandular cysts in the stomach may occur in the setting of polyposis syndromes. These lesions are occasionally observed at VCE (◘ Figs. 8.2-16, 8.2-18, and 8.2-19) but are defined much more reliably by conventional gastroscopy (◘ Fig. 8.2-17). VCE is also less than completely reliable in the detection of gastric tumors (◘ Fig. 8.2-20). If VCE is applied in patients with known gastric lymphoma in the search for intestinal manifestations, gastric tumor may cause temporary gastric retention (◘ Fig. 8.2-21).

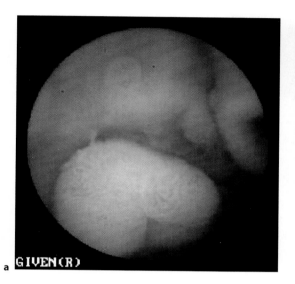

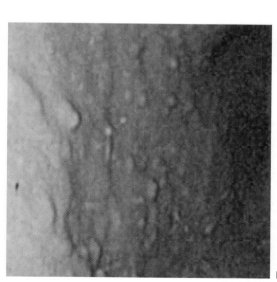

◘ **Fig. 8.2-16a, b.** Gastric polyp in Peutz-Jeghers syndrome. **a** VCE. **b** Gastroscopy

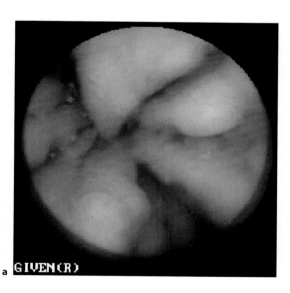

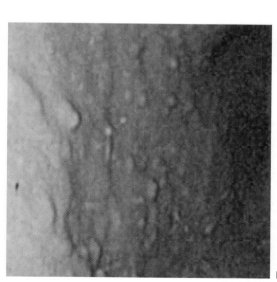

◘ **Fig. 8.2-17a, b.** Glandular cysts. **a** VCE. **b** Multiple cysts at gastroscopy. Biopsy-confirmed. Known familial adenomatous polyposis

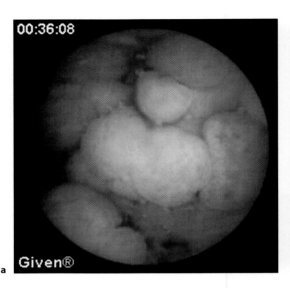

a

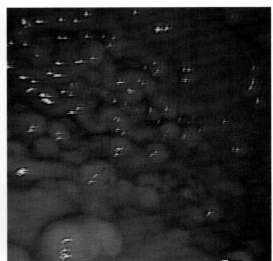

b

■ **Fig. 8.2-18.** Familial adenomatous polyposis: multiple hyperplastic polyps. **a** VCE. **b** Gastroscopy. **c** Histology (courtesy of Renate Höhne, M.D.)

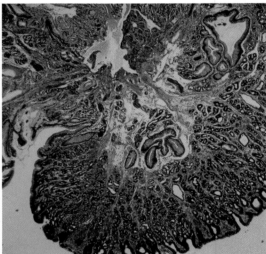

c

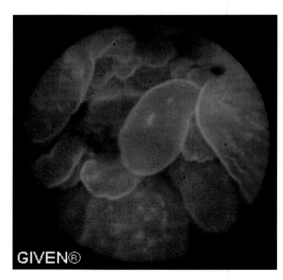

■ **Fig. 8.2-19.** Familial adenomatous polyposis. Giant hyperplastic gastric polyp with a corral-like appearance surrounding the capsule (courtesy of Virender Sharma, M.D.)

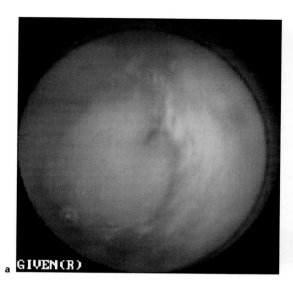

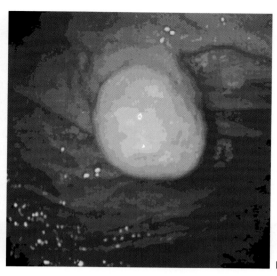

Fig. 8.2-20a, b. Gastric leiomyoma. **a** VCE shows a very subtle bulging of the mucosa. **b** Gastroscopy with air insufflation clearly demonstrates a tumor in the gastric body protruding into the lumen

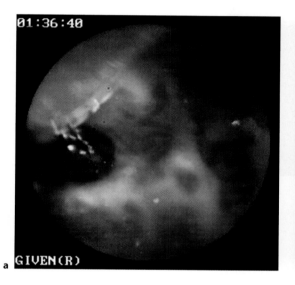

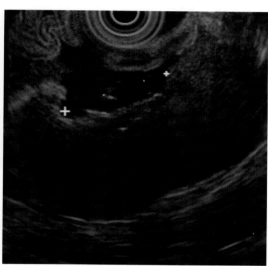

Fig. 8.2-21a, b. NK/T-cell lymphoma of the stomach. VCE shows the necrotic tumor (**a**), but is entrapped in the necrotic cavern (▪ Fig. 1.2-6). Using a second recording system after 1 h, retention of the capsule in the stomach could be detected. The capsule was then endoscopically placed into the duodenum (see Chap. 1.4.1) (**b**). Endosonography demonstrates the large tumor with central necrosis. VCE was performed to rule out intestinal involvement of lymphoma

References

Adler S, Fireman T (2003) Evaluation of the performance of the video capsule system for screening of the stomach. Gastrointest Endosc 57:AB167

Delvaux M, Fassler I, Gay G (2004) Clinical usefulness of the endoscopic video capsule as the initial intestinal investigation in patients with obscure digestive bleeding: validation of a diagnostic strategy based on the patient outcome after 12 months. Endoscopy 36:1067–1073

Mascarenhas-Saraiva M, Lopes L, Mascarenhas-Saraiva A (2003) Watermelon stomach seen by wireless-capsule endoscopy. Endoscopy 35:100

Raju GS, Morris K, Boening S, Carpenter D, Gomez G (2003) Capillary refilling sign demonstrated by capsule endoscopy. Gastrointest Endosc 58:936–937

Van Gossum A, Hittelet A, Schmit A, Francois E, Devière J (2003) A prospective comparative study of push and wireless-capsule enteroscopy in patients with obscure digestive bleeding. Acta Gastroenterol Belg 66:199–205

8.3   Colon

M. Appleyard, M. Keuchel, F. Hagenmüller

To date, VCE has not proven feasible for examinations of the colon, even with technical modifications (Schreiber et al. 2001; Fireman et al. 2002). This is due to the prolonged transit time of the capsule in the colon, the usual inability to image past the ascending colon, inadequate illumination of the larger lumen and the obscuring effect of fecal residues. Since the video capsule does not permit endoscopic irrigation, suction, or air insufflation, the images are not comparable to those obtained with flex-ible colonoscopy, even after bowel cleansing. Nevertheless, attention should still be given to any lesions that happen to be detected in the colon (Gay et al. 2002). The initial images of the cecum should be identified to make certain that the small bowel has been completely examined.

The colonic mucosa (■ Fig. 8.3-1a) is paler than that of the ileum (■ Fig. 8.3-1b), has a more prominent vascular pattern, is haustrated (■ Fig. 8.3-2), and is devoid of villi. The orifice of the appendix can often be identified (■ Fig. 8.3-3). The colon is rarely imaged distal to the right colic flexure (■ Fig. 8.3-4), and imaging of the rectum is very rare (■ Fig. 8.3-5). Nevertheless, in occasional cases, excretion of the capsule may be visualized (■ Fig. 8.3-6).

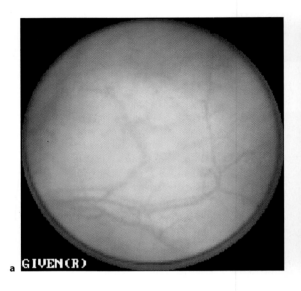

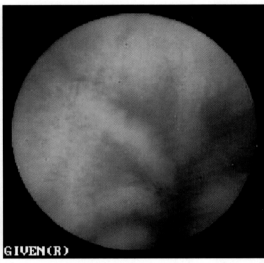

a GIVEN(R)

b GIVEN(R)

■ **Fig. 8.3-1.** **a** Colon: mucosa is paler than in the small bowel, has more prominent blood vessels, and no valvulae conniventes. **b** Ileum with villi

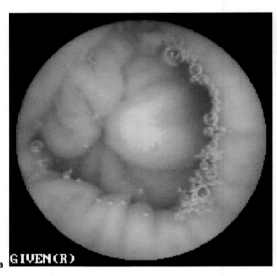

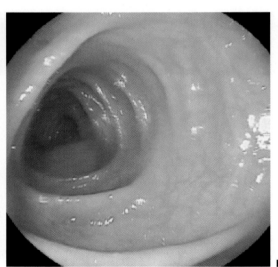

a GIVEN(R)

b

■ **Fig. 8.3-2a, b.** Colonic haustrae. **a** VCE. **b** Colonoscopy

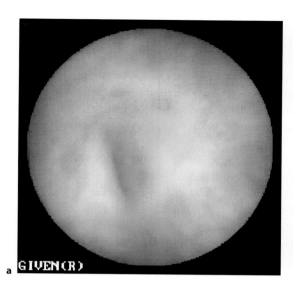

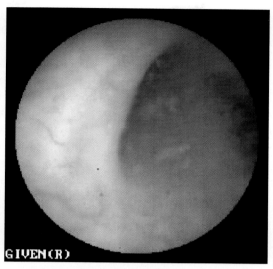

Fig. 8.3-3a, b. The orifice of the appendix is occasionally visible in the cecum as a diverticulum-like outpouching in the lower right quadrant

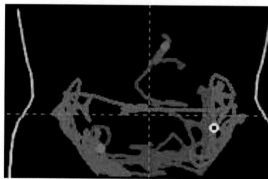

Fig. 8.3-4. Localization software traces the path of the capsule through the limbs of the colon (yellow-green: colon, blue-green: small bowel, blue: stomach)

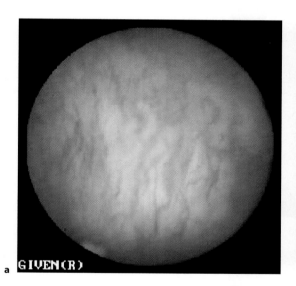

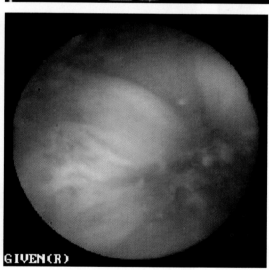

Fig. 8.3-5a–d. Rectum, anus. **a** Longitudinal vessels of the rectum. **b** Sphincter. **c** Hemorrhoidal plexus. **d** For comparison, flexible rectoscopy from the oral side via colostomy

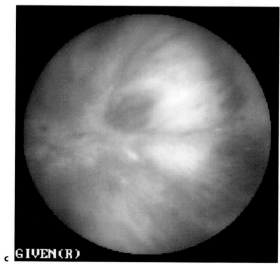

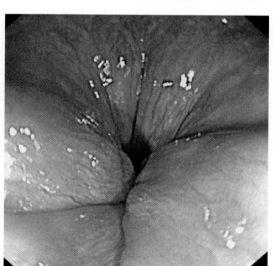

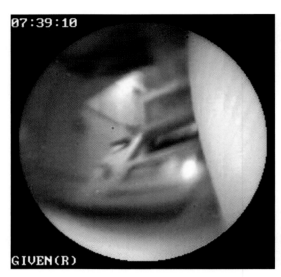

◻ Fig. 8.3-6. Capsule excreted after 7.5 h shows patient's bathroom view out of the toilet

Diverticula (◻ Figs. 8.3-7–8.3-9), angiectasias (◻ Fig. 8.3-10), or polyps (◻ Fig. 8.3-12) are occasionally detected in the cecum with VCE. They cannot be excluded, however. VCE should not be used to complete an incomplete colonoscopy (Rösch and Ell 2004).

Colonic images should not be ignored, however. Selby presented five patients in whom the bleeding originated from bleeding cecal angiectasias, cecal carcinomas (◻ Fig. 8.3-13), and cecal inflammation (Kitiyakara and Selby 2004).

Patients with known colonic disease may benefit from capsule endoscopy. Capsule endoscopy in patients with problematic indeterminate colitis (◻ Fig. 8.3-11a) may help differentiate a large proportion with a Crohn's disease phenotype (◻ Fig. 8.3-11b) when ileoscopy and radiology have been nondiagnostic (Mow et al. 2003; Whittaker et al. 2004). This has obvious implications for management.

Diverticula

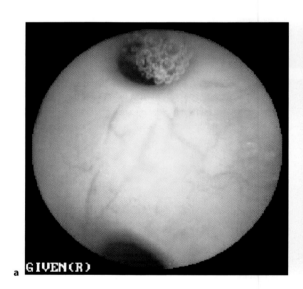

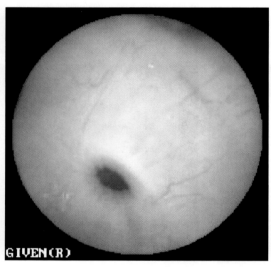

◻ Fig. 8.3-7. Uninflamed colonic diverticulum detected incidentally

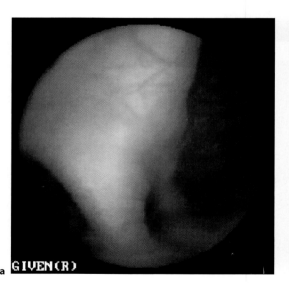

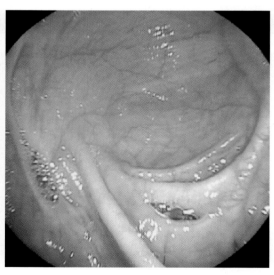

◻ Fig. 8.3-8a, b. Cecal diverticulum. **a** VCE. **b** Colonoscopy in the same patient

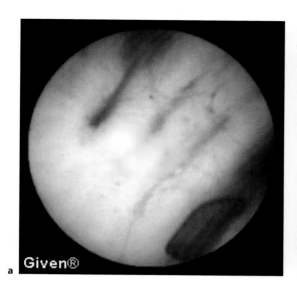
a

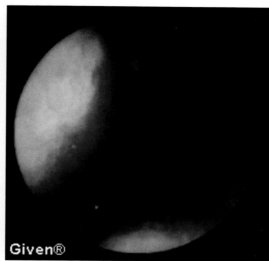
b

Fig. 8.3-9a, b. Colonic diverticula (**a**) and blood in the colon (**b**) together with normal VCE of the small intestine and prior exclusion of other colonic lesions by lower endoscopy ensure the assumption of colonic diverticula as source of relapsing bleeding

Angiectasias

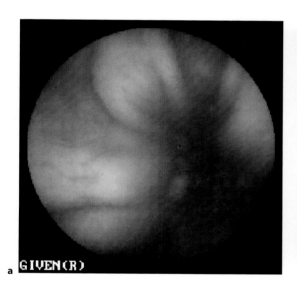
a

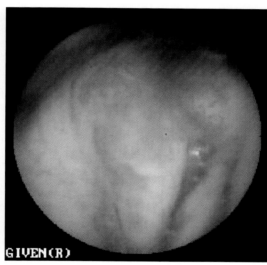
b

Fig. 8.3-10a–c. Known large angiectasias of the cecum and ascending colon (**a, b**), preoperative VCE to evaluate the small bowel. **c** Colonoscopy (courtesy of Rainer Porschen, M.D.). The patient presented clinically with overt bleeding and a transfusion reaction

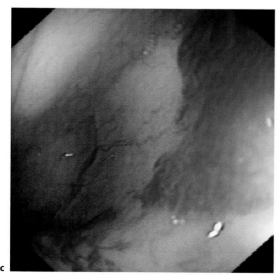
c

Colitis

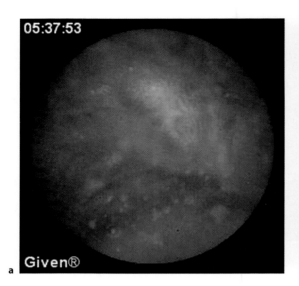

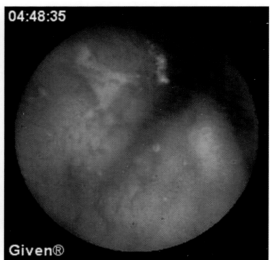

Fig. 8.3-11. a Cecal inflammation in a patient with indeterminate colitis. **b** Ulceration in the ileum consistent with Crohn's disease

Polyps

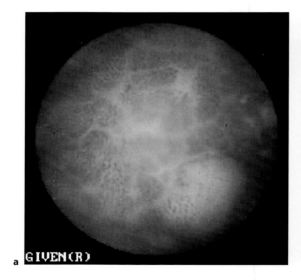

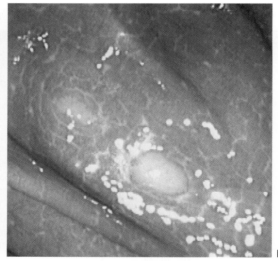

Fig. 8.3-12a, b. Hyperplastic colonic polyp confirmed by biopsy. Pseudomelanosis noted as an incidental finding. **a** VCE. **b** Colonoscopy in the same patient

Carcinoma

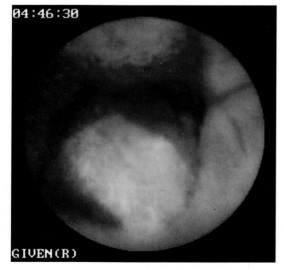

Fig. 8.3-13. Cecal cancer detected at VCE (courtesy of Warwick Selby, M.D.)

References

Fireman Z, Kopelman Y, Jacob H et al (2002) Wireless capsule colonoscopy. J Gastroenterol Hepatol 17 [Suppl]:A976

Gay G, Delvaux M, Fassler I et al (2002) Localization of colonic origin of obscure bleeding with the capsule endoscope: a case report. Gastrointest Endosc 56:758–762

Kitiyakara T, Selby W (2004) Non-small intestinal causes of blood loss found at capsule endoscopy in patients with obscure GI bleeding. 3rd International Conference on Capsule Endoscopy, p 47

Mow WS, Lo SK, Targan SR et al (2004) Initial experience with wireless capsule enteroscopy in the diagnosis and management of inflammatory bowel disease. Clin Gastroenterol Hepatol 2:31–40

Rösch T, Ell C (2004) Position paper on capsule endoscopy for the diagnosis of small bowel disorders. Z Gastroenterol 42:247–259

Schreiber R, Fischer D, Frisch M et al (2001) The use of gastrographin in advancing the GIVEN M2A capsule endoscope through the colon. Gastrointest Endosc 53:AB178

Whitaker D, Hume G, Radford-Smith GL Appleyard MN (2004) Can capsule endoscopy help differentiate the aetiology of indeterminate colitis? Gastrointest Endosc 59:AB177

Postoperative and Postinterventional Changes

M. Keuchel, R. De Franchis, W. Teichmann

As postoperative changes can cause difficulties in the interpretation of video capsule endoscopy, knowledge of these differences is as important as in radiology (Lappas 2004). It is not uncommon to examine patients who have had a previous fundoplication, some type of gastrectomy, a partial small bowel resection, or an ileocecal resection (Wu et al. 2003). The findings obtained with VCE, especially at anastomotic sites, are often less than spectacular, at most demonstrating portions of the anastomosis.

Esophagus

Fundoplication

Today, fundoplication is usually performed laparoscopically in selected patients with a hiatal hernia and significant reflux. This procedure can lead to relative stenosis of the gastroesophageal junction, causing a delay in capsule passage (■ Fig. 9-1).

Esophagojejunostomy

An esophagojejunostomy is performed after a total gastrectomy (■ Fig. 9.2), usually constructing an end-to-side anastomosis with a terminolateral pouch and an efferent loop. A Roux-en-Y anastomosis is also necessary for the bile-carrying limb of small bowel.

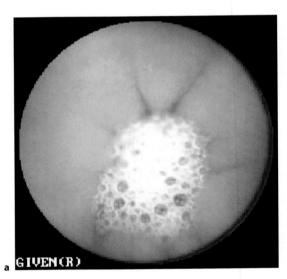

a

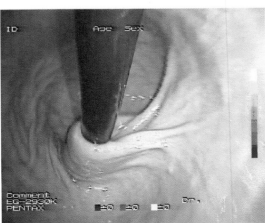

b

■ **Fig. 9-1a, b.** Fundoplicated stomach: **a** VCE shows a relative stenosis of the gastroesophageal junction within the hiatal hernia, evidenced by the gastric folds; some secretion is also present. **b** Retroflexed gastroscopic view of the tight plication cuff

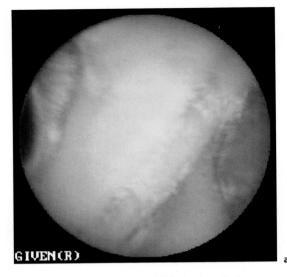

a

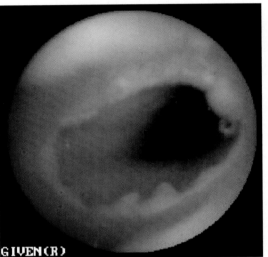

b

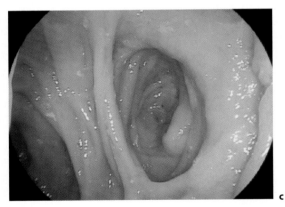

c

■ **Fig. 9-2a–c.** Esophagojejunostomy with an end-to-side anastomosis. **a** Anastomotic septum viewed from the esophagus. **b** Reverse view of the anastomosis and esophagus from the small bowel. **c** Endoscopic view

Stomach

Partial or Total Gastrectomy

Billroth I. In this most commonly used reconstruction technique, the end of the distally resected stomach is anastomosed to the end of the duodenum (◻ Fig. 9-3), leaving passage through the stomach and duodenum essentially intact. Biliary reflux into the stomach may occur.

Billroth II. The Billroth II operation is an end-to-side gastrojejunostomy with afferent and efferent loops of jejunum (◻ Fig. 9-4). A Braun side-to-side anastomosis can be added distally between the afferent and efferent loops (◻ Fig. 9-7) to prevent biliary reflux (◻ Fig. 9-5) into the stomach.

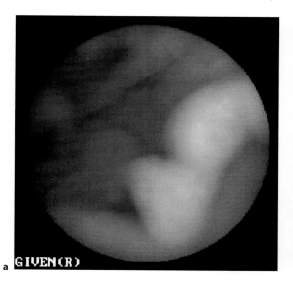
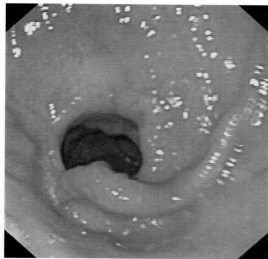

◻ **Fig. 9-3a, b.** Billroth I anastomosis: **a** partially displayed by VCE, **b** corresponding endoscopic view

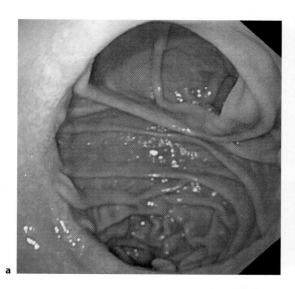
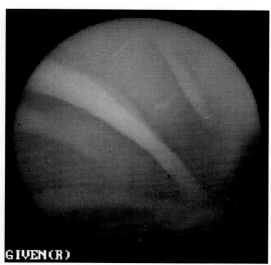
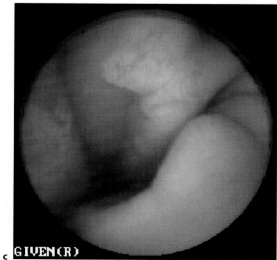
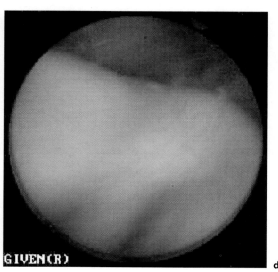

◻ **Fig. 9-4a–d.** Billroth II anastomosis. **a** Endoscopic appearance. **b** VCE: (efferent?) small bowel loop. **c** White area on the anastomotic rim as in intestinal metaplasia. **d** Anastomotic septum

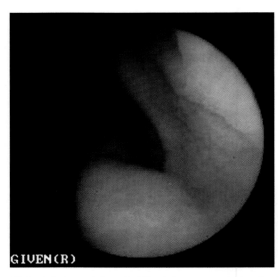

▣ Fig. 9-5. Lateral view of a Billroth II anastomosis showing bile reflux into the stomach

Gastroenterostomy

A jejunal loop is fixed terminolaterally to the stomach, mainly at the posterior wall (▣ Fig. 9-6a, b), combined with a distal Roux-en-Y anastomosis (▣ Fig. 9-6c, d) if the regular passage through the distal stomach or duodenum is not assured and the underlying benign or malignant disease is not resolvable by definitive surgery. The presence of a gastroenterostomy should alert the examiner to a high risk of impeded capsule passage.

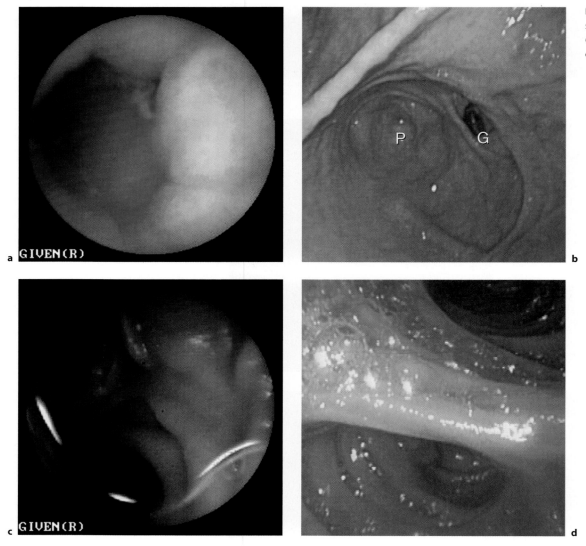

▣ Fig. 9-6a–d. Posterior gastroenterostomy. **a** VCE. **b** Gastroscopy: *P* pylorus, *G* gastroenterostomy. **c, d** Distal Roux-en-Y anastomosis

Small Intestine

Besides a total gastrectomy or distal gastric resection, small intestinal anastomoses are most commonly found after partial resections of the intestine (◘ Fig. 9-10), ileocecal resections, or colectomy (◘ Figs. 9-16 and 9-17). Rare postoperative situations include previous diverticulectomy (◘ Fig. 9-14) and mesenteric plication (◘ Fig. 9-15).

Braun Side-to-Side Anastomosis

The endoscopic appearance of a distal side-to-side anastomosis consists of two lumina separated by a narrow septum (◘ Fig. 9-7).

Roux-en-Y

This technique involves an end-to-end gastrojejunostomy with a Y-shaped distal anastomosis of the bile-carrying loop of the jejunum (◘ Fig. 9-8).

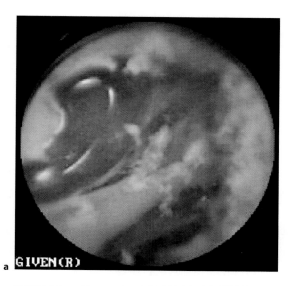

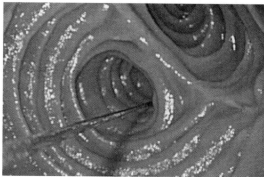

◘ **Fig. 9-7a, b.** Braun side-to-side anastomosis. **a** Two lumina with an intervening septum, food retention due to a more distal stenosis (not seen at VCE). **b** Push enteroscopy

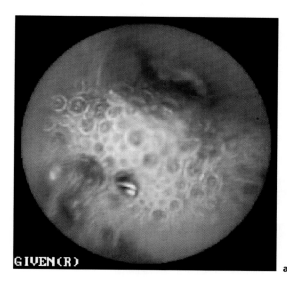

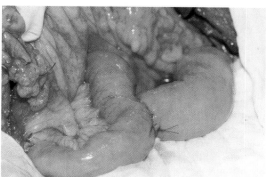

◘ **Fig. 9-8a, b.** Roux-en-Y anastomosis: **a** bile draining from the upper lumen, **b** appearance at operation

Enteroenteral Anastomoses

In patients with previous partial small bowel resection, often the anastomoses are not demonstrated or only partially demonstrated at VCE. End-to-end anastomoses are predominant (◘ Fig. 9-9), while side-to-side anastomoses are rare (◘ Fig. 9-10).

VCE can show scars, sewing material or staples (◘ Fig. 9-11), and diverticula at the anastomosis (◘ Fig. 9-12). Suture granulomas may have a tumorlike appearance (◘ Fig. 7.1-1).

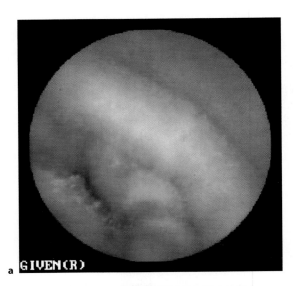

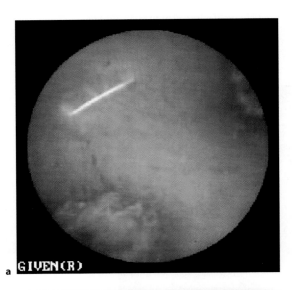

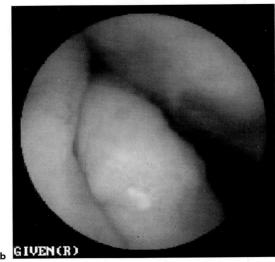

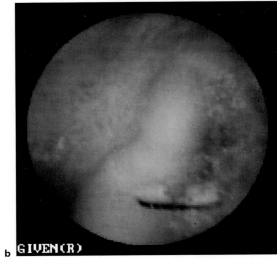

◘ **Fig. 9-9a.** Raised scar at an end-to-end jejunoileostomy. **b** Small ulcer on a duodenojejunostomy

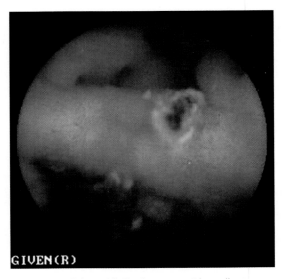

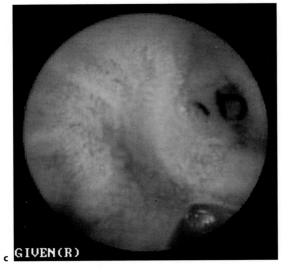

◘ **Fig. 9-11a–c.** Surgical fixation materials: **a** staple, **b** and **c** suture

◘ **Fig. 9-10.** Side to side ileoileostomy with small suture granuloma

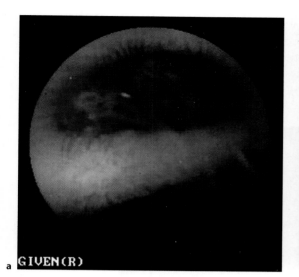

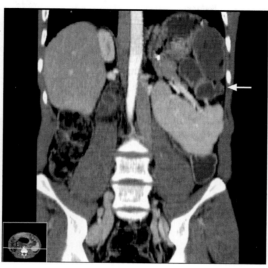

Fig. 9-12a, b. Small diverticulum at an anastomosis demonstrated by VCE (**a**) and CT (**b**) (↑, courtesy of Ernst Malzfeldt, M.D.)

Anastomotic Strictures

Rarely, stricturing anastomotic ulcers may be seen (❑ Fig. 9-13). Stenotic anastomoses can lead to capsule impaction (de Franchis et al. 2003a). It may be prudent, therefore, to include imaging procedures in the initial work-up. After exclusion of stenoses by small bowel X-ray series, VCE was performed safely in a group of ten patients with prior small bowel resection (De Palma et al. 2004). However, normal radiologic findings do not guarantee uncomplicated passage of the capsule. In doubtful cases, application of the Patency Capsule (Chap. 1.5) prior to VCE might be helpful to exclude relevant stenoses.

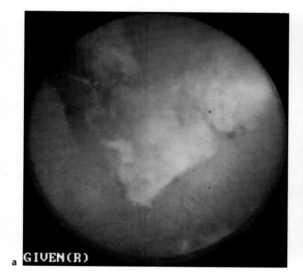

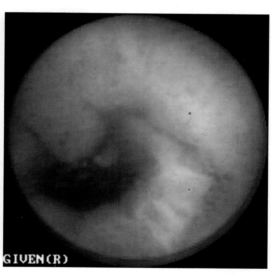

Fig. 9-13a, b. Ulcerated lesions at an anastomotic stricture in the ileum (reprinted from de Franchis et al. 2003b with permission from Editrice Gastroenterologica Italiana S.r.l.)

9

Previous Diverticulectomy

Especially after resection of a Meckel's diverticulum (■ Fig. 9-14a) rather than segmental small intestinal resection, persisting ulcers (■ Fig. 9-14b, c) rarely may cause relapsing bleeding.

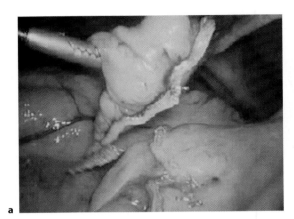

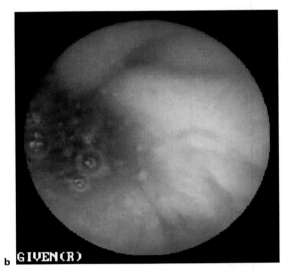

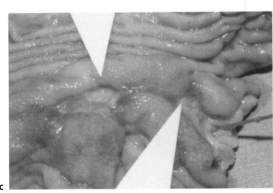

■ **Fig. 9-14a–c.** Diverticulectomy. **a** Initial laparoscopic removal with a GIA stapler. A second capsule endoscopy was done 1 year later for recurrence of intestinal blood loss (■ Figs. 4-9). **b** Shallow ulcers approximately 2 cm from the diverticulectomy site. **c** Surgical specimen with two ulcers (courtesy of Jörg Caselitz, M.D.)

Mesenteric Plication

Mesenteric plication itself or the underlying disease may hamper the passage of the capsule. Endoscopy can show sharply bent small bowel loops (■ Fig. 9-15).

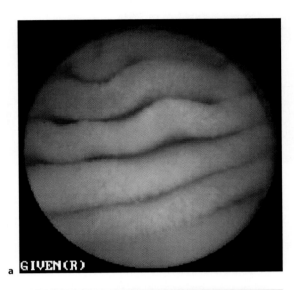

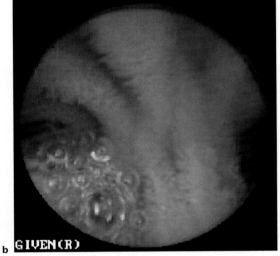

■ **Fig. 9-15a, b.** Patient had a previous Noble operation with a meandering arrangement of the small bowel loops followed by a Child-Philipps mesenteric plication. **a** Closely spaced valvulae conniventes. **b** Sharp bend of the small bowel lumen with a 360° loop

Ileocolostomy

Anastomoses after right-sided colectomy or ileocecal resection (◙ Figs. 9-16 and 9-17) are sometimes difficult to visualize by VCE if the capsule passes quickly through a wide anastomosis or if reflux of feces from the colon reduces the quality of images. However, these anastomoses are inspected routinely at colonoscopy prior to VCE.

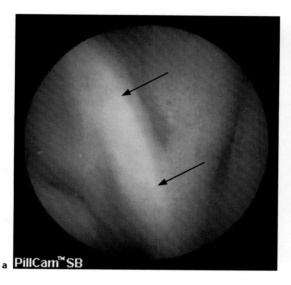

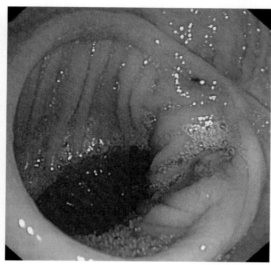

◙ **Fig. 9-16a, b.** Ileocolostomy. **a** Smooth, relatively pale colonic mucosa is visible on the left side of the image, separated by a scar (*arrow*) from the darker ileal mucosa with villi on the right side. **b** Colonoscopy

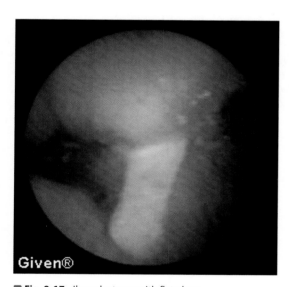

◙ **Fig. 9-17.** Ileocolostomy with flat ulcer

Adhesions

At present it does not appear that VCE is a reliable tool for the diagnosis of adhesions. Suspicious indirect signs include strangulation (◘ Fig. 9-18), sharp angulation, segmental dilation of small intestinal loops, and the arrest of capsule progression. Minor changes seen at capsule endoscopy (◘ Fig. 9-19a) may be associated with severe adhesions (◘ Fig. 9-19b). Moreover, dilatation of the small bowel in some cases may be due entirely to bowel cleansing with lavage. In other cases adhesions can lead to capsule retention (◘ Fig. 10-15).

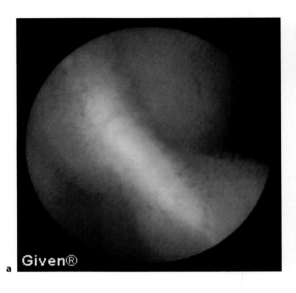

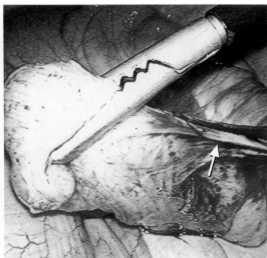

◘ **Fig. 9-18a, b.** Adhesion after prior resection of a Meckel's diverticulum. **a** Strangulation of an ileal loop. **b** Laparoscopic view of adhesion (↑). A 24-year-old women with crampy abdominal pain

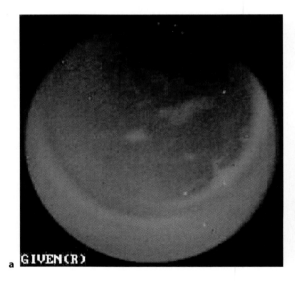

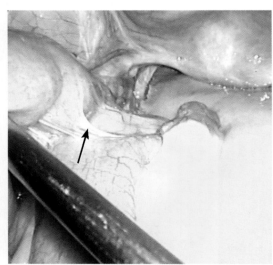

◘ **Fig. 9-19.** **a** Dark images with fluid-filled small bowel loops appearing in only a few frames. **b** Laparoscopy showed extensive adhesions (*arrow*). Abdominal pain persisted after surgery. Recurrence of retroperitoneal leiomyosarcoma was detected months later

Vascular Surgery

Personal experience shows no problems concerning passage of the video capsule after prior graft implantation for abdominal aortic aneurysm or after aortofemoral bypass. However, aortoduodenal fistula is a rare, but hazardous complication after aortic graft surgery. A case of such a fistula demonstrated by VCE has already been described (González-Suárez et al. 2002) (■ Fig. 9-20).

Ileostomy, Ileoanal Pouch, Ileorectostomy

If the ileum must perform a reservoir function after removal or exclusion of the colon, the mucosa is sometimes affected by edematous changes (■ Fig. 9-21a). Small residual polyps are occasionally found in patients with polyposis (■ Fig. 9-21b). Special attention should be paid to polyps in patients with familial adenomatous polyposis and remaining rectum after colectomy (■ Fig. 9-22).

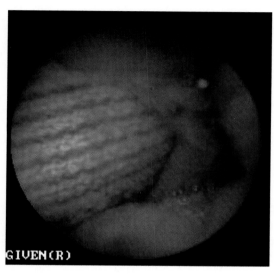

■ Fig. 9-20. Aortoduodenal fistula after aortic graft for aneurysm repair. VCE showing vascular prosthesis from the duodenum (courtesy of Begoña González-Suárez, M.D., reprinted from González-Suárez et al. 2002 with permission from Georg Thieme Verlag, Stuttgart)

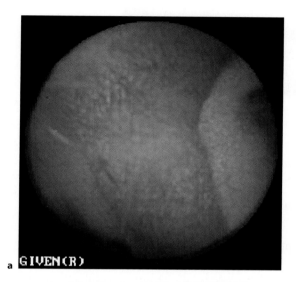

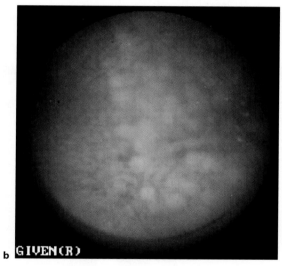

■ Fig. 9-21. a Ileostomy: slight edema. **b** Ileoanal pouch after colectomy for FAP, multiple small polyps (confirmed by biopsy)

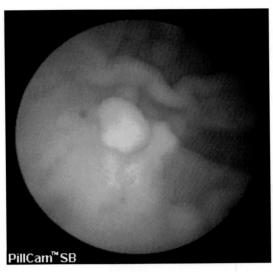

■ **Fig. 9-22.** Small rectal polyp in a patient with familial adenomatous polyposis and prior colectomy. Histology revealed tubular adenoma

Previous Small Intestinal Transplantation

Small bowel transplantation may be indicated in patients with a short-bowel syndrome that necessitates parenteral nutrition for the patient's lifetime. With modified operating techniques and recent advances in immunosuppressant drugs, patient and transplant survival rates have

been improved markedly (Fishbein et al. 2003). Regular endoscopic examinations should be performed initially through an ileostomy placed temporarily for easy access, so that complications such as rejection or infection can be detected at an early stage. VCE can be used in selected patients with normal ileoscopy to detect abnormalities in inaccessible portions of the small bowel (■ Fig. 9-23; de Franchis et al. 2003b).

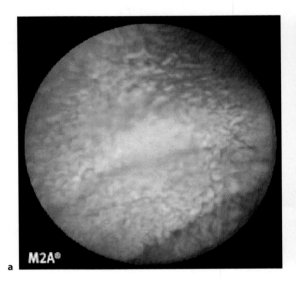

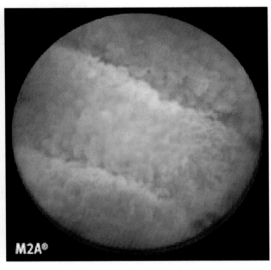

■ **Fig. 9-23a, b.** Previous small bowel transplantation. **a** Swollen, whitish villi and circumscribed hyperemia 20 days after transplantation. **b** Diffuse edema, thickened villi 64 days postoperatively (reprinted from de Franchis et al. 2002 with permission from Given Imaging)

Findings Following Endoscopic Intervention

As video capsule endoscopy is used as a diagnostic tool in concert with upper and lower gastrointestinal (GI) endoscopy, changes following endoscopic intervention may be seen at VCE. Most frequently, small focal lesions are seen after endoscopic biopsy of the duodenum (■ Fig. 9-24a) or terminal ileum (■ Fig. 9-24b). These small reddish

or ulcerated lesions may persist for a longer time. Knowledge of previous biopsy helps to avoid confusion with ulcers caused by inflammatory bowel disease. Other findings may be ulcer following coagulation (■ Fig. 9-25), scars after mucosectomy (■ Fig. 9-26a), or hemoclips (■ Fig. 9-26b). Ink mark is sometimes injected during double-balloon enteroscopy to document the extent of investigation (■ Fig. 9-27).

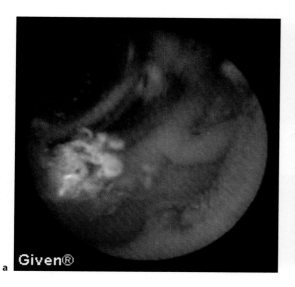

a

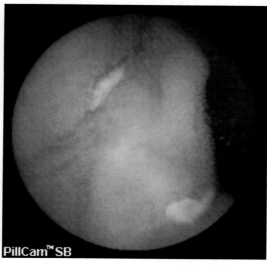

b

■ **Fig. 9-24a, b.** Findings after endoscopic biopsy. **a** Small duodenal defect with minimal mucosal hemorrhage. **b** Ulcers in the terminal ileum

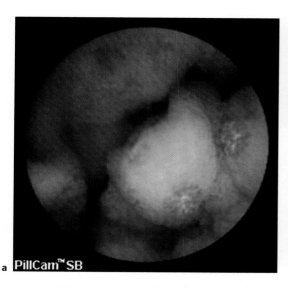

a

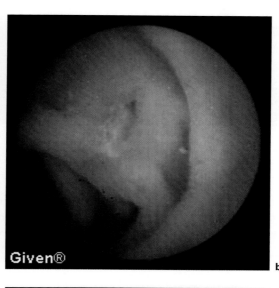

b

■ **Fig. 9-25a–d.** Findings after prior argon plasma coagulation. **a** Superficial lesions after coagulation of multiple angiectasias. **b** Small ulcer. **c** Ulceration, edema, lymphangiectasia, and erythema and **d** large deep defect after coagulation of multiple confluent angiectasias in a patient with hereditary hemorrhagic teleangiectasia

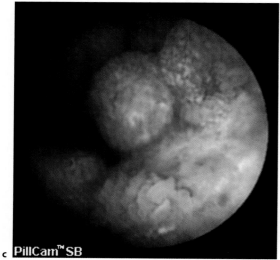

c

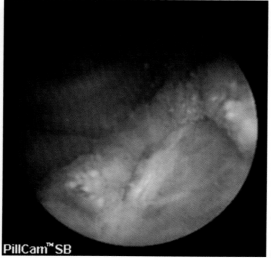

d

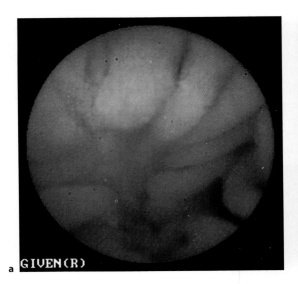

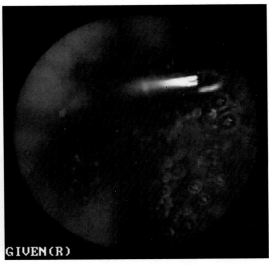

Fig. 9-26. a Scar with focal loss of folds as a consequence of endoscopic mucosa resection in the duodenum. **b** Hemoclip in the terminal ileum

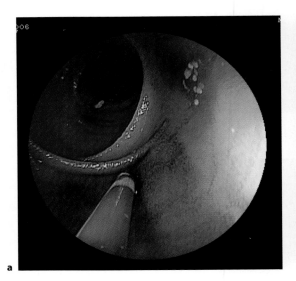

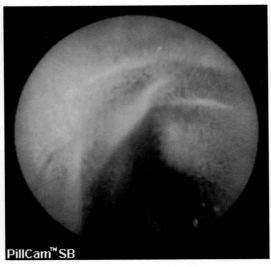

Fig. 9-27a, b. Ink mark. **a** Injection during double-balloon enteroscopy. **b** Image of the »tattoo« at VCE

Internet

www.intestinaltransplant.org: International Intestine Transplant Registry

References

de Franchis R, Rondonotti E, Abbiati C et al (2002) Transplantation. In: Halpern M, Jacob H (eds) Atlas of capsule endoscopy. Given Imaging, Norcross, GA, USA

de Franchis R, Avesani EM, Abbiati C et al (2003a) Unsuspected ileal stenosis causing obscure GI bleeding in patients with previous abdominal surgery – diagnosis by capsule endoscopy: a report of two cases. Dig Liver Dis 35:577–584

de Franchis R, Rondonotti E, Abbiati C et al (2003b) Capsule enteroscopy in small bowel transplantation. Dig Liver Dis 35:728–731

De Palma GD, Rega M, Puzziello A et al (2004) Capsule endoscopy is safe and effective after small-bowel resection. Gastrointest Endosc 60:135–138

Fishbein TM, Gondolesi GE, Kaufman SS (2003) – Intestinal transplantation for gut failure. Gastroenterology 124:1615–1628

Gonzalez-Suarez B, Guarner C, Escudero JR, Viver E, Palmer J, Balanzo J (2002) Wireless capsule video endoscopy: a new diagnostic method for aortoduodenal fissure. Endoscopy 34:938

Lappas JC (2004) Imaging of the postsurgical small bowel. Radiol Clin N Am 41:305–326

Wu GY, Aziz K, Whalen GF (2003) An internist's illustrated guide to gastrointestinal surgery. Humana Press, Totowa, NJ

Complications: Prevention and Management

J. Barkin, M. Cheng, M. Keuchel, G. Gay

VCE is a noninvasive procedure with few side effects. Knowledge of possible complications will further improve the safety of the method. As the use of VCE has increased, more is being understood as to the safety of VCE, including its risks, complications, and contraindications and this list is decreasing (Barkin and O'Loughlin 2004). Present contraindications to VCE are listed in ◻ Table 10-1.

Pharyngeal Dysphagia

VCE is initiated by swallowing the capsule endoscope (CE), and complications may be seen in patients with oropharyngeal transfer dysphagia. Inability to adequately swallow may result in misplacement of the CE into the pyriform sinuses (Fleischer et al. 2003) (◻ Fig. 10-1).

◻ **Table 10-1.** Contraindications to VCE

Contraindications
- Known or suspected gastrointestinal obstruction, strictures, or fistulae – unless surgery is warranted or patency is proven
- Pseudo-obstruction

Relative contraindications
- Pregnancy
- Cardiac pacemaker or defibrillator
- Extensive Crohn's disease
- Prior pelvic or abdominal surgery – if signs of chronic obstruction
- Prior pelvic or abdominal radiotherapy – unless patency is proven
- Severe adhesions – unless patency is proven

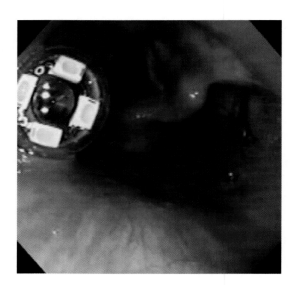

◻ **Fig. 10-1.** Capsule in the pyriform recess (courtesy of David Fleischer, M.D., reprinted from Fleischer et al. 2003 with permission from the American Society for Gastrointestinal Endoscopy). The capsule was retrieved with a Roth net, while the airways were protected with a balloon

Aspiration

Single cases of aspiration into the trachea have been described (◻ Fig. 10-2). Some events were either of brief duration, because patients expectorated the capsule (Schneider et al. 2003) (◻ Fig. 10-2a, b), while in others, aspiration was asymptomatic (Morandi et al. 2003) or causing only minor symptoms such as mild respiratory distress or foreign body sensation (Buchkremer at al. 2004; Sinn et al. 2004;Tabib et al. 2004). However, emergent rigid or flexible bronchoscopy has been necessary for extraction of these capsules. Interestingly, review of capsule transit studies has shown instances of asymptomatic aspiration and subsequent coughing up into the mouth with re-swallowing into the esophagus.

Cave		
The risks of aspiration and of capsule impaction should be explained to the patient during preprocedure counseling and written consent should be obtained.		

❶ X-ray of the chest should be considered in any case of coughing, dyspnea, or foreign body sensation after ingestion of the capsule.

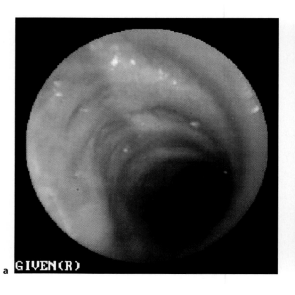

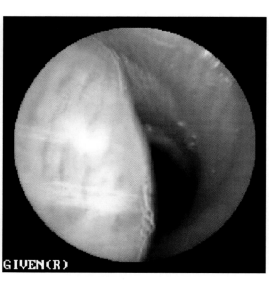

◻ **Fig. 10-2a, b.** Aspiration. View into the trachea (**a**), prolapse of the membranous trachea on coughing (**b**)

Difficult Capsule Passage

A transient delay in passage of the CE through physiologic sphincters, for example, the lower esophageal sphincter, pylorus, and ileocecal valve, has been noted.

Esophagus

Older patients are more likely to have a cricopharyngeal bar and subsequent development of Zenker's diverticulum. Retention of the CE in a Zenker's diverticulum requiring endoscopic removal and placement into the stomach has been reported (Knapp and Ladetsky 2005). Esophageal transport dysphagia may also potentially complicate passage of the CE due to abnormalities in esophageal motility (◘ Figs. 8.1-18–8.1-19). Leung and Sung (2004) reported esophageal retention of the CE in an elderly diabetic woman due presumably to impaired esophageal motility and cardiomegaly compressing on the esophagus (◘ Fig. 10-3). Other risk factors for esophageal transport abnormalities are epiphrenic diverticula (◘ Fig. 10-4) or surgical procedures such as resections (◘ Fig. 10-5) or fundoplication (◘ Fig. 9-1). These cases are in general asymptomatic.

Because of the potential complications with the CE in patients with dysphagia, it is recommended to exclude swallowing problems by taking a detailed history. Moreover, patients with dysphagia should undergo further evaluation with video esophagograms in conjunction with swallowing a 13-mm barium pill prior to VCE to rule out any potential lesions that may cause retention of the CE.

These conditions are not contraindications for VCE and can be overcome by endoscopic placement of the capsule in the stomach or duodenum.

Risk factors for impaired esophageal capsule transport:

- Abnormalities in esophageal motility
- Diverticula (Zenker's diverticulum, epiphrenic diverticulum)
- Compression from outside (e.g., cardiomegaly)
- Prior esophageal surgery (resection, fundoplication)

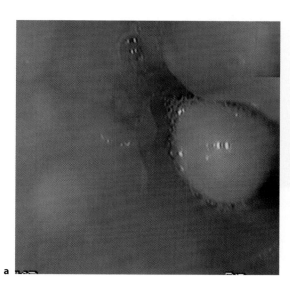
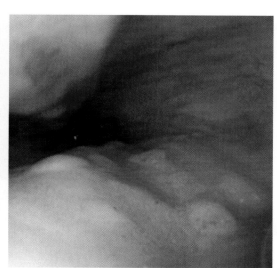
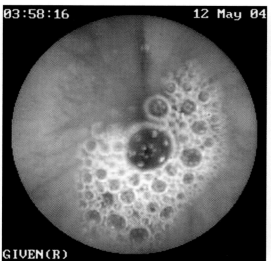
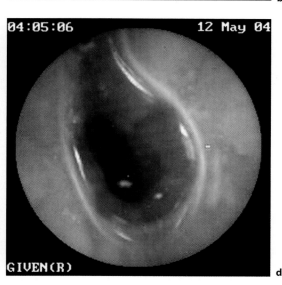

◘ **Fig. 10-3.** **a** The video capsule is retained in front of an esophageal narrowing caused by the thoracic aorta for 4.5 h. Endoscopic view with (**a**) and without (**b**) capsule. View from the video capsule (**c**, **d**). The capsule could easily be pushed endoscopically into the stomach

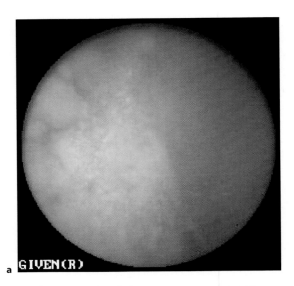

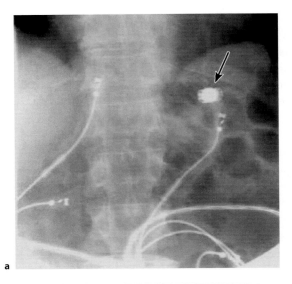

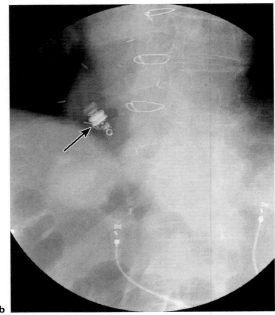

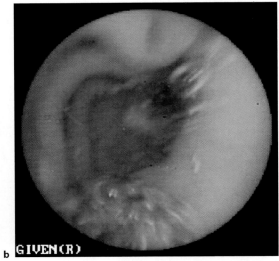

Fig. 10-5a, b. Capsule (*arrow*) temporarily retained in the curved limb of an esophagojejunostomy, later passed spontaneously: **a** radiograph, **b** VCE

Fig. 10-4a, b. Capsule retention in an epiphrenic diverticulum throughout the examination. **a** VCE. **b** Fluoroscopy. Capsule in air-filled diverticulum (*arrow*), also electrodes for VCE and cerclage wires after sternotomy (Fig. 8.1-16)

Stomach and Duodenum

Gastric retention of the CE may occur in patients with gastroparesis, with upside-down stomach, after vagotomy, or with anatomic narrowing of the pylorus or duodenum (❏ Figs. 10-6–10-9). Various techniques have been described for endoscopically assisted VCE in these instances. The capsule may either be inserted endoscopically or grasped after the patient has swallowed the capsule (Chap. 1.4.1). In one patient, the capsule had to be extracted endoscopically from the stomach after 2 weeks, although the endoscope could be easily passed to the duodenum (Mow et al. 2004). Strictured areas need to be dilated in patients with pyloric or duodenal narrowing.

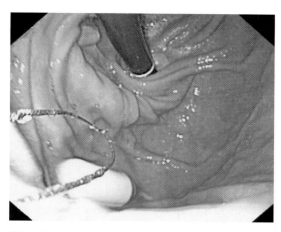

❏ **Fig. 10-6.** Retroflexed endoscopic view of a large hiatal hernia. The capsule had to be pushed from the hernia into the duodenum with a polypectomy snare

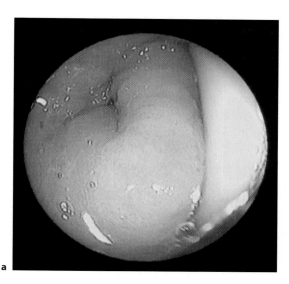

a

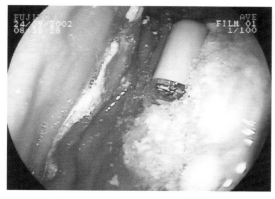

❏ **Fig. 10-7.** Diabetic gastroparesis. Video capsule, food, and tablet residues retained in the stomach

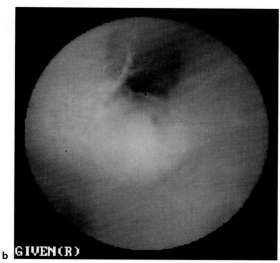

b GIVEN(R)

❏ **Fig. 10-9.** **a** Scarred bulb with a pouch that entrapped the capsule. **b** VCE. The capsule could not be placed endoscopically into the duodenum with a Dormia basket. Capsule passage resumed after treatment with i.v. erythromycin

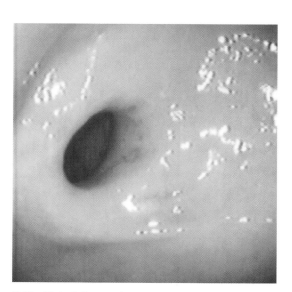

❏ **Fig. 10-8.** Relative pyloric stenosis in a young patient. Small hemorrhagic areas after endoscope passage indicate the relative stenosis. The capsule did not leave the stomach spontaneously until the end of the transmission period

Capsule Retention in the Small Intestine

Incidence

Small bowel retention of the CE can also occur. Anatomic narrowings in the small bowel can cause retention or non-natural passage of the CE. Barkin and Friedman (2002) have reported the incidence of non-natural capsule passage that occurred in the initial worldwide VCE studies. Surgical intervention was required in 0.75% (7 of 934 patients). An endoluminal process was found in all seven of these patients that explained the patients' presentation of obscure gastrointestinal bleeding. Six of seven of our patients had normal small bowel series.

However, in a later series on 20 patients with suspected Crohn's disease, the rate of impaction was as high as 15% (Ge et al. 2004).

Retention of the CE usually occurs proximal to the small bowel lesion, whether endoluminal or extraluminal. Retention has also been reported secondary to Meckel's diverticulum (Gortzak et al. 2003), adhesions (Keuchel et al. 2003; ◻ Fig. 10-15), and even in an appendiceal stump (Van Gossum et al. 2003; ◻ Fig. 10-19).

> 🛈 The impaction of a capsule proximal to a stenosis is a complication only if neither the clinical features (◻ Fig. 10-14) nor the diagnosis (◻ Fig. 7-2.3) justify an operation or endoscopic intervention

Discovery of Retention

Patients who retain the CE in the small bowel usually display no clinical signs or symptoms of obstruction. Transient pain may occur as the capsule passes through a stenosis. Discovery of capsule non-passage is elicited by findings of an obstructing lesion on review of the VCE study, or by patients' history that the capsule has not been excreted. Non-visualization of the cecum may be the only evidence of stenosis during review of the video, if the capsule approaches the stenosis with the blind back (Madisch et al. 2003). The presumed degree of stenosis does not furnish definite information on whether the lumen is still passable (◻ Fig. 10-10). The CE is expelled naturally after an average time of 72 h (range: 24–222 h) (De Luca et al. 2003). If retention of the CE is suspected, an abdominal flat plate radiograph can be done to verify CE retention and to follow its progression (◻ Fig. 10-11). The timing of this radiograph has been suggested by consensus to be 2 weeks after CE ingestion in asymptomatic patients (Lewis 2005). If the CE is present at 48 h but has passed at 96 h, then the patient is designated to have delayed passage. If the CE is still present at a minimum of 2 weeks post ingestion, then the patient is deemed to have a retained CE. Ultrasound (◻ Fig. 10-12) can demonstrate the capsule with an associated acoustic shadow (Girelli et al. 2004) but is not reliable enough to exclude capsule retention. Computed tomography (CT) scan can provide additional information on extraluminal changes (◻ Fig. 10-13).

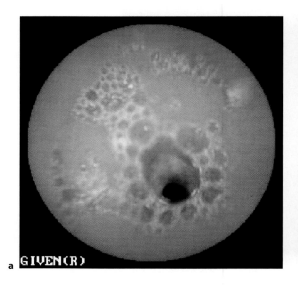
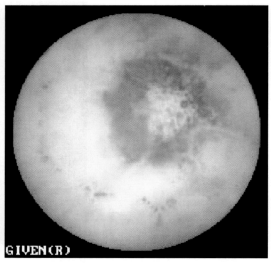

◻ Fig. 10-10. a High-grade stenosis in the mid-small bowel. **b** The capsule is pressed against the stenosis. Nevertheless, the capsule passed spontaneously on the evening after the examination, with associated transient abdominal pain

a GIVEN(R) GIVEN(R) b

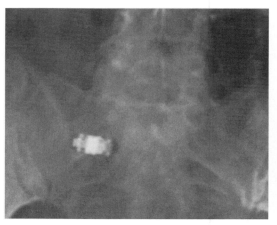
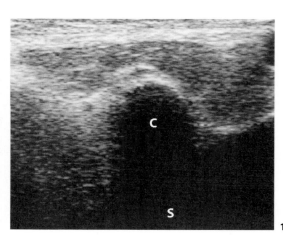

◻ Fig. 10-11. Capsule retained for 4 weeks: radiographic detection

◻ Fig. 10-12. Capsule retained for 4 weeks: sonographic detection of a video capsule (*C*) with acoustic shadow (*S*)

C

S

10-11   10-12

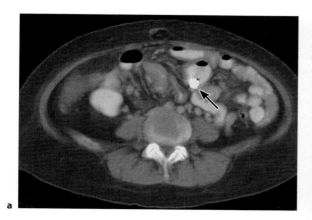

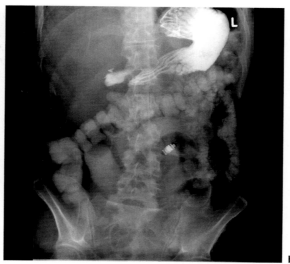

Fig. 10-13a, b. Capsule (*arrow*) retained for 6 months. **a** CT detection (courtesy of Ernst Malzfeldt, M.D.). Crohn's disease with stricture, fistulae, and conglomerate mass (VCE performed elsewhere). **b** Small bowel follow through (courtesy of Uwe-Paul Eggers, M.D.)

Management of Retention

The management of a retained capsule is evolving. The most reasonable approach to a retained capsule in an asymptomatic patient depends on the finding of the image by the CE. If a lesion is seen on review of the capsule images, it is reasonable to initiate therapy. This can include a medical course of steroids, endoscopic attempt at removal of the capsule, or surgical approach. The medical approach with a course of corticosteroids is to decrease inflammation, thus allowing capsule passage. This has been utilized in patients with Crohn's disease and ulcerative jejunitis complicating celiac disease. The endoscopic approach with retrieval of the capsule is feasible if the obstruction is within reach of an endoscope, whether it is in the proximal small bowel or in the distal small bowel (■ Fig. 10-16). Previous endoscopic dilation of a stricture might be necessary before retrieval (Arifuddin et al. 2005; Keuchel and Hagenmüller 2002) (■ Fig. 10-17a–c). If the capsule is not within reach of an endoscope, then surgery with laparotomy may be indicated to retrieve the capsule (Fry et al. 2005) (■ Fig. 10-18). In future, double-balloon endoscopy (Chap. 2.2) is a true alternative for removal of impacted capsules (■ Fig. 10-17d, e) (May et al. 2005). Moreover, asymptomatic patients with a retained CE proximal to a partially obstructing lesion have been observed for over 2 years without sequelae (Sears et al. 2004). Whether this will prove to be a viable approach remains to be seen.

> ❗ The risk of capsule retention with possible requirement of surgical or endoscopic retrieval is the major issue of the informed consent

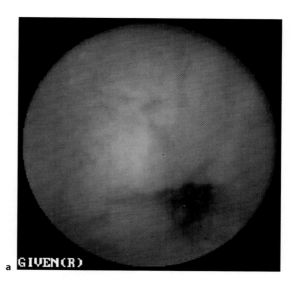

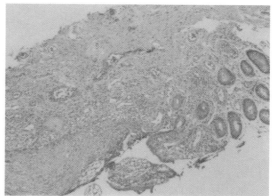

Fig. 10-14. a Symptomatic stricture in the jejunum in a patient with known Crohn's disease. Enteroclysis was normal, and complaints persisted after laparoscopic lysis of adhesions. Capsule passed at 14 days. **b** Based on VCE findings, four strictures were resected and histologically examined (courtesy of Michael Heine, M.D.). Afterward the patient was free of complaints

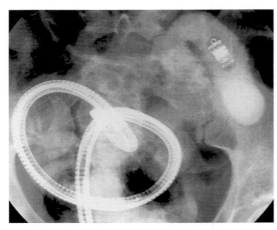

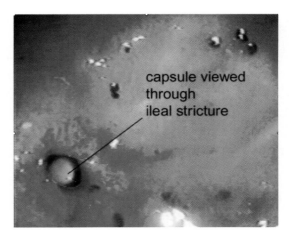

Fig. 10-15. Adhesions. The patient had a previous partial small bowel resection and colectomy for familial adenomatous polyposis. The capsule became impacted proximal to a sharp bend caused by an adhesion. It was out of endoscopic range and finally was removed surgically, at which time intra-abdominal desmoids were also diagnosed

Fig. 10-16. Endoscopic view of retained capsule endoscope

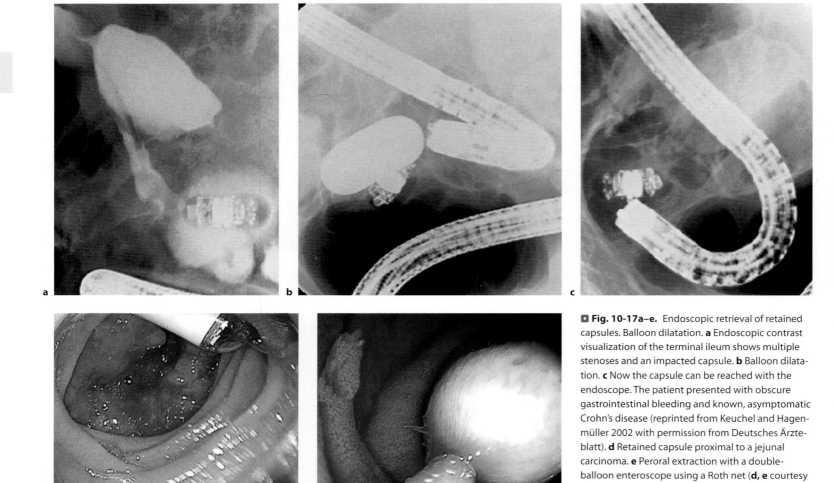

Fig. 10-17a–e. Endoscopic retrieval of retained capsules. Balloon dilatation. **a** Endoscopic contrast visualization of the terminal ileum shows multiple stenoses and an impacted capsule. **b** Balloon dilatation. **c** Now the capsule can be reached with the endoscope. The patient presented with obscure gastrointestinal bleeding and known, asymptomatic Crohn's disease (reprinted from Keuchel and Hagenmüller 2002 with permission from Deutsches Ärzteblatt). **d** Retained capsule proximal to a jejunal carcinoma. **e** Peroral extraction with a double-balloon enteroscope using a Roth net (**d, e** courtesy of Horst Neuhaus, M.D.)

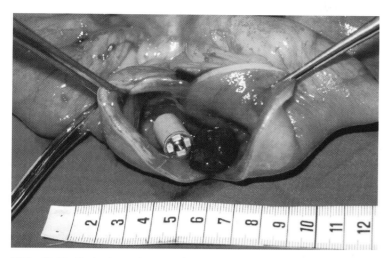

■ **Fig. 10-18.** Ileal stricture due to Crohn's disease seen at operation. The capsule was surgically retrieved proximal to the stricture. Capsule endoscopy was done to exclude additional proximal stenoses with a known stenosis requiring surgical treatment (courtesy of Dirk Hartmann, M.D. and Jürgen Riemann, M.D.)

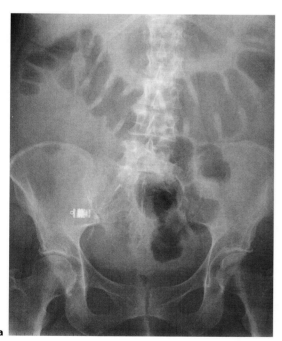

■ **Fig. 10-19a–c.** Video capsule entrapped in an appendiceal stump (courtesy of André Van Gossum, M.D., reprinted from Van Gossum et al. 2003 with permission from Acta Gastroenterol Belg). **a** X-ray shows the capsule near the ileocecal valve. The patient was asymptomatic. **b** The video capsule is trapped in the appendiceal stump (colonoscopy image). **c** Video capsule after removal from the appendiceal stump

a

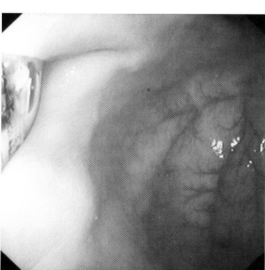

b

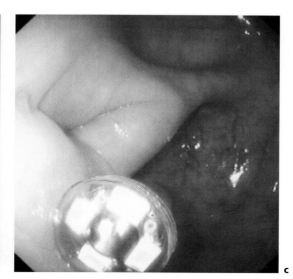

c

Prevention of Retention

A small bowel series is recommended prior to VCE to exclude anatomic narrowing that potentially can cause capsule retention in patients at risk. Enteroclysis, CT, magnetic resonance imaging, or ultrasound may also be used, depending on local expertise. However, CE retention may occur at anatomical narrowing not seen on the radiographic studies. Most patients with CE retention secondary to small bowel narrowing have been asymptomatic.

In patients with documented stenosis or with underlying conditions predisposing for intestinal stenosis, a biodegradable Patency Capsule (Given Imaging Ltd., Yoqneam, Israel) can be helpful to demonstrate intestinal patency (Chap. 1.5). However, it should be noted that in patients with long tight stenosis of the small intestine, especially in established Crohn's disease, even this biodegradable Patency Capsule may cause symptomatic obstruction (◘ Figs. 10-20 and 10-21) (Boivin et al. 2005; Gay et al. 2005). A modified Agile Patency Capsule with two plugs – one at each pole – is under evaluation.

> ❗ A normal X-ray examination of the small bowel does not guarantee uneventful passage of the capsule.

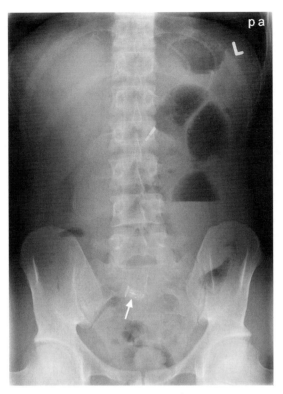

◘ **Fig. 10-20.** Intact patency capsule (↑) causing small intestinal obstruction. Note decompression tube (courtesy of Winfried Voderholzer, M.D. and Patrick Hein, M.D.)

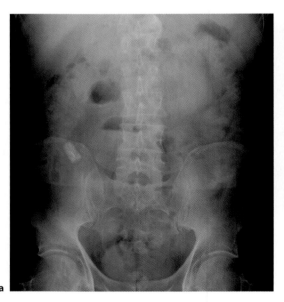

a

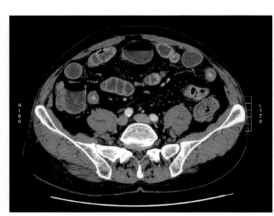

b

◘ **Fig. 10-21a–d.** Long stricture of the ileum with remnants of the Patency Capsule within the stenosis. **a** Plain abdominal X-ray with intact Patency Capsule. **b** CT scan with partially dissolved Patency Capsule proximal to an ileal stenosis. **c** Surgical situs with ileal stenosis. **d** Remnants of the dissolved Patency Capsule within the stenosis

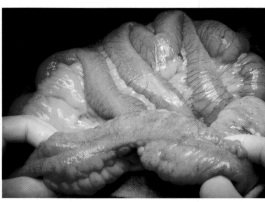

c

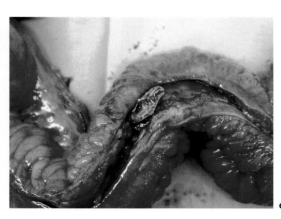

d

Pacemakers

The use of VCE has been contraindicated in patients with cardiac pacemakers. Unfortunately, pacemakers are being used in an increasing percentage of our population that subsequently will be excluded from the benefits of VCE. Our approach is to explain the risks and benefits of the procedure and consult the patient's cardiologist for approval of the procedure. The patient can be hospitalized in the telemetry unit for the duration of the procedure or it can be performed on an outpatient basis. As per the general experience, we have had no problems with using VCE in patients with pacemakers (Lewis 2002). A recent prospective study on 100 patients with cardiac pacemakers revealed that four of the patients had CE electromagnetic interference as determined by using an external Test Cap (Given Imaging Ltd., Yoqneam, Israel) (Dubner et al. 2005). The interference was clinically insignificant, and the patients had no adverse outcomes. The study concluded that VCE appears to be safe in patients with pacemakers. They suggested that an external Test Cap should be used to exclude any possible adverse interference between the CE and pacemaker before initiating the VCE study (◘ Fig. 10-22). The Test Cap is a device that reproduces the effect of the CE by transmitting the same frequency. Leighton's studies have shown the safety of CE in patients with pacemakers and cardiac defibrillators (Leighton et al. 2004, 2005), as well as a study by Payeras et al. 2005, which confirm our clinical experience.

The performance of VCE in patients with pacemakers and defibrillators is still a relative contraindication. In practice we hospitalize these patients for telemetry monitoring during the exam. We have not had any adverse events during VCE in patients with pacemakers. The use of endoscopic-assisted capsule endoscopy to avoid close approximation of the capsule to the pacemaker and the use of the »cap test« in patients with a pacemaker deserves further study.

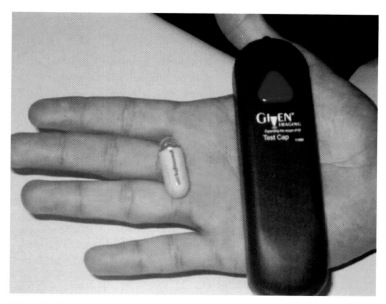

◘ **Fig. 10-22.** Capsule endoscope and Test Cap

References

Arifuddin RM, Baichi MM, Mantry PS (2005) Small bowel capsule impaction and successful endoscopic retrieval. Clin Gastroenterol Hepatol 3:A34

Barkin JS, Friedman S (2002) Wireless capsule endoscopy requiring surgical intervention: the world's experience. Am J Gastroenterol 97 [Suppl]:S298

Barkin JS, O'Loughlin C (2004) Capsule endoscopy contraindications: complications and how to avoid their occurrence. Gastrointest Endosc Clin N Am 14:61–65

Boivin ML, Voderholzer W, Lochs H (2005) Does passage of a Patency Capsule indicate small bowel patency? A prospective trial. Endoscopy 37:808–815

Buchkremer F, Herrmann T, Stremmel W (2004) Mild respiratory distress after wireless capsule endoscopy. Gut 53:472

De Luca L, Di George P, Rivellini G et al (2003) Capsule endoscopy: experience in southern Italy. 2nd International Conference on Capsule Endoscopy, Berlin, 23–25 March 2003

Dubner S, Dubner Y, Gallino S et al (2005) Electromagnetic interference with implantable cardiac pacemakers by video capsule. Gastrointest Endosc 61:250–254

Fleischer DE, Heigh R, Nguyen CC et al (2003) Videocapsule impaction at the cricopharyngeus: first report of this complication and its successful resolution. Gastrointest Endosc 57:427–428

Fry LC, De Petris G, Swain JM, Fleischer DE (2005) Impaction and fracture of a video capsule in the small bowel requiring laparotomy for removal of the capsule fragments. Endoscopy 37:674–676

Gay G, Delvaux M, Laurent V, Reibel N et al (2005) Temporary intestinal occlusion induced by a »patency capsule« in a patient with Crohn's disease. Endoscopy 37:174–177

Ge ZZ, Hu YB, Xiao SD (2004) Capsule endoscopy in diagnosis of small bowel Crohn's disease. World J Gastroenterol 10:1349–1352

Girelli CM, Amato A, Rocca F (2004) Easy ultrasound detection of retained video endoscopy capsule. J Gastroenterol Hepatol 19:241

Gortzak Y, Lantsberg L, Odes HS (2003) Video Capsule entrapped in a Meckel's diverticulum. J Clin Gastroenterol 37:270–271

Keuchel M, Hagenmüller F (2002) Small bowel endoscopy with the wireless video capsule. Dtsch Ärztebl 99:A2702–2710

Keuchel M, Thaler C, Csomós G et al (2003) Video capsule endoscopy: technical and medical failures. Endoscopy 35 [Suppl]:A6

Knapp AB, Ladetsky L (2005) Endoscopic retrieval of a small bowel enteroscopy capsule lodged in a Zenker's diverticulum. Clin Gastroenterol Hepatol 3:xxxiv

Leighton JA, Sharma VK, Srivathsan K et al (2004) Safety of capsule endoscopy in patients with pacemakers. Gastrointest Endosc 59:567–569

Leighton JA, Srivathsan K, Carey EJ et al (2005) Safety of wireless capsule endoscopy in patients with implantable cardiac defibrillators. Am J Gastroenterol 100:1728–1731

Leung WK, Sung JJY (2004) Endoscopically assisted video capsule endoscopy. Endoscopy 36:562–564

Lewis BS (2002) Complications and contraindications in capsule endoscopy. Gastroenterology 122:A330

Lewis BS (2005) How to prevent endoscopic capsule retention. Endoscopy 37:852–853

Madisch A, Schimming W, Kinzel F et al (2003) Locally advanced small-bowel adenocarcinoma missed primarily by capsule endoscopy but diagnosed by push enteroscopy. Endoscopy 35:861–864

May A, Nachbar L, Ell C (2005) Extraction of entrapped capsules from the small bowel by means of push-and-pull enteroscopy with the double-balloon technique. Endoscopy 37:591–593

Morandi E, Passoni GR, Stillittano D et al (2003) An unusual complication: capsule endoscopy in the bronchial tree. 2nd International Conference on Capsule Endoscopy, Berlin, 23–25 March 2003

Mow WS, Lo SK, Targan SR et al (2004) Initial experience with wireless capsule enteroscopy in the diagnosis and management of inflammatory bowel disease. Clin Gastroenterol Hepatol 2:31–40

Payeras G, Piqueras J, Moreno VJ et al (2005) Effects of capsule endoscopy on cardiac pacemakers. Endoscopy 37:1181–1185

Schneider AR, Hoepffner N, Rösch W, Caspary WF (2003) Aspiration of an M2A capsule. Endoscopy 35:713

Sears DM, Avots-Avotins A, Culp K, Gavin MW (2004) Frequency and clinical outcome of capsule retention during capsule endoscopy for GI bleeding of obscure origin. Gastrointest Endosc 60:822–827

Sinn I, Neef B, Andus T (2004) Aspiration of a capsule endoscope. Gastrointest Endosc 59:926–927

Tabib S, Fuller C, Daniels J, Lo SK (2004) Asymptomatic aspiration of a capsule endoscope. Gastrointest Endosc 60:845–848

Van Gossum A, Hittelet A, Schmit A et al (2003) A prospective comparative study of push and wireless-capsule enteroscopy in patients with obscure digestive bleeding. Acta Gastroenterol Belg 66:199–205

10

Pediatric Findings

E.G. Seidman, G.L. De' Angelis, M. Thomson, F. Costea, A.M.G.A. Sant'Anna, M.H. Dirks

Introduction

Almost all but the most proximal and distal segments of the small bowel are essentially out of range of current endoscopes and enteroscopes. In adults, push enteroscopy can theoretically visualize the small bowel, but generally only the proximal areas of the jejunum, up to about 150 cm distal to the pylorus. Moreover, the need of an overtube (15 mm) limits the applicability of this relatively invasive technique in children (MacKenzie 1999). Alternatively, the entire small bowel can be visualized using intraoperative enteroscopy. However, this necessitates abdominal laparotomy or laparoscopy, with potential complications such as prolonged postoperative ileus, obstruction, perforation, and fistula formation (Waye 2003). Double-balloon enteroscopy is a novel method which has shown promising initial results for achieving complete enteroscopy and providing therapy without requiring laparotomy (Yamamoto et al. 2004). However, this technique requires a long period of manipulation and its availability is limited, with no experience in pediatric patients reported to date. Thus, the small bowel has justifiably been deemed the last uncharted frontier in terms of endoscopic visualization in pediatric patients (Seidman et al. 2004).

The recent invention of an ingestible, wireless capsule endoscope has, for the first time, enabled the visualization of the entire small bowel in a noninvasive manner. This ingenious technological discovery was achieved by scientists in Israel who miniaturized the components necessary to transmit video signals to an external data recorder (Iddan et al. 2000) (Chap. 1.1). The ultrashort focal length of the lens (1 mm) permits highly detailed imaging of the intestinal mucosa as the capsule transits along in a forward or backward orientation through the lumen, without requiring insufflation of air. »Red-outs« are thus not problematic, as in the case of standard endoscopic procedures. The remarkable resolution of the lens (0.1 mm) yields extraordinarily detailed, high-quality images of the mucosa, including the ability to visualize normal villi (◘ Fig. 11-1a). Consequently, the clear identification of areas of villous atrophy is made possible as never before seen by any endoscopic device (◘ Fig. 11-1b, c). The goals of this review are to provide representative images that illustrate the key indications and findings of video capsule endoscopy in the pediatric age group.

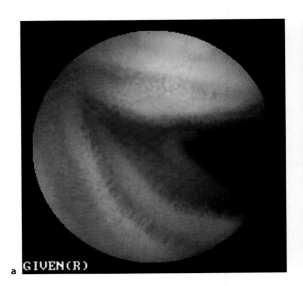

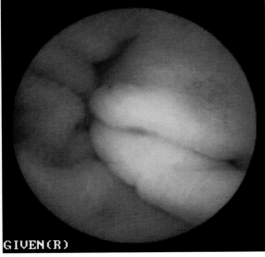

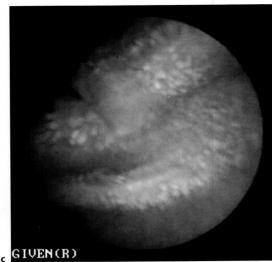

◘ **Fig. 11-1. a** The extraordinary resolution of the capsule endoscope is capable of revealing the minute features of normal small bowel mucosa, such as the feathery, hair-like microvilli. **b** Capsule study in a child with atopic dermatitis and food allergies, showing discrete changes in the small bowel mucosa, not detected by other endoscopic or imaging studies: edematous proximal jejunal folds, atrophy of microvilli, and focal erythema. **c** Capsule study reveals focal inflammatory changes in the small bowel mucosa in an adolescent with indeterminate colitis. The microvilli are broad and »white-tipped« and focally atrophied, with a small linear mucosal break

Clinical Indications in Pediatrics

Several studies in adult populations have demonstrated that video capsule endoscopy is a highly effective and safe method to explore the small bowel for obscure causes of bleeding, inflammatory disorders such as Crohn's and celiac disease, as well as tumors (Costamagna et al. 2002; Ell et al. 2002; Pennazio et al. 2004; Triester et al. 2004; Petroniene et al. 2005; de Mascarenhas-Saraiva and da Silva Araujo Lopes 2003). To date, relatively few studies have been carried out in children. On the basis of our recent trial in Montreal (Sant'Anna et al. 2005), the Given M2A capsule was approved for the investigation of disorders of the small bowel in children and adolescents above age 10 by both the Food and Drug Administration in the USA and Health Protection Branch of Health and Welfare Canada. Potential indications of video capsule endoscopy in the pediatric age group are summarized in ◘ Table 11-1.

◘ **Table 11-1.** Potential indications for video capsule endoscopy in pediatric patients

Small bowel inflammatory disorders

Crohn's disease; celiac disease; food allergic or eosinophilic enteropathies; intestinal vasculitis; Henoch-Schönlein purpura; drug-induced mucosal injury (nonsteroidal anti-inflammatory or chemotherapy); radiation entero-pathy; graft-versus-host disease; intestinal transplantation

Small bowel polyps and tumors

Peutz-Jeghers syndrome, other familial and nonfamilial polyposes; lymphoma, leiomyoma, carcinoid and other tumors; suspected Kaposi's sarcoma in AIDS

Occult or obscure intestinal bleeding

Including vascular malformations, portal hypertension, and small bowel varices

Abnormal findings on small bowel imaging

Unexplained malabsorption and protein-losing enteropathies

Intestinal lymphangiectasia, allergic or congestive enteropathies, etc.

Chronic abdominal pain with high suspicion of small bowel pathology

Motility disorders

Esophageal disorders[a]

Esophagitis, Barrett's esophagus, esophageal varices

[a] Requires use of the two-sided ESO capsule with placement of chest leads

Inflammatory Disorders

Whereas in adults, obscure bleeding is the most common indication for video capsule endoscopy, ruling out Crohn's disease accounted for the majority of studies in the pediatric age group (Sant'Anna and Seidman 2003). In our recent prospective study (Sant'Anna et al. 2005), video capsule endoscopy was found to be highly useful for the investigation of »obscure« small bowel Crohn's disease. The latter was defined as Crohn's disease which is clinically suspected, but not proven by conventional methods such as complete ileocolonoscopy with biopsies and barium imaging of the upper gastrointestinal (GI) tract and small bowel (Sant'Anna et al. 2005). The diagnostic yield was high (60%) in this inflammatory category, with Crohn's disease or eosinophilic gastroenteropathy diagnosed only by capsule (vs 0% for conventional imaging) (Sant'Anna et al. 2005). Another study in adolescents yielded similar results (58.3 vs 0%) for Crohn's disease missed by conventional imaging (Arguelles-Arias et al. 2004). In some cases, identification of lesions compatible with Crohn's disease by video capsule endoscopy (◘ Fig. 11-2a, b) precluded laparoscopic assessment to rule out a possible intestinal lymphoma. Moreover, in the approximately 40% of cases with negative exams, Crohn's disease of the small bowel could be definitively excluded by video capsule endoscopy. Other imaging techniques have been shown to have higher false-positive results. Video capsule endoscopy is also potentially useful for the reassessment of small bowel Crohn's disease after therapy to objectively demonstrate the degree of mucosal healing of the small bowel or to diagnose a relapse (◘ Fig. 11-2c) in a noninvasive manner.

Findings of obscure small bowel Crohn's disease uncovered by video capsule endoscopy included inflammatory strictures in addition to typical mucosal ulcerations (◘ Fig. 11-2d) and other inflammatory changes such as pseudopolyps (◘ Fig. 11-2e) or the presence of white-tipped villi (◘ Fig. 11-1c). In our experience, a normal barium study does not exclude one or more small bowel stenoses resulting in capsule retention (Seidman et al. 2004; Sant'Anna et al. 2005). Video capsule endoscopy has also been helpful in identifying (as well as excluding) small bowel lesions in patients with »indeterminate« colitis, allowing for a change in diagnosis and precluding colectomy for the wrong indication (◘ Figs. 11-1c and 11-2f).

The findings found to be most characteristic of eosinophilic gastroenteropathy included marked focal villous atrophy, with clearly delineated areas of erythematous, glossy mucosa adjacent to normal villi. Focal areas of mucosal edema and denudation were also commonly seen (◘ Fig. 6.3-1a), but are less specific findings. Strictures and polyps were also found in this disorder (◘ Fig. 6.3-1b, c). The children with eosinophilic gastroenteropathy diagnosed by video capsule endoscopy presented with a protein-losing enteropathy. Video capsule endoscopy in this latter clinical setting in pediatric patients has also been reported to yield a diagnosis of obscure Crohn's disease (Barkay et al. 2005).

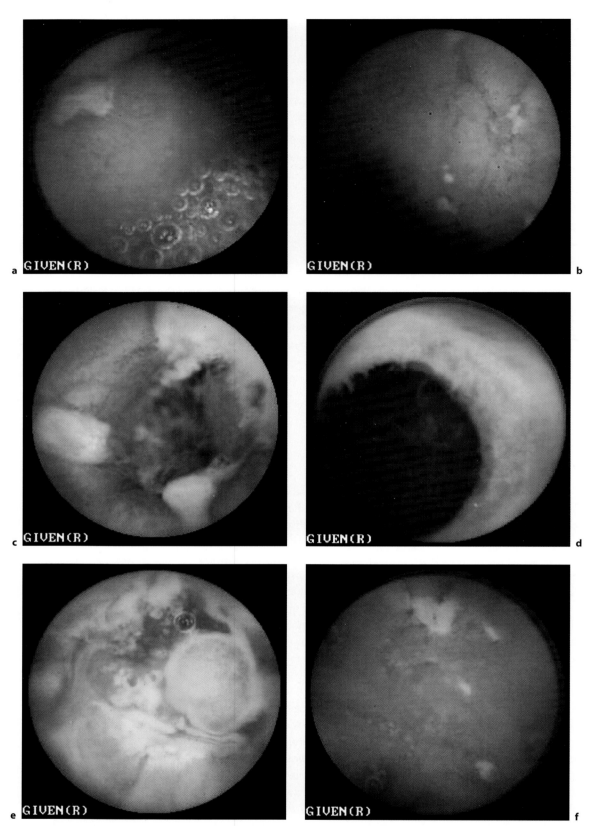

■ **Fig. 11-2.** **a** Capsule image of one of numerous small bowel ulcerations in an 11-year-old male with »obscure« Crohn's disease. Despite suggestive characteristic symptoms and signs, as well as biological markers (anemia, high CRP, positive ASCA serology), all other imaging, endoscopic, and even histopathological evidence of Crohn's disease had been lacking. The focal ulceration is covered with exudates and surrounded by erythema. **b** Focal ulcerations and mucosal fissuring in an adolescent female whose initial presentation of Crohn's disease was massive obscure GI bleeding. The capsule exam was able to establish the diagnosis of Crohn's disease and avoided a laparotomy. A prior colonoscopy had only revealed active bleeding coming from the small bowel. The barium small bowel follow through was normal. **c** Relapse of Crohn's disease diagnosed at the ileocolonic anastomosis in an 18-year-old male patient with abdominal pain. The capsule was evacuated spontaneously. **d** Inflammatory stricture of the non-terminal ileum in an 18-year-old female with known Crohn's disease who presented with persistent abdominal pain and anemia. She had undergone a previous resection of the terminal ileum, and repeat colonoscopy as well as barium imaging of the small bowel had failed to reveal any recurrence of Crohn's disease. **e** A follow-up study in a 16-year-old male treated for Crohn's disease shows inflammatory pseudopolyps in the ileum. **f** Video capsule endoscopy in an 8-year-old girl with steroid-resistant indeterminate colitis revealed numerous lesions of the small bowel suggestive of Crohn's disease. A colectomy was averted in view of these findings, in favor of further medical therapy with infliximab

Although nonsteroidal anti-inflammatory drugs are less commonly employed in children, they commonly cause mucosal injury, including ulcerations that mimic Crohn's disease (Maiden et al. 2005; Goldstein et al. 2005). The drug-induced lesions may include mucosal breaks, focal ulcerations (⬛ Fig. 11-3a, b) as well as circumferential, ulcerated strictures (⬛ Fig. 11-3c). Histological confirmation of specific diagnoses suggested by video capsule endoscopy should thus always be considered, where feasible.

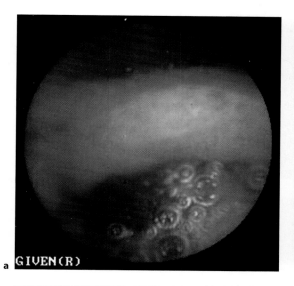

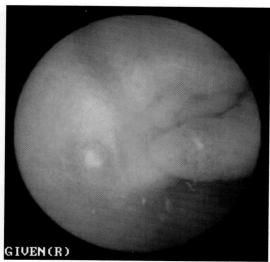

⬛ **Fig. 11-3a–c.** Small bowel lesions due to use of nonsteroidal anti-inflammatory drugs (NSAIDs) in pediatric patients. **a** Focal lesion on an ileal fold in a 15-year-old boy with spina bifida and use of NSAIDs for back pain. **b** Small aphthous-like ulcers in the proximal jejunum of an 11-year-old female with NSAID use for juvenile rheumatoid arthritis. **c** Ulcerated, circumferential stricture in an adolescent patient on chronic NSAIDs and methotrexate for polyarticular arthritis. The lesion is similar to that caused by Crohn's disease

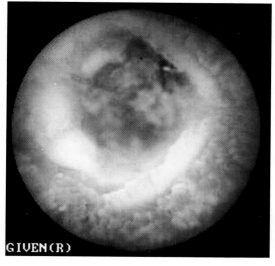

Polyposis Syndromes and Other Intestinal Tumors

Among adult patients, video capsule endoscopy has been shown to be highly efficient in detecting small bowel tumors that were missed by conventional endoscopic and imaging methods, including push enteroscopy (de Mascarenhas-Saraiva and da Silva Araujo Lopes 2003; Mata et al. 2004). Although small bowel malignancies are rare in children, inherited gastrointestinal polyposis disorders such as Peutz-Jeghers syndrome are not uncommonly seen by pediatric gastroenterologists and surgeons. Complications of these tumors include small bowel intussusception, bleeding, and less commonly malignancy. Surveillance of the small bowel for polyps in these disorders is difficult and current recommendations for management of these syndromes are ambiguous. In our recent pediatric capsule study (Sant'Anna et al. 2005), intestinal polyposes such as Peutz-Jeghers syndrome constituted the second most common indication for video capsule endoscopy. We observed 100% concordance between capsule identification of the presence or absence of small bowel polyps compared to previous imaging modalities (endoscopic and radiological) (Sant'Anna et al. 2005). Video capsule endoscopy was able to identify a far greater number of polyps per patient than the other imaging and endoscopic procedures in a noninvasive manner and without exposure to radiation (Sant'Anna et al. 2005). Others have reported similar results in familial adenomatous polyposis and Peutz-Jeghers syndrome (Soares et al. 2004; Caspari et al. 2004; Schulmann et al. 2005). Polyps less than 15 mm are better detected with video capsule endoscopy than magnetic resonance imaging (MRI) or other imaging studies (Caspari et al. 2004). Furthermore, 24% of patients with hereditary polyposis had jejunal or ileal polyps that were only detected by video capsule endoscopy (Schulmann et al. 2005). The available data thus suggest that video capsule endoscopy should replace barium X-rays, MRI, and push enteroscopy for the identification of small bowel polyps in the pediatric age group. The localization software can also guide the clinician to the possibility of reaching a polyp for removal endoscopically. Representative images are shown in ⬛ Figs. 11-4–11-7.

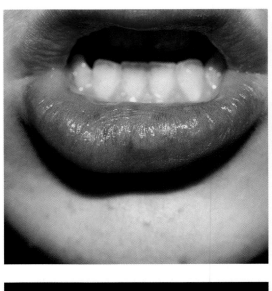

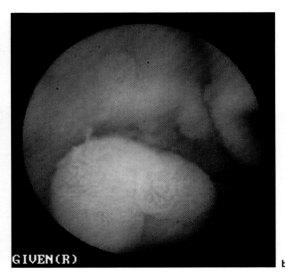

■ **Fig. 11-4a–d.** Peutz-Jeghers syndrome (PJS). A 13-year-old boy with perioral pigmentation (**a**), hyperplastic gastric polyps (**b**), pedunculated hamartomatous polyps in the jejunum and ileum (**c**) and colon (**d**)

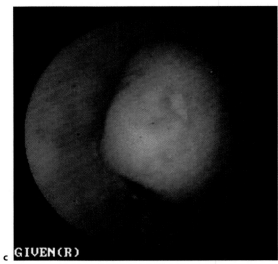

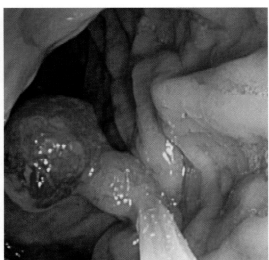

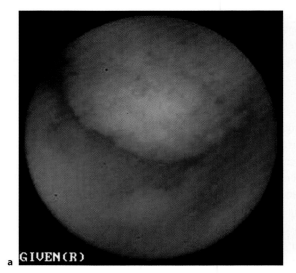

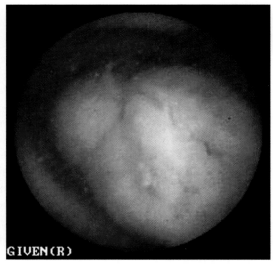

■ **Fig. 11-5. a** Large PJS polyp in the ileum of a 17-year-old male revealed by video capsule endoscopy. **b** Jejunal PJS polyp in another patient

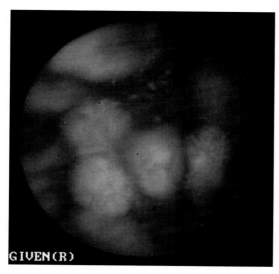

⬛ Fig. 11-6. Several small colonic PJS polyps in an 11-year-old girl seen at video capsule endoscopy

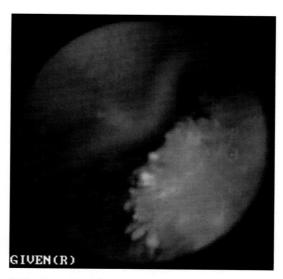

⬛ Fig. 11-7. Distal duodenal polyp discovered by video capsule endoscopy in a 12-year-old patient with a familial polyposis syndrome, missed at upper GI endoscopy and barium series. The capsule study directed the endoscopic removal and retrieval of the polyp

Occult or Obscure Intestinal Bleeding

The first and still most common indication for video capsule endoscopy in adult studies has been the identification of a source of bleeding in patients with visible blood loss of obscure origin (Costamagna et al. 2002; Ell et al. 2002; Pennazio et al. 2004). Obscure bleeding is defined as bleeding of unknown origin that persists or recurs (recurrent or persistent visible bleeding, iron-deficiency anemia with positive fecal occult blood testing) after a negative initial or primary endoscopy (upper and/or lower endoscopy) (Pennazio et al. 2005). The source of bleeding is frequently located in the small bowel and may result from a number of conditions, including vascular lesions and inflammatory lesions, or tumors. Imaging techniques for evaluation of the small bowel are relatively insensitive for intestinal bleeding lesions that are flat, small, infiltrative, or inflammatory. Angiography and radioisotope bleeding scans are insensitive in the absence of brisk active bleeding. As noted above, intraoperative enteroscopy is the most thorough, but also the most invasive means to visualize the small bowel. Although push enteroscopy is an effective diagnostic procedure, it is time consuming and only allows the exploration of the proximal jejunum. Double-balloon enteroscopy is the newest method that offers the possibility of achieving complete small bowel enteroscopy and providing therapy without the need of laparotomy. However, accessibility to this method is not widespread and pediatric experience is highly limited. The key advantages of video capsule endoscopy for patients with obscure intestinal bleeding have recently been reviewed (Pennazio et al. 2005). They include the ability to image the entire small bowel noninvasively, with-

out radiation exposure, the superior clarity of the images compared to other endoscopic devices, the ability to review and share images, patient preference, safety profile, and the ability to conduct the testing in a variety of settings.

Little pediatric experience has been published to date in terms of experience with video capsule endoscopy in the clinical setting of pediatric patients with obscure GI bleeding. In our recent study (Sant'Anna et al. 2005), a diagnosis of arteriovenous malformations or angiectasia as the source of obscure bleeding in the small bowel was confirmed using the capsule in 3/4 of children and adolescents. Other imaging techniques (upper and lower endoscopies as well as selective mesenteric angiography) had failed to identify the source of bleeding in any of these cases. Video capsule endoscopy has been found to be a useful tool for diagnosing and monitoring the effects of therapy in patients with blue rubber bleb nevus syndrome (De Bona et al. 2005). We have also diagnosed cases of bleeding from small bowel varices in pediatric cases with portal hypertension (⬛ Fig. 11-8) and from ulcers due to Crohn's disease or NSAIDs (⬛ Figs. 11-2b and 11-3). Other bleeding lesions can include angiodysplastic lesions, erosions, and Meckel's diverticulum (⬛ Figs. 11-9–11-11).

Despite the limited pediatric data to date, studies in adults have supported the use of video capsule endoscopy in order to reduce the number of diagnostic procedures in such cases and has been recommended as the initial diagnostic choice in the face of chronic GI bleeding after negative upper and lower colonoscopies (Costamagna et al. 2002; Ell et al. 2002; Pennazio et al. 2004; Pennazio et al. 2005).

11

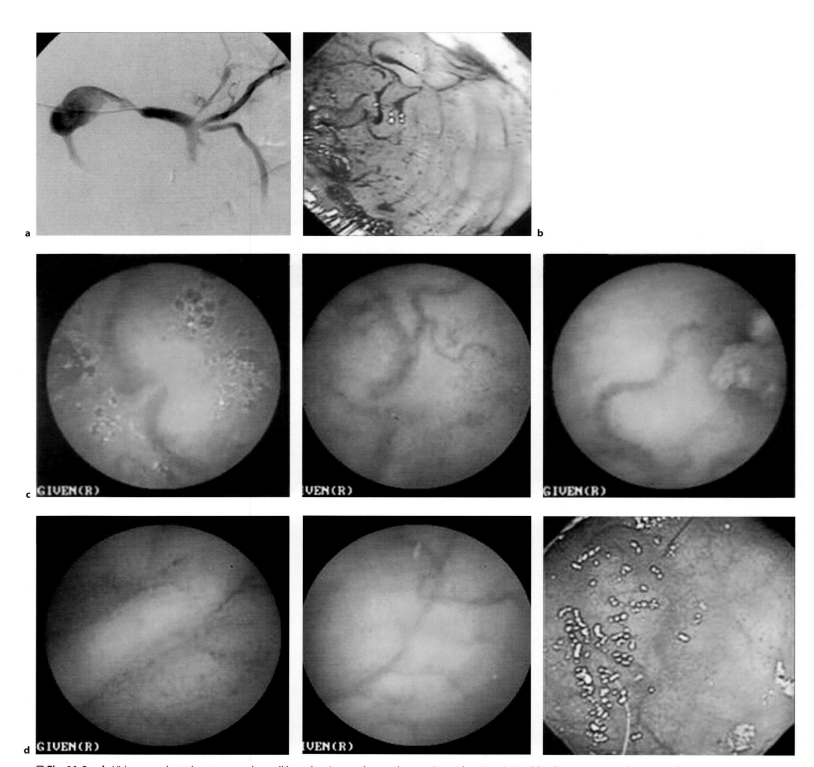

■ **Fig. 11-8a–d.** Video capsule endoscopy reveals small bowel varices undetected by other endoscopic and imaging tests. The patient is a 15-year-old female with Alagille syndrome, presenting with obscure GI bleeding 12 years post liver transplant. **a** Transhepatic portography revealing portal vein stenosis with poststenotic dilatation. Contrast demonstrates perigastric and perisplenic varices (portal and mesenteric pressures 18 mmHg). **b** Colonoscopy revealed non-bleeding recto-sigmoid varices. Active bleeding was seen to be coming from proximal to the ileo-cecal valve. **c** Video capsule endoscopy revealed several varices in the distal small bowel. The portal vein stenosis was dilated angiographically and a stent was placed. Small bowel bleeding subsequently stopped. **d** Repeat video capsule endoscopy revealed only one slightly prominent small bowel vein (*left*), and colonoscopy confirmed disappearance of the rectosigmoid varices (*right*)

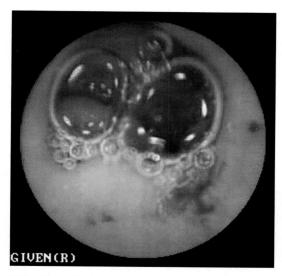

Fig. 11-9. Bleeding erosion in the ileum of an 8-year-old boy with anemia and positive fecal occult blood tests

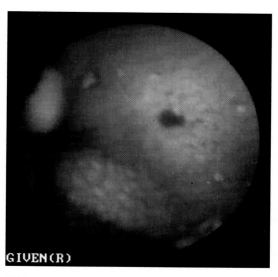

Fig. 11-10. Angiectasia in the ileum in a 3-year-old child with anemia and occult GI bleeding. Previous investigations had failed to reveal a source of bleeding

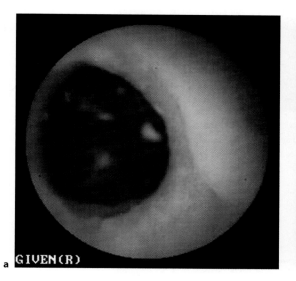

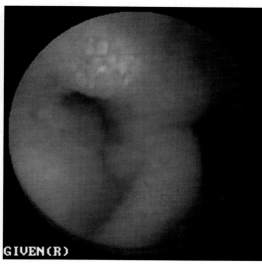

Fig. 11-11. a Meckel's diverticulum in a 14-year-old boy with iron deficiency anemia (hemoglobin 6.4 g/dl) and positive fecal occult blood tests. The patient was referred to surgery without prior scintigraphy, and the diagnosis was confirmed. **b** Orifice of a Meckel's diverticulum with small ulcer in another patient

Celiac Disease

A pilot study (Petroniene et al. 2005) showed that video capsule endoscopy, as interpreted by an experienced observer, was highly sensitive and specific for the diagnosis of untreated celiac disease in adult patients with moderate to severe villous atrophy. However, little prospective data have been reported. Murray et al. (2004) reported 38 adult patients ultimately shown to have celiac disease, in whom approximately 90% had changes suggestive of atrophy on capsule study. This was substantially higher than the rate of atrophic changes on prior upper endoscopy. Recently, a group of highly regarded experts published a consensus report on the role of video capsule endoscopy in celiac disease (Cellier et al. 2005). It was felt that there was adequate evidence to support the use of video capsule endoscopy in patients who have treated, previously confirmed celiac disease who had developed alarm symptoms. However, such cases of »efractory sprue« or lymphoma compli-

cating celiac disease are exceedingly rare in pediatrics. The consensus panel did feel that video capsule endoscopy may have a future role as an initial diagnostic test for confirming atrophy in patients who are seropositive. Video capsule endoscopy was recommended as an alternative to biopsy in selected patients who are unwilling or unable to undergo upper endoscopy for confirmation of villous atrophy (Cellier et al. 2005). The findings that are characteristic of celiac disease are summarized in ◘ Table 11-2, and a representative case is illustrated in ◘ Fig. 11-12.

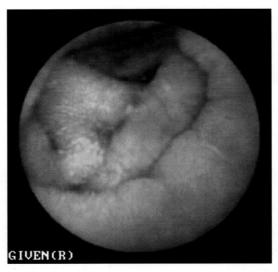

◘ **Table 11-2.** Video capsule endoscopy findings of the small bowel mucosa suggestive of celiac disease[a]

Fissuring
Scalloping
Mosaic pattern
Nodularity
Late appearance of villi (absence of villi detected in the duodenum and proximal jejunum)
Loss of circular folds

[a] The identification of at least two of these findings, confirmed by experienced observers, is considered suggestive of celiac disease

◘ **Fig. 11-12.** Video capsule endoscopy in an adolescent with an uncertain diagnosis of celiac disease, undergoing a gluten challenge (3 months). Video capsule endoscopy revealed scalloped fold in the distal duodenum (D3-4) with focal villous atrophy

Other Indications

In addition to the more common indications that have been tested and discussed above, video capsule endoscopy is likely to prove clinically useful for a variety of other potential disorders of the small bowel in the pediatric age group (◘ Table 11-1). The identification of abnormal but undiagnosed findings on small bowel imaging is a worthwhile indication for capsule study. Pathologies that have been uncovered include small bowel lymphomas (◘ Fig. 11-13). In our experience (Peretti et al. 2005), video capsule endoscopy represents the diagnostic imaging method of choice to detect intestinal lymphangiectasia (◘ Fig. 11-14). We have also diagnosed chronic intussusception and ischemic bowel disease as causes of recurrent abdominal pain by video capsule endoscopy in adolescent patients (◘ Fig. 11-15). Video capsule endoscopy can also be useful to ascertain the intestinal manifestations of immunodeficiency disorders (Mihaly et al. 2005) (◘ Fig. 6.5-8) as well as graft-versus-host disease (Yakoub-Agha et al. 2005) (Chap. 6.7). It is not uncommon to observe lymphoid hyperplasia of the distal ileum in normal children and adolescents (◘ Figs. 11-16 and 11-17). However, an immunodeficiency was evoked by a capsule study that showed extensive multifocal lymphoid hyperplasia of the duodenum and ileum (◘ Fig. 11-18). The ultimate diagnosis was IgA deficiency. The timed movement of the capsule through various segments of the GI tract (gastric emptying time, small bowel transit time) can also serve as a useful tool in the assessment of children with motility disorders.

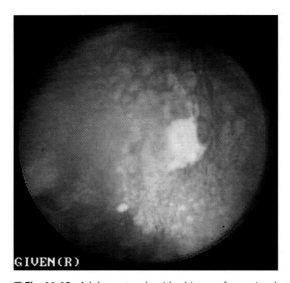

◘ **Fig. 11-13.** Adolescent male with a history of a previously treated lymphoma presents with abdominal pain of uncertain etiology. Video capsule endoscopy revealed an ulcerated »bulge« in the distal ileum. Surgical resection confirmed a recurrence of the lymphoma

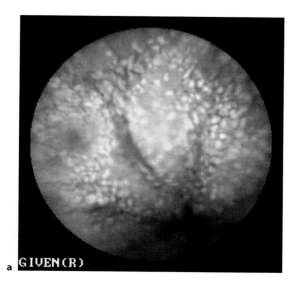

a GIVEN(R)

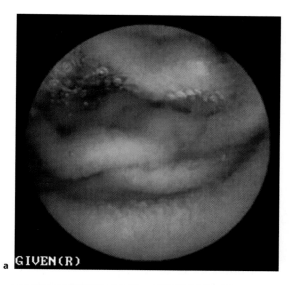

a GIVEN(R)

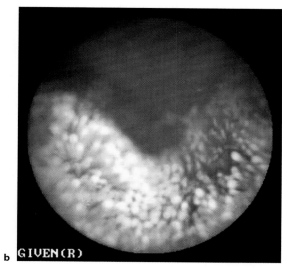

b GIVEN(R)

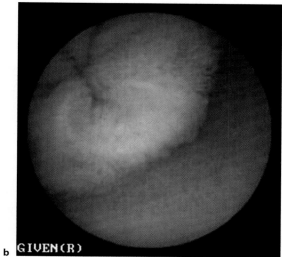

b GIVEN(R)

■ **Fig. 11-14a, b.** **a** Intestinal lymphangiectasia diagnosed by video capsule endoscopy in a 30-month-old child referred for a protein-losing enteropathy and anasarca. An incidental phlebectasia was noted. **b** Example from another patient with intestinal lymphangiectasia

■ **Fig. 11.15.** **a** Jejunal intussusception, with a small mucosal erosion on the lead point. **b** Persistence of the same intussusception for well over an hour, as recorded by video capsule endoscopy. The patient is an adolescent male who presented with abdominal pain, of uncertain relation to the intussusception. The small bowel was otherwise normal

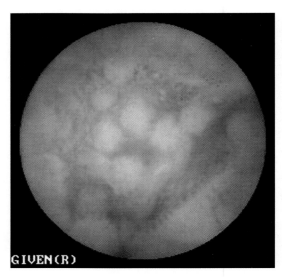

■ **Fig. 11-16.** Lymphoid follicular hyperplasia in a 9-year-old boy observed at video capsule endoscopy

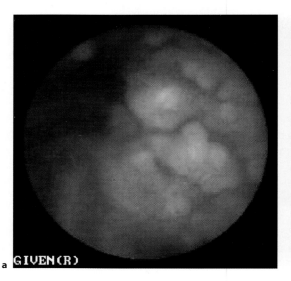

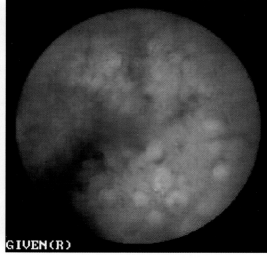

■ **Fig. 11-17a, b.** Lymphoid follicular hyperplasia in an 18-year-old male with rectal bleeding. Small prominent vessels are seen in **b**

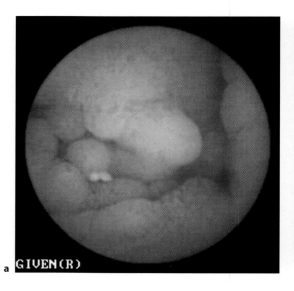

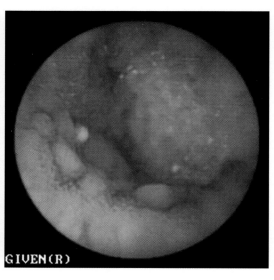

■ **Fig. 11-18a, b.** Lymph node hyperplasia in atypical locations revealed by capsule study (duodenum in **a**, mid small bowel in **b**) was a tip-off that this 9-year-old had an immunodeficiency. Selective IgA deficiency was subsequently confirmed

Practical Issues

Video capsule endoscopy is very well tolerated in children able to swallow the capsule, usually above the age of 9. It is far better appreciated by young patients than other imaging techniques, as patients can even return to school or go about their usual daily activities, even during the exam. In our experience, video capsule endoscopy does not routinely require a bowel preparation or the use of a prokinetic drug in children. However, the clinician should ascertain if there is any history suggestive of gastroparesis or if medications are being used (e.g., narcotics) which may interfere with gastric emptying. Patients should be fasting for at least 8 h prior to the test. We generally permit patients to drink clear fluids 1–2 h after the study has begun and to eat a light meal about 2 h after ingesting the capsule.

One of the key considerations prior to undertaking video capsule endoscopy in a child is to ascertain the patient's ability to swallow the relatively large capsule. Although a common problem in children under the age of 8, this may even be encountered in older children and adolescents. For individuals judged unable to swallow the capsule, or for patients with gastroparesis, severe dysphagia, or swallowing disorders, the study can be safely undertaken by introducing the capsule into the proximal duodenum endoscopically under direct vision, as discussed in Chap. 1.4.1. Currently, our preferred method is to »front load« the capsule on a gastroscope (Seidman et al. 2004; Barth et al. 2004), holding it in place using either a Dormia basket, the Roth net, or a specific device designed for the PillCam video capsule, as shown in ◘ Figs. 11-19 and 11-20.

Another important consideration is the limiting age or size that will permit the capsule to pass through the pylorus and ileocecal valve. While guidelines are not yet available, we have successfully employed

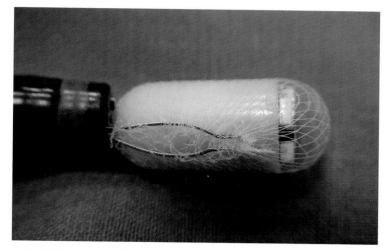

◘ **Fig. 11-19.** Method of »front loading« the PillCam onto a gastroscope using a Roth net

the capsule in children as young as 3 years of age. The critical limiting factor appears to be the size, rather than the age of the child. In our experience, the lower weight limit is approximately 17 kg.

Finally, intestinal strictures or other obstructing lesions (tumors, adhesions) are a contraindication to study, as they may preclude the capsule's passage and a bowel obstruction may theoretically ensue. It is advisable to demonstrate luminal patency in patients with Crohn's disease or in those with obstructive symptoms prior to capsule study. However, stenoses are not always excluded despite negative barium studies. We have had success in predicting tolerance to and passage of the PillCam by first employing a same sized, dissolvable »Patency« Capsule for such cases.

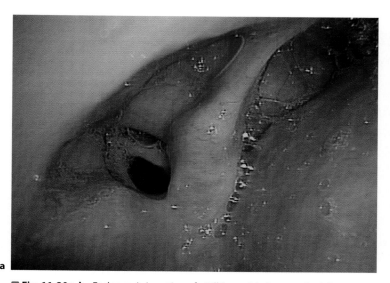

a

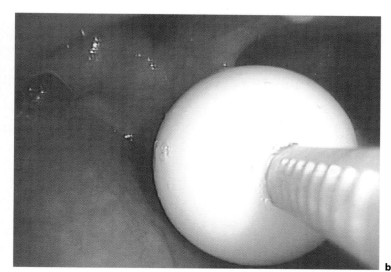

b

◘ **Fig. 11-20a, b.** Endoscopic insertion of a PillCam with the capsule delivery device in a 17-year-old female unable to swallow the capsule. **a** Endoscopic view of the larynx. **b** The front-loaded capsule is advanced under direct visualization into the esophagus

Summary

Wireless capsule endoscopy represents an extraordinary technical innovation in diagnostic gastrointestinal endoscopy. As in adult patients, it opens new horizons that permit an accurate and noninvasive approach to identify occult lesions in the small bowel in children and adolescents. A limitation in children is the size of the capsule, precluding its use in infants and very young children. In school-age children unable to swallow the capsule, »front loading« the gastroscope to introduce it into the duodenum is a suitable alternative approach.

References

Arguelles-Arias F, Caunedo A, Romero J et al (2004) The value of capsule endoscopy in pediatric patients with a suspicion of Crohn's disease. Endoscopy 36:869–873

Barkay O, Moshkowitz M, Reif S (2005) Crohn's disease diagnosed by wireless capsule endoscopy in adolescents with abdominal pain, protein-losing enteropathy, anemia and negative endoscopic and radiologic findings. Isr Med Assoc J 7:262–263

Barth BA, Donovan K, Fox VL (2004) Endoscopic placement of the capsule endoscope in children. Gastrointest Endosc 60:818–821

Caspari R, von Falkenhausen M, Krautmacher C et al (2004) Comparison of capsule endoscopy and magnetic resonance imaging for the detection of polyps of the small intestine in patients with familial adenomatous polyposis or with Peutz-Jeghers' syndrome. Endoscopy 36:1054–1059

Cellier C, Green PH, Collin P, Murray J (2005) ICCE consensus for celiac disease. Endoscopy 37:1055–1059

Costamagna G, Shah SK, Riccioni ME et al (2002) A prospective trial comparing small bowel radiographs and video capsule endoscopy for suspected small bowel disease. Gastroenterology 123:999–1005

De Bona M, Bellumat A, De Boni M (2005) Capsule endoscopy for the diagnosis and follow-up of blue rubber bleb nevus syndrome. Dig Liver Dis 37:451–453

de Mascarenhas-Saraiva MN, da Silva Araujo Lopes LM (2003) Small-bowel tumors diagnosed by wireless capsule endoscopy: report of five cases. Endoscopy 35:865–868

Ell C, Remke S, May A et al (2002) The first prospective controlled trial comparing wireless capsule endoscopy with push enteroscopy in chronic gastrointestinal bleeding. Endoscopy 34:685–689

Goldstein JL, Eisen GM, Lewis B et al (2005) Video capsule endoscopy to prospectively assess small bowel injury with celecoxib, naproxen plus omeprazole, and placebo. Clin Gastroenterol Hepatol 3:133–141

Iddan G, Meron G, Glukhovsky A, Swain P (2000) Wireless capsule endoscopy. Nature 405:417

MacKenzie JF (1999) Push enteroscopy. Gastrointest Endosc Clin N Am 9:29–36

Maiden L, Thjodleifsson B, Theodors A et al (2005) A quantitative analysis of NSAID-induced small bowel pathology by capsule enteroscopy. Gastroenterology 128:1172–1178

Mata A, Bordas JM, Feu F et al (2004) Wireless capsule endoscopy in patients with obscure gastrointestinal bleeding: a comparative study with push enteroscopy. Aliment Pharmacol Ther 20:189–194

Mihaly F, Nemeth A, Zagoni T et al (2005) Gastrointestinal manifestations of common variable immunodeficiency diagnosed by video- and capsule endoscopy. Endoscopy 37:603–604

Murray JA, Brogan D, Van dyke C et al (2004) Mapping the extent of untreated celiac disease with capsule enteroscopy. Gastrointest Endosc 59:AB101

Pennazio M, Eisen G, Goldfarb N (2005) ICCE consensus for obscure intestinal bleeding. Endoscopy 37:1046–1050

Pennazio M, Santucci R, Rondonotti E et al (2004) Outcome of patients with obscure gastrointestinal bleeding after capsule endoscopy: report of 100 consecutive cases. Gastroenterology 126:643–653

Peretti N, Sant'Anna AMGA, Dirks MH, Seidman EG (2005) Capsule endoscopy detects lymphangiectasia missed by other means. 4th International Conference on Capsule Endoscopy, Miami, FL, 7–8 March 2005, p 189

Petroniene R, Dubenco E, Baker JP et al (2005) Given capsule endoscopy in celiac disease: evaluation of diagnostic accuracy and interobserver variation. Am J Gastroenterol 100:685–694

Sant'Anna AMGA, Seidman EG (2003) Wireless capsule endoscopy: comparison study in pediatric and adult patients. J Pediatr Gastroenterol Nutr 37:332

Sant'Anna AMGA, Dubois J, Miron MJ, Seidman EG (2005) Wireless capsule endoscopy for obscure small bowel disorders: final results of the first pediatric controlled trial. Clin Gastroenterol Hepatol 3:264–270

Schulmann K, Hollerbach S, Kraus K et al (2005) Feasibility and diagnostic utility of video capsule endoscopy for the detection of small bowel polyps in patients with hereditary polyposis syndromes. Am J Gastroenterol 100:27–37

Seidman EG, Sant'Anna AMGA, Dirks MH (2004) Potential applications of wireless capsule endoscopy in the pediatric age group. Gastrointest Endosc Clin N Am 14:207–218

Soares J, Lopes L, Vilas Boas G, Pinho C (2004) Wireless capsule endoscopy for evaluation of phenotypic expression of small-bowel polyps in patients with Peutz-Jeghers syndrome and in symptomatic first-degree relatives. Endoscopy 36:1060–1066

Triester SL, Leighton JA, Gurudu SR et al (2004) A meta-analysis of capsule endoscopy (CE) compared to other modalities in patients with non-stricturing small bowel Crohn's disease (NSCD). Am J Gastroenterol 99:S271–S272

Waye JD (2003) Small-bowel endoscopy. Endoscopy 35:15–21

Yakoub-Agha I, Maunoury V, Wacrenier A et al (2005) Impact of small bowel exploration using video-capsule endoscopy in the management of acute gastrointestinal graft-versus-host disease. Transplantation 79:1767

Yamamoto H, Kita H, Sunada K et al (2004) Clinical outcomes of double-balloon endoscopy for the diagnosis and treatment of small-intestinal diseases. Clin Gastroenterol Hepatol 2:1010–1016

12

Influence of VCE on Clinical Outcome

L.C. Fry, F. Hagenmüller, D.E. Fleischer

Introduction

Video capsule endoscopy (VCE) has been demonstrated to be superior when compared with small bowel follow through (SBFT) and push enteroscopy for the evaluation of obscure gastrointestinal bleeding (OGIB) and clinically suspected Crohn's disease (CD) (Lewis and Swain 2002; Ell et al. 2002; Mylonaki et al. 2003; Saurin et al. 2003; Costamagna et al. 2002; Fireman et al. 2003; Herrerias et al. 2003; Triester et al. 2005, 2006). However, the usefulness of VCE for conditions such as chronic diarrhea, chronic abdominal pain, polyposis syndromes, and celiac disease has not been established (Bardan et al. 2003; Keuchel and Hagenmüller 2004). Because VCE is a new technique there are few prospective data evaluating clinical outcomes (Penazzio et al. 2004; Delvaux et al. 2004; Rastogi et al. 2004; Neu et al. 2005; Saurin et al. 2005). In this chapter we will review the evidence as to whether the use of this technology improves health outcomes, focusing on the two major established clinical indications for VCE, OGIB and suspected Crohn's disease.

Definition of Clinical Outcome

One measure of clinical outcome is the impact of this diagnostic technique on subsequent patient management and the patient's health. The findings of VCE may result in a therapeutic consequence or intervention, which can be active (i.e., invasive or medical therapy) or nonactive (no therapy). Negative as well as positive findings on VCE could minimize further examinations, resulting in improved patient's quality of life, less economic costs, and prompt treatment. The evaluation of clinical outcome must also include the evaluation of side effects and complications, which could have a negative impact on patient health and quality of life (Barkin and O'Loughlin 2004; Fleischer et al. 2003; Fry et al. 2005; Leighton et al. 2004). There are very few data on clinical outcomes in most diagnostic areas of gastroenterology. Nevertheless, many of the large studies using VCE have enough variables to analyze patients' clinical outcomes.

Outcome in Obscure Gastrointestinal Bleeding

Patients with OGIB represent approximately 5% of patients with gastrointestinal (GI) bleeding (Lewis 1994). Patients who have OGIB present diagnostic and therapeutic challenges because the source of bleeding is not identified by conventional radiological or endoscopic evaluation. Since the introduction of VCE, several publications have concluded that VCE has a better diagnostic yield than other techniques and is currently recommended as the first line in the work-up of OGIB patients (Penazzio et al. 2004; Delvaux et al. 2004; Triester et al. 2005). The most common lesions reported in patients with OGIB are angiectasia (◘ Figs. 12-1 and 12-2), ulcers, erosions, nonsteroidal anti-inflammatory drug (NSAID)-induced ulcers, and tumors (◘ Fig. 12-3). VCE has been compared mainly with push enteroscopy (PE) with all but one report revealing a higher yield of VCE, and in most of them with a significant statistical difference (Ell et al. 2002; Buchman and Wallin 2003; Hartmann et al. 2003; Mylonaki et al. 2003; Saurin et al. 2003; Mata et al. 2004; Van Gossum et al. 2003; Adler et al. 2004; Delvaux et al. 2004; Penazzio et al. 2004; Rastogi et al. 2004). Ell et al. (2002) found that VCE identified a definite source of bleeding in 21 of 32 (66%) patients studied and provided additional information not detected by push enteroscopy in 16 of 32 (50%) cases. In addition, all of their patients had undergone small bowel enteroclysis, which did not reveal any abnormality in any case (Ell et al. 2002). The most important studies evaluating the usefulness of VCE in OGIB are summarized in ◘ Table 12-1.

Of the published studies there are five that have included long-term follow-up data and evaluation of clinical outcome (Penazzio et al. 2004; Delvaux et al. 2004; Rastogi et al. 2004; Neu et al. 2005; Saurin et al. 2005). Penazzio et al. (2004) reported that the subsequent therapeutic approach after the findings on VCE led to a resolution of the clinical problem in 87% of patients with ongoing overt OGIB, in 41% of patients with previously overt OGIB, and in 69% of patients with occult OGIB. Delvaux et al. (2004) reported a positive predictive value of VCE of 94.4% in patients with intestinal lesions, and the negative predictive value was 100% in patients with normal VCE findings. In addition, the outcome of 77.3% of patients in this study was influenced by the findings of VCE. After

◘ **Table 12-1.** Yield of VCE compared with other techniques in patients with obscure gastrointestinal bleeding (OGIB). *A* angiectasia, *T* tumors, *IBD* aphthae, erosions, *B* blood, *U* ulcers, *PE* push enteroscopy

Author	Pts	Yield VCE (%)	Yield PE (%)	p	Complications	Findings during VCE
Lewis and Swain (2002)	20	55	30	NS	No	
Ell et al. (2002)	32	66	28	p<0.001	1 retention	A=53%, T=6%, IBD=6%
Buchman and Wallin (2003)	20	60	15	p=0.02	No	A=40%, IBD=10%, U=5%
Hartmann et al. (2003)	33	76	21	Not reported	No	A=46%, U=21%, T=3%
Mylonaki et al. (2003)	50	68	32	p<0.05	No	A=32%, B=16%, IBD=6%, T=4%
Saurin et al. (2003)	58	69	38	p<0.04	No	A=29, U=10, T=3%
Mata et al. (2004)	42	74	19	p=0.05		A=45%, B=23%, U=10%, T=6%
Van Gossum et al. (2003)	21	52	61	NS	1 retention in appendical stump	A=19%, T=4%, ileal varices=4%
Adler et al. (2004)	20	70	25	Not reported	No	B=25%, A=20, red spots 15%, U=5%

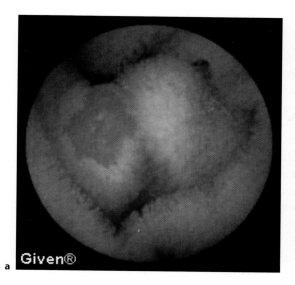

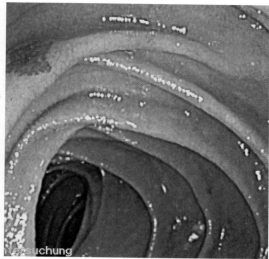

Fig. 12-1a, b. Large angiectasia. **a** VCE. **b** Push enteroscopy

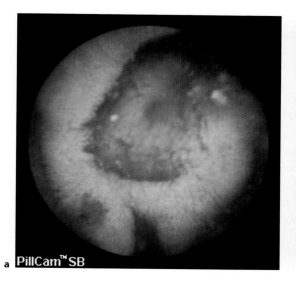

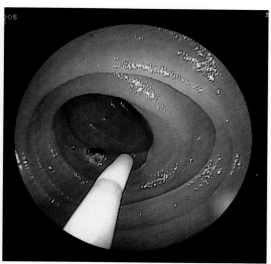

Fig. 12-2a, b. One of multiple angiectasias seen at VCE (**a**). After argon plasma coagulation of multiple angiectasias at double-balloon enteroscopy (**b**), bleeding stopped

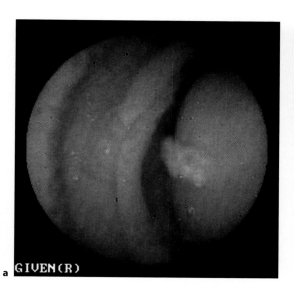

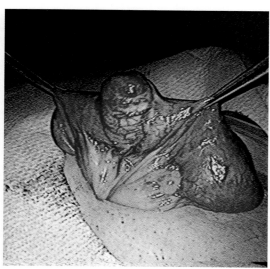

Fig. 12-3a, b. Jejunal gastrointestinal stromal tumor responsible for transfusion-dependent overt bleeding and detected by VCE (**a**). Guided by VCE finding, the tumor was removed by laparoscopically assisted minilaparotomy and segmental resection (**b**) (courtesy of Wolfgang Teichmann, M.D.)

appropriate endoscopic, medical, or surgical therapy, recurrent bleeding was observed in only one patient after a follow-up of 1 year. Also, they reported an important reduction of further endoscopies after VCE. A different plausible cause for anemia was found in all of the patients with negative VCE, resulting in a negative predictive value of 100% (Delvaux et al. 2004). Saurin et al. (2003) reported an additional diagnostic yield of VCE over PE of 36%. Not all of the authors report a significant number of patients with improved clinical outcome when studied with VCE. Rastogi et al. (2004) evaluated 44 patients with OGIB. The overall diagnostic yield was 42% (18 of 43) including angiodysplasias (n=13), intestinal ulcers (n=2), Crohn's disease (n=2), and a tumor (n=1). A specific intervention was carried out in 12 of 18 patients with positive findings. The authors followed the patients for a mean period of 6.7 months and considered the clinical outcome to be positive in only 16%.

A major deficiency in these studies is the failure to compare the outcomes of VCE to other methods. Neu et al. (2005) compared the impact of VCE vs push enteroscopy, angiography, and enteroclysis in 56 patients with OGIB. As the diagnostic yield was 68% for VCE and 38% for all other tests, it is concluded that VCE might be able to replace the other tests in decision making.

Maieron et al. (2004) reported therapy was altered, stopped, or initiated after VCE was performed in 58% of patients. It is evident that VCE results in a decreased number of endoscopic procedures when evaluating OGIB. In the study of Delvaux et al. (2004), the use of VCE as the first-line examination in patients with OGIB resulted in an important reduction of endoscopic procedures performed, not only in patients with positive findings but also in patients with negative findings avoiding future examinations.

Long-term follow-up of 47 patients with OGIB after VCE followed by intraoperative enteroscopy with argon plasma coagulation or resection showed a rebleeding rate of 26%, mainly due to angiectasias. None of the six patients with negative VCE examination had signs of rebleeding (Schmidt et al. 2005).

In several studies, VCE findings, especially angiectasias, were treated only in part (◘ Table 12-2). This therapy mainly involved coagulation

of angiectasias or surgical resection. In some cases, hormone therapy was started, which has no proven effect on outcome. With double-balloon enteroscopy becoming ever more available for the treatment of lesions detected during VCE (◘ Fig. 12-2), outcome data might change in the future.

Sometimes it may be necessary to repeat endoscopies in patients referred for VCE. Tang et al. (2004) found that 27% of lesions (8 of 29) were within reach of conventional endoscopy but that they had not been identified during the initial investigation. The percentage of patients with a bleeding source within reach of routine endoscopy but missed during pre-capsule endoscopy was significantly higher for those patients undergoing endoscopy only in the community (30%, 8 of 27) versus in the authors' center (0%, 0 of 19). In the landmark study of Costamagna et al. (2002) and the study of Rastogi et al. (2004), 14–30% of lesions found with VCE were within the reach of the endoscope. These three studies suggest that a »second-look« endoscopy may be considered before ordering VCE for obscure GI bleeding when local expertise is available (Tang et al. 2004). Saunders et al. (2004) have shown that the diagnostic yield of push enteroscopy for a small intestinal source following a negative VCE was zero, further supporting the use of VCE as the test of choice after initial negative upper and lower endoscopic evaluation in patients with OGIB.

Clinical Outcome in IBD

Another important indication for VCE is for the diagnosis of suspected inflammatory bowel disease (IBD) or the evaluation of patients with known IBD (◘ Fig. 12-4). VCE has proved to be an effective diagnostic procedure for patients with suspected IBD when previous conventional studies showed negative results [i.e., SBFT, computed tomography (CT) enterography]. The most important published clinical trials reported a diagnostic yield of VCE of 43–71% for lesions suggestive of CD (Eliakim et al. 2003; Fireman et al. 2003; Voderholzer et al. 2003; Costamagna et al. 2002; Liangpunsakul et al. 2003; Herrerias et al. 2003).

◘ **Table 12-2.** Long-term follow-up after VCE for obscure gastrointestinal bleeding (OGIB). *PE* push enteroscopy, *IOE* intraoperative enteroscopy

Authors	Follow-up		Diagnostic VCE				Neg. VCE	Comments
	n	Months	Yield	Angiectasias	Therapy	Rebleed	Rebleed	
Delvaux et al. (2004)	44	12	61%	50%	100%	12%	0%	1 death after surgery
Pennazio et al. (2004)	91	18	47%	46%	88%[a]	22%	54%	5 retentions
			92%		100%	14%	0%	Overt ongoing
			13%		50%	50%	62%	Overt previous
			44%		74%	20%	50%	Occult
Rastogi et al. (2004)	41	6.7	42%	72%	67%[b]	38%	80%	
Neu et al. (2005)	56	13	68%	71%	45%	56%	22%	VCE vs PE, radiology
								2 deaths after surgery
Saurin et al. (2005)	58	12	72%	71%	40%	19%	23%	
					61%			High bleeding potential
					28%			Intermediate bleeding potential
Schmidt et al. (2005)	47	11.5	70%	63%	100%	29%	0%	VCE and IOE; abstract

[a] Hormone therapy and iron supplementation included
[b] Hormone therapy included

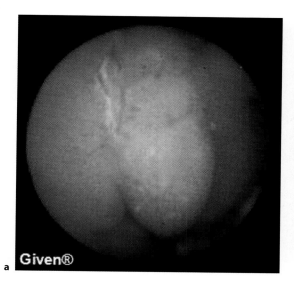
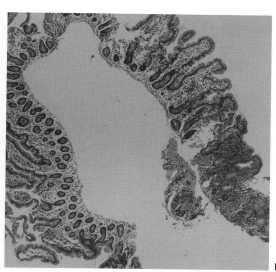

Fig. 12-4a, b. Crohn's disease. **a** Fissural ulcer of the jejunum seen at VCE. **b** Biopsy obtained at enteroscopy (H&E, courtesy of Wilhelm-Wolfgang Höpker, M.D.)

Eliakim et al. (2003) compared the yield of VCE vs SBFT and CT enterography in patients with suspected CD. VCE detected all the lesions detected by other methods and diagnosed lesions not detected by other modalities in 47% of cases. Patients diagnosed as CD patients were treated [5-aminosalicylic acid (5-ASA) or steroids] with significant clinical improvement. Fireman et al. (2003) were able to diagnose CD in 12 of 17 patients with suspected CD. Subsequently all of the patients were treated with 5-ASA and steroids with some or good clinical improvement in all of them. Voderholzer et al. (2003) reported a therapeutic impact of VCE of 24% overall: 17% in patients with established diagnosis of CD and 100% in patients with suspected CD. The change in treatment, based on VCE findings, led to clinical improvement in all patients. Liangpunsakul et al. (2003) found 3 of 40 patients (who underwent VCE for all indications) with multiple small bowel ulcers (with negative previous small bowel barium studies). All three patients improved after therapy for CD, having normal endoscopies and enteroclysis. Herrerias et al. (2003) confirmed CD in 9 of 21 patients studied with VCE. All of them clinically improved after treatment with steroids and mesalazine. Chong et al. (2005) detected ulcers in 4 of 21 patients with suspected CD. Management was changed in 14 cases, with an improvement of symptoms in 8 patients after a mean follow-up of 8.4 months. In 22 patients with known CD, positive VCE findings were recorded in 17, leading to changes in management in 16 and improvement in 9 cases. Mow et al. (2004) analyzed 50 patients with known or suspected IBD. Symptoms improved after increased specific therapy in 17 of 20 patients with diagnostic and in 7 of 10 patients with suspicious findings during VCE.

Since the introduction of VCE, it has been possible to decrease the time for the diagnosis in CD, specifically in those patients with negative previous work-up, but the most important finding is the number of patients who improved based on VCE results.

Voderholzer at al. (2005) found small intestinal lesions with VCE in 25 of 41 patients with known Crohn's disease, but only in 12 of these 41 with CT enteroclysis ($p<0.004$). Therapy was changed in ten patients due to VCE findings, with consecutive clinical improvement in all. However, 15 patients (27%) had to be excluded from the study because of strictures seen at CT enteroclysis. In those patients with suspected or known CD, it is important to consider a small bowel contrast study in order to avoid capsule retention due to strictures or fistulae. The role of the Patency Capsule for such patients is discussed in Chap. 1.5.

Outcome in Abdominal Pain – Diarrhea/Irritable Bowel Syndrome

Patients with chronic abdominal pain or diarrhea usually undergo several diagnostic procedures until a final diagnosis is reached. The likelihood of positive findings of VCE in those patients has been low (Keuchel and Hagenmüller 2004). In one published study involving 20 patients that examined the diagnostic yield of VCE in persons with chronic abdominal pain, none of the subjects had significant findings on VCE (Bardan et al. 2003). In our own experience we reviewed 64 patients with chronic abdominal pain and/or diarrhea and the yield of VCE was 6% in patients with abdominal pain, 14% in patients with diarrhea, and 13% in patients with both symptoms (Fry et al. 2006). Despite the low incidence of positive findings of VCE, it should be considered, because it may avoid further noninvasive and invasive diagnostic procedures. Abnormal transit time of VCE was reported as a possible positive finding which can cause abdominal pain or diarrhea, but future studies are required to determine whether abnormal transit time can be considered pathologic and causing symptoms (Mele et al. 2003). Future studies evaluating the outcome of VCE in patients with abdominal pain or diarrhea are required.

Polyposis Syndromes

When compared with SBFT, CT, and magnetic resonance imaging (MRI), VCE identified a considerably higher number of polyps with lesion sizes ranging between 1 and 30 mm (Fig. 12-5). MRI was more accurate in terms of localization whereas VCE was more arbitrary (Caspari et al. 2004). Soares et al. (2004) found VCE an effective method for evaluation of the small bowel in patients with Peutz-Jeghers syndrome. There are no studies addressing the outcome of VCE in this group of patients. Nevertheless, given that Peutz-Jeghers syndrome has a high prevalence of small intestinal polyps and risks of obstruction and malignant degeneration of those polyps, VCE appears to be a useful test for initial staging and also for regular follow-up. The use of VCE in patients with familial adenomatous polyposis (FAP) is less well substantiated, given the fact that, with the exception of the duodenum, polyps of the remaining small bowel are very rare (Chap. 7.3).

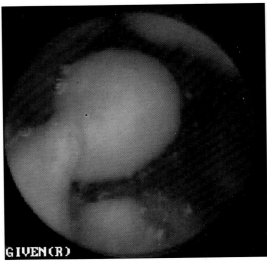
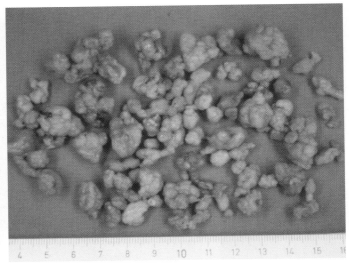

Fig. 12-5a, b. One of multiple polyps seen at VCE (**a**). A total of 100 polyps were removed during intraoperative enteroscopy (**b**) (courtesy of Jörg Caselitz, M.D.)

Celiac Disease

The main role of VCE in celiac disease is for patients with known celiac disease who are symptomatic despite gluten-free diet, in whom there is a suspected complication such as ulcerative jejunitis and associated T-cell lymphoma. Data exist only for diagnostic outcome, showing a high rate of persisting villous atrophy in these patients, but also a significant number of unexpected findings such as erosions and even tumors (Culliford et al. 2005). Data on health outcome are still pending.

Miscellaneous

Several case reports have shown unsuspected lesions diagnosed by VCE and missed by other techniques. Whipple's disease involving the entire small intestine, autoimmune enteropathy (**Fig. 12-6**), Meckel's diverticulum, helminthiasis (*Ascaris, Enterobius, Taenia saginata*), tuberculosis of the small bowel, Dieulafoy's lesion of the colon, radiation-induced enteritis, ileal ulcers in a long-distance runner, varices of the small bowel as well as NSAID-induced diaphragms of the intestine are among the pathologies discovered by VCE that led to an important change in the therapeutic approach.

Summary

VCE has become an established method for the diagnosis of small bowel diseases. The diagnostic yield of VCE has ranged from 43 to 92%. In OGIB VCE is superior to other methods. The usefulness of VCE for the diagnosis of suspected IBD is also high. The usefulness of VCE for the diagnosis of the other small bowel disorders or chronic conditions such as abdominal pain and diarrhea is less well established. There is insufficient evidence to permit conclusions concerning the effect of VCE on health outcomes in all other clinical indications. The practicing clinician needs to take into consideration that even negative results can influence patient therapies and outcomes. A definite diagnosis has led to a change in management in up to 87% of patients studied with VCE, which in turn has an impact on patient outcomes. The issues of patient reassurance at having reached a diagnosis, patient preferences, and quality of life also need further evaluation in clinical outcomes. It has become clear that patient outcomes are a very relevant standard for assessment of the utility of VCE. Clinical outcomes have rarely been examined for other diagnostic procedures such as radiography, nuclear medicine, and endoscopy. Therefore, comparative clinical outcome studies would be useful.

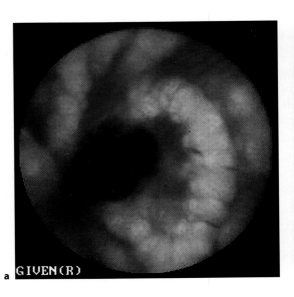
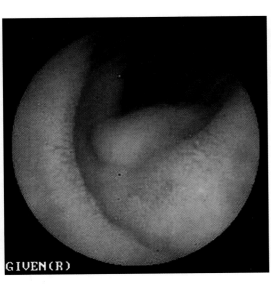

Fig. 12-6a, b. Severe diffuse intestinal bleeding. VCE diagnosed villous atrophy (**a**). Initiation of steroids for suspected autoimmune enteropathy led to rapid, sustained cessation of bleeding and partial recovery of villi (**b**)

References

Adler DG, Knipschield M, Gostout C (2004) A prospective comparison of capsule endoscopy and push enteroscopy in patients with GI bleeding of obscure origin. Gastrointest Endosc 59:492–498

Bardan E, Nadler M, Chowers Y et al (2003) Capsule endoscopy for the evaluation of patients with chronic abdominal pain. Endoscopy 35:688–689

Barkin JS, O'Loughlin C (2004) Capsule endoscopy contraindications: complications and how to avoid their occurrence. Gastrointest Endosc Clin N Am 14: 61–65

Buchman AL, Wallin A (2003) Videocapsule endoscopy renders obscure gastrointestinal bleeding no longer obscure. J Clin Gastroenterol 37:303–306

Caspari R, von Falkenhausen M, Krautmacher C et al (2004) Comparison of capsule endoscopy and magnetic resonance imaging for the detection of polyps of the small intestine in patients with familial adenomatous polyposis or with Peutz-Jeghers' syndrome. Endoscopy 36:1054–1059

Chong AK, Taylor A, Miller A et al (2005) Capsule endoscopy vs. push enteroscopy and enteroclysis in suspected small-bowel Crohn's disease. Gastrointest Endosc 61:255–261

Costamagna G, Shah SK, Riccioni ME et al (2002) A prospective trial comparing small bowel radiographs and video capsule endoscopy for suspected small bowel disease. Gastroenterology 123:999–1005

Culliford A, Daly J, Diamond B et al (2005) The value of wireless capsule endoscopy in patients with complicated celiac disease. Gastrointest Endosc 62:55–61

Delvaux M, Fassler I, Gay G (2004) Clinical usefulness of the endoscopic video capsule as the initial intestinal investigation in patients with obscure digestive bleeding: validation of a diagnostic strategy based on the patient outcome after 12 months. Endoscopy 36:1067–1073

Eliakim R, Fischer D, Suissa A et al (2003) Wireless capsule video endoscopy is a superior diagnostic tool in comparison to barium follow-through and computerized tomography in patients with suspected Crohn's disease. Eur J Gastroenterol Hepatol 15:363–367

Ell C, Remke S, May A et al (2002) The first prospective controlled trial comparing wireless capsule endoscopy with push enteroscopy in chronic gastrointestinal bleeding. Endoscopy 34:685–689

Fireman Z, Mahajna E, Broide E et al (2003) Diagnosing small bowel Crohn's disease with wireless capsule endoscopy. Gut 52:390–392

Fleischer DE, Heigh RI, Nguyen CC et al (2003) Videocapsule impaction at the cricopharyngeus: a first report of this complication and its successful resolution. Gastrointest Endosc 57:427–428

Fry LC, Carey EJ, Shiff AD et al (2006) The yield of capsule endoscopy in patients with abdominal pain or diarrhea. Endoscopy (in press)

Fry LC, De Petris G, Swain JM, Fleischer DE (2005) Impaction and fracture of a video capsule in the small bowel requiring laparotomy for its removal. Endoscopy 37:674–676

Hartmann D, Schilling D, Bolz G et al (2003) Capsule endoscopy versus push enteroscopy in patients with occult gastrointestinal bleeding. Z Gastroenterol 41:377–382

Herrerias JM, Caunedo A, Rodriguez-Tellez M et al (2003) Capsule endoscopy in patients with suspected Crohn's disease and negative endoscopy. Endoscopy 35:564–568

Keuchel M, Hagenmüller F (2004) Video capsule endoscopy in the work-up of abdominal pain. Gastrointest Endosc Clin N Am 14:195–205

Leighton JA, Sharma VK, Srivathsan K et al (2004) Safety of capsule endoscopy in patients with pacemakers. Gastrointest Endosc 59:567–569

Lewis BS (1994) Small intestinal bleeding. Gastroenterol Clin North Am 23:67–91

Lewis BS, Swain P (2002) Capsule endoscopy in the evaluation of patients with suspected small intestinal bleeding: results of a pilot study. Gastrointest Endosc 56:349–353

Liangpunsakul S, Chadalawada V, Rex DK et al (2003) Wireless capsule endoscopy detects small bowel ulcers in patients with normal results from state of the art enteroclysis. Am J Gastroenterol 98:1295–1298

Maieron A, Hubner D, Blaha B et al (2004) Multicenter retrospective evaluation of capsule endoscopy in clinical routine. Endoscopy 36:864–868

Mata A, Bordas JM, Feu F et al (2004) Wireless capsule endoscopy in patients with obscure gastrointestinal bleeding: a comparative study with push enteroscopy. Aliment Pharmacol Ther 20:189–194

Mele C, Infantolino A, Conn M et al (2003) The diagnostic yield of wireless capsule endoscope in patients with unexplained abdominal pain. Am J Gastroenterol 98: S298

Mow WS, Lo SK, Targan SR et al (2004) Initial experience with wireless capsule enteroscopy in the diagnosis and management of inflammatory bowel disease. Clin Gastroenterol Hepatol 2:31–40

Mylonaki M, Fritscher-Ravens A, Swain P (2003) Wireless capsule endoscopy: a comparison with push enteroscopy in patients with gastroscopy and colonoscopy negative gastrointestinal bleeding. Gut 52:1122–1226

Neu B, Ell C, May A et al (2005) Capsule endoscopy versus standard tests in influencing management of obscure digestive bleeding: results from a German multicenter trial. Am J Gastroenterol 100:1736–1742

Pennazio M, Santucci R, Rondonotti E et al (2004) Outcome of patients with obscure gastrointestinal bleeding after capsule endoscopy: report of 100 consecutive cases. Gastroenterology 126:643–653

Rastogi A, Schoen RE, Slivka A (2004) Diagnostic yield and clinical outcomes of capsule endoscopy. Gastrointest Endosc 60:959–964

Saunders M, Nietsch H, Lee SD et al (2004) Capsule endoscopy versus push enteroscopy for obscure GI bleeding: a randomized, single-blind, cross-over study. Gastrointest Endosc 59:AB100

Saurin JC, Delvaux M, Gaudin JL et al (2003) Diagnostic value of endoscopic capsule in patients with obscure digestive bleeding: blinded comparison with video push-enteroscopy. Endoscopy 35:576–584

Saurin JC, Delvaux M, Vahedi K et al (2005) Clinical impact of capsule endoscopy compared to push enteroscopy: 1-year follow-up study. Endoscopy 37:318–323

Schmidt H, Hartmann D, Kinzel F et al (2005) Capsule endoscopy followed by intraoperative enteroscopy and therapy in patients with chronic gastrointestinal bleeding: long term results of a prospective controlled multicentric trial. Gastrointest Endosc 61:AB181

Soares J, Lopes L, Vilas Boas G, Pinho C (2004) Wireless capsule endoscopy for evaluation of phenotypic expression of small-bowel polyps in patients with Peutz-Jeghers' syndrome and in symptomatic first-degree relatives. Endoscopy 36:1060–1066

Tang SJ, Christodoulou D, Zanati S et al (2004) Wireless capsule endoscopy for obscure gastrointestinal bleeding: a single-centre, one-year experience. Can J Gastroenterol 18:559–565

Triester SL, Leighton JA, Leontiadis GI et al (2005) A meta-analysis of the yield of capsule endoscopy compared to other diagnostic modalities in patients with obscure gastrointestinal bleeding. Am J Gastroenterol 100:2407–2418

Triester SL, Leighton JA, Leontiadis GI et al (2006) A meta-analysis of the yield of capsule endoscopy (CE) compared to other diagnostic modalities in patients with non-stricturing small bowel Crohn's disease. Am J Gastroenterol (in press)

Van Gossum A, Hittelet A, Schmit A et al (2003) A prospective comparative study of push and wireless-capsule enteroscopy in patients with obscure digestive bleeding. Acta Gastroenterol Belg 66:199–205

Voderholzer WA, Ortner M, Rogalla P et al (2003) Diagnostic yield of wireless capsule enteroscopy in comparison with computed tomography enteroclysis. Endoscopy 35:1009–1014

Voderholzer WA, Beinhoelzl J, Rogalla P et al (2005) Small bowel involvement in Crohn's disease: a prospective comparison of wireless capsule endoscopy and computed tomography enteroclysis. Gut 54:369–373

Esophageal Capsule Endoscopy (PillCam ESO)

R. Eliakim, V.K. Sharma, M.B. Fennerty

Technique and Application

The esophageal video capsule is a newly developed esophageal imaging system similar in design to the small bowel capsule (developed by Given Imaging, Ltd. in Yoqneam, Israel) for visualization of esophageal disorders. A feasibility study found it to have high sensitivity, specificity, positive predictive value (PPV), and negative predictive value (NPV) and led to a prospective international seven-center study which confirmed the earlier results (Eliakim et al. 2005). These studies led to U.S. Food and Drug Administration clearance of the new capsule for clinical use in 2004. Recently two studies have demonstrated similar sensitivity and specificity rates in detecting esophageal varices (Eisen et al. 2006).

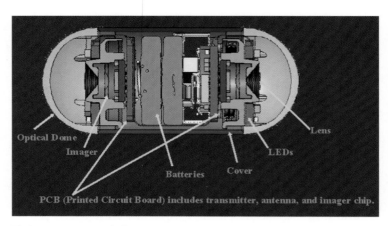

■ **Fig. 13-1.** A view of PillCam ESO (courtesy of Given Imaging)

Technology

The new capsule differs from the conventional small bowel capsule in that it has two optical domes at either end of the capsule (■ Fig. 13-1), which when activated emit from light-emitting diodes (LEDs) a strobe light at the rate of 7 flashes/s from each end (14 total/s) (■ Fig. 13-2). All the other elements and transmission techniques of this capsule are similar to the small bowel capsule. Normal esophageal capsule operating time is 30 min.

> Technical specifications of PillCam ESO (Given Imaging):
>
> - Height 11 mm, width 27 mm, weight 3.7 g
> - Field of view 140°, magnification 1:8 at both sides
> - Operating time 30 min

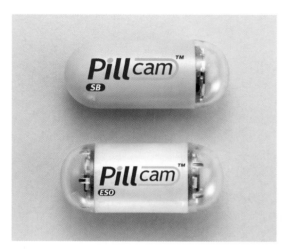

■ **Fig. 13-2.** A view of both the PillCam Small Bowel and the new PillCam ESO capsule (courtesy of Given Imaging)

Procedure

The application of the new esophageal capsule is markedly different from the traditional small bowel capsule. There is no need for more than an hour of fasting. Three sensors are attached to the patient's chest, from the xiphoid upwards (■ Fig. 13-3). After first drinking water, the patient swallows the PillCam ESO in the supine position in order to prolong esophageal passage time (■ Figs. 13-4 and 13-5). The supine swallowing portion of the procedure lasts 5 min after which the patient then initially sits and then stands; after 20 min the sensors and recorder are then disconnected and discharged. The recorder is downloaded into a computer analysis program (Rapid 3 system) and is then read with the two separate camera images simultaneously displayed on the screen (■ Fig. 13-6). During the review process one can mark specific image frames (thumbnails) and save them as in the small bowel procedure. The same images can be saved to the final written report and provide a complete summary for the patient file. Additionally the entire video image can be saved in an audio video interleave (AVI) format.

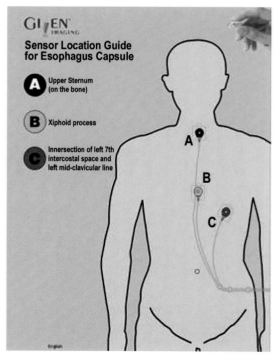

■ **Fig. 13-3.** Sensor location guide for PillCam ESO (courtesy of Given Imaging)

- Drink a glass of water
- Ingest the capsule in flat position
- Gradual body inclination up to sitting position 5 min procedure
- Sip of water
- Wait 15 more min in waiting room

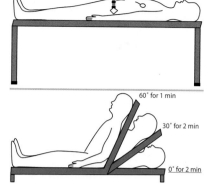

60° for 1 min

30° for 2 min

0° for 2 min

◘ Fig. 13-4. The swallowing procedure for PillCam ESO (courtesy of Given Imaging)

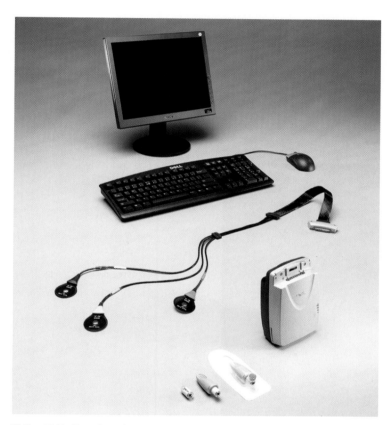

◘ Fig. 13-5. Capsule endoscopy equipment. *Front left*: ESO capsule, capsule in holder, blister. *Front right*: DR 2 data recorder with integrated power supply. *Middle*: three sensor areas. *Rear*: workstation (courtesy of Given Imaging)

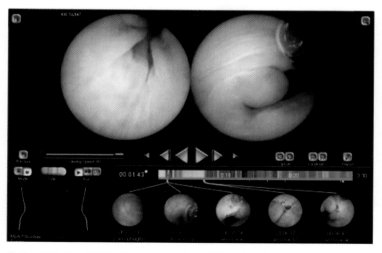

◘ Fig. 13-6. The RAPID 3.0 screen (courtesy of Given Imaging)

Application of PillCam ESO

This is a new type of the capsule and only a few studies have been completed with it as of today confirming its efficacy and high diagnostic accuracy when compared to a gold standard of imaging with traditional endoscopy in patients with chronic gastroesophageal symptoms or Barrett's esophagus (Eliakim et al. 2004, 2005). In the multicenter trial 55 of 80 patients had positive esophageal findings, and PillCam ESO identified esophageal abnormalities in 51 (sensitivity 93%, specificity 100%). The per protocol sensitivity, specificity, PPV, and NPV of the capsule for Barrett's esophagus were 97, 100, 100, and 98%, respectively, and for esophagitis 90, 100, 100, and 95%, respectively. PillCam ESO was preferred over traditional endoscopy by all patients. There were no adverse events related to PillCam ESO. Pilot studies assessing the accuracy of the new capsule in visualizing varices in patients with chronic liver disease revealed very promising results (Eisen et al. 2006).

Indications for PillCam ESO:

- Patients being screened for esophagitis
- Patients being screened for Barrett's esophagus
- Patients being screened for esophageal varices

The patient should be informed about the conduct. Contraindications and risks associated with the procedure, which are no different from those of the small bowel capsule, ought to be explained. A printed information sheet should be provided and a written informed consent form signed prior to the beginning of the procedure.

Contraindications to PillCam ESO:

- Dysphagia
- Zenker's diverticulum
- Strictures of the gastrointestinal tract
- Electronic implants
- Pregnancy
- Planned magnetic resonance imaging (MRI) within the near future

All limitations and possible complications mentioned in Chaps. 1.3.1 and 10 are also relevant to the esophageal capsule.

Interpretation

During the procedure a mean of 680 images are captured from the esophagus and transmitted and recorded in the hard disk of the recording unit. The data are downloaded to a computer using a special software system (Rapid 3 or higher) and a digital video is created. The video playback can be controlled on the computer much the same as a VCR. Images from both camera heads are seen simultaneously on the screen (◘ Fig. 13-6), potentially allowing measurement of the length of suspected Barrett's, or of a hiatus hernia, although the use of the device for this purpose has yet to be established. Clear views of the esophagus (◘ Fig. 13-7), Z line (squamocolumnar junction, ◘ Fig. 13-8), and pathologies such as esophagitis and suspected Barrett's esophagus can often be obtained (◘ Figs. 13-10, 13-12, and 13-14a, b), similar to those seen in conventional endoscopy (◘ Figs. 13-9, 13-11, 13-13, and 13-14c). Similarly, clear views of esophageal varices can be seen (◘ Fig. 13-15). Even rare diseases such as papilloma may be detected (◘ Fig. 13-16).

Review of the esophageal procedure generally takes the physician about 8-10 min. The water swallowed just prior to the procedure and breathing through an open mouth after swallowing (to prevent swallowing more saliva) is meant to reduce the number of bubbles during the procedure. The use of simethicone is currently being evaluated as a means of decreasing the number of procedures where the view is obscured by bubbles.

> **Impediments to visualization with PillCam ESO:**
> - Bubbles
> - Food residue
> - Rapid transit across the esophagogastric junction

Space requirements for PillCam ESO are similar as for the small bowel capsule. The only additional equipment needed is a bed that can be inclined allowing the upper part of the body to be lifted to 30–60°. The patient is discharged 20 min after swallowing the capsule, returning to the doctor's office only to consult with the physician about the results of the examination.

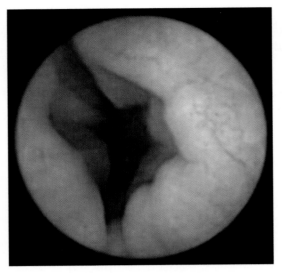

Fig. 13-7. A longitudinal view of a normal esophagus captured by PillCam ESO

Fig. 13-8a–d. Images of a normal Z line captured by PillCam ESO

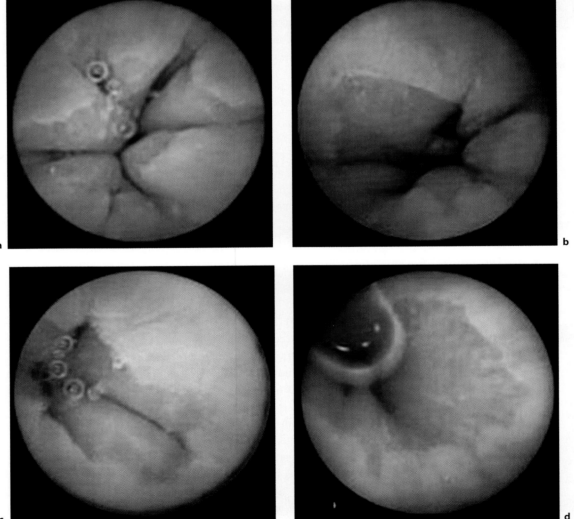

a

b

c

d

13

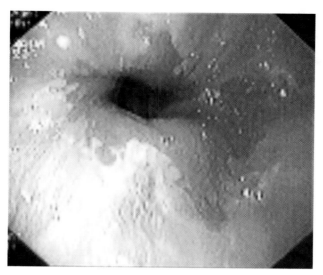

◘ Fig. 13-9. A normal Z line as seen on traditional endoscopy

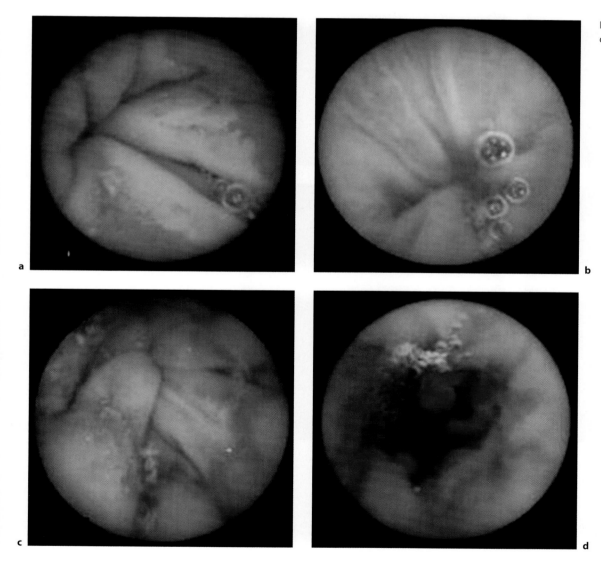

◘ Fig. 13-10a–d. Images of esophagitis captured by PillCam ESO

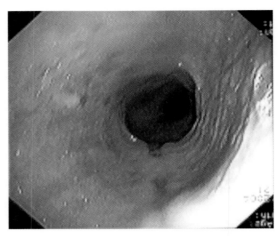

◘ Fig. 13-11. Grade A esophagitis seen on traditional endoscopy

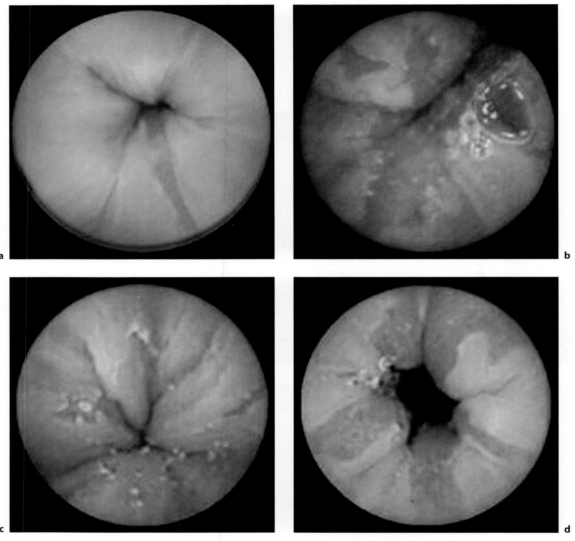

◘ Fig. 13-12a–d. Images of suspected Barrett's metaplasia captured by PillCam ESO

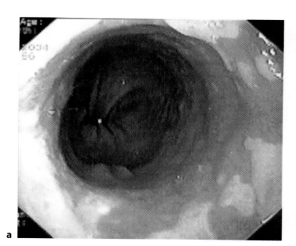
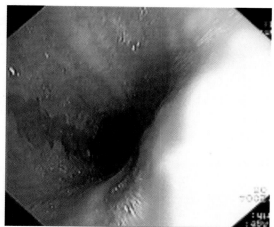

Fig. 13-13a, b. Barrett's metaplasia seen on traditional endoscopy

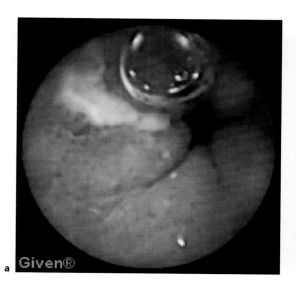
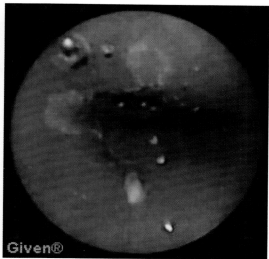

Fig. 13-14a–d. Barrett's metaplasia and erosion. **a, b** Images captured by PillCam ESO. **c** Zoom endoscopy. **d** Histology showing Barrett's intestinal metaplasia (Alcian blue stain; courtesy of Jörg Caselitz, M.D.)

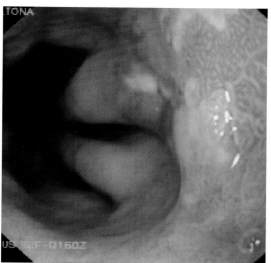
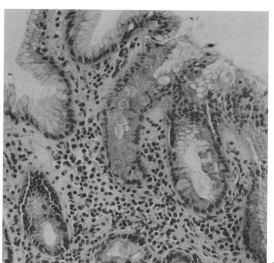

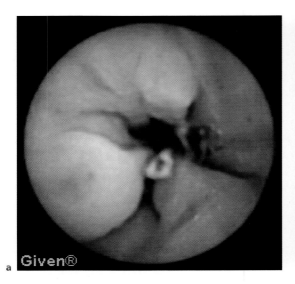 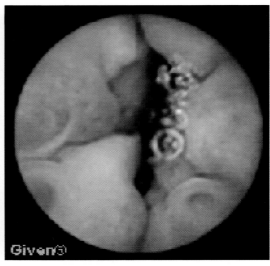

■ **Fig. 13-15a, b.** Esophageal varices captured by PillCam ESO

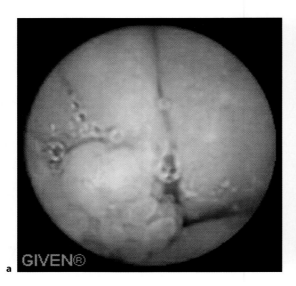 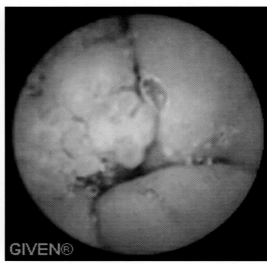

■ **Fig. 13-16a, b.** Papilloma of the esophagus (proven by histology)

References

Eisen GM, Eliakim R, Zaman A, Schwartz J, Faigel D, Rondonotti E, Villa F, Weizman E, Yassin K, de Franchis R (2006) The accuracy of PillCam ESO capsule endoscopy versus conventional upper endoscopy for the diagnosis of esophageal varices: a prospective three-center pilot study. Endoscopy 38:31–35

Eliakim R, Yassin K, Shlomi I, Suissa A, Eisen GM (2004) A novel diagnostic tool for detecting oesophageal pathology: PillCam oesophageal video capsule. Aliment Pharmacol Ther 20:1083–1089

Eliakim R, Sharma VK, Yassin K, Adler SN, Jacob H, Cave DR, Sachdev R, Mitty RD, Hartmann D, Schilling D, Riemann JF, Bar-Meir S, Bardan E, Fennerty B, Eisen GM, Faigel D, Lewis BS, Fleischer DE (2005) A prospective study of the diagnostic accuracy of Given® esophageal capsule endoscopy versus conventional upper endoscopy in patients with chronic gastroesophageal reflux diseases. J Clin Gastroenterol 39:572–578

Future Developments of Capsule Endoscopy

C.P. Swain

Introduction

The advent of wireless video capsule endoscopy has released the endoscopist from the requirement to exert force on a long floppy cable type endoscope to examine relatively short segments of small intestine. The key to the development of the wireless capsule endoscopy was miniaturization of electronic components and especially the development of very small video cameras and wireless transmitters (◘ Table 14-1)

(◘ Fig. 14-1). Miniaturization of electrical components has allowed the manufacture of a capsule-sized endoscope without wires which can take video images (◘ Fig. 14-2) of the gastrointestinal (GI) tract and transmit this information to a recorder, which is worn by the patient on a belt. Perhaps the most difficult problem with the development of wireless capsule endoscopy was thinking that it was possible and risking the time and money on making it to see how well it might work.

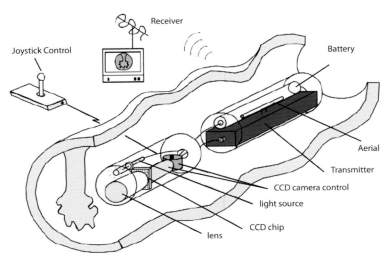

◘ **Fig. 14-1.** This illustration shows an early concept drawing of wireless endoscopy from 1994. A CCD camera, microwave transmitter, aerial, light source, and battery are combined to form a small endoscope. An aerial, microwave signal receiver, and color monitor receive the signal. A joystick control to communicate with and control the wireless endoscope is still a futuristic idea. Reprinted from Gong et al. 2000 with permission from the American Society for Gastrointestinal Endoscopy

◘ **Table 14-1.** Milestones in development of wireless capsule endoscopy

1949	Invention of transistor – Bardeen, Brattain, and Shockley (Nobel Prize 1956)
1954	Fiberoptic image transmission – Hopkins
1957	Radio pills (temperature, pressure, pH) – Zworkin, Mackay, and Noller
1969	Charge coupled device (CCD) – Smith and Boyle
1994	CMOS improvements – Fossum
1994	First publication on feasibility – Swain, Gong, Mills
1996	First live pictures from pig GI tract with a wireless device – Swain, Gong, Mills
1997	Codevelopment with Israeli group (Given Imaging)
1999	Ethical Committee approval for human use – Swain
2000	Publication in *Nature* – Iddan, Meron, Glukhovsky, Swain, *N Engl J Med* 2001 – Appleyard, Glukhovsky, Swain
2001	CE mark and FDA approval
2005	200,000 patients examined

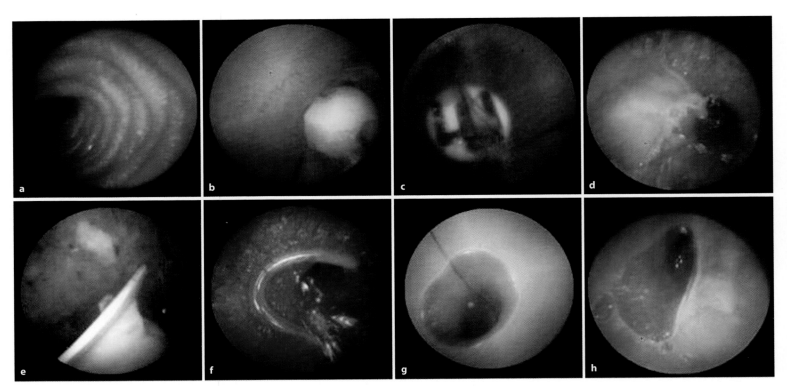

◘ **Fig. 14-2a–h.** Early images from wireless capsule endoscopy in dogs. Capsules identified significantly more beads beyond the reach of the push enteroscope. An *Ascaris* worm was the first small intestinal pathology found using wireless capsule endoscopy. **a** Normal small intestine; **b** round bead sutured to small intestine; **c** flat bead with black marks sutured to small intestine; **d** inflammatory nodule; **e** ingested white plastic material in the cecum; **f** ascaris worm; **g** ingested black hair; **h** small intestinal ulcers. Reprinted from Appleyard et al. 2000 with permission from the American Gastroenterological Association

Future Innovations

Wireless capsule technology is an incompletely developed technology and might change endoscopy forever and has the capacity to replace a good deal of conventional endoscopy. Will capsule endoscopy replace much of conventional gastroscopy and colonoscopy? The answer is probably yes but the time frame is unclear. Will capsule endoscopy be able to deliver therapy? This is also possible.

There are two major challenges to the expansion of capsule technology into a position where it can challenge conventional diagnostic gastroscopy and colonoscopy. The first challenge is power management. At present the PillCam capsule contains two small 3-V hearing aid batteries which allow about 8 h of continuous imaging. The use of complementary metal oxide semiconductor (CMOS) technology for the video has the advantage of requiring extremely low power levels. Slowing the video frame rate to two frames/s increased the life span of the capsule. More batteries or more efficient batteries would help but might increase the size and weight of the capsule. The development of external power transmission methods using electrical field induction, radio frequency, microwave, or ultrasound technology would free the capsule from the requirement for batteries. This would substantially lighten the capsule, allow space and power for other functions such as biopsy or drug delivery but above all would allow the capsule to be powered for infinite periods which would make the problem of capsule colonoscopy much easier to solve (Table 14-2).

The development of capsule endoscopy was made possible by miniaturization of digital chip camera technology especially CMOS chip technology. The continued reduction in size, increases in pixel numbers, and improvements in imaging with the two rival technologies – CCD and CMOS – are likely to change the nature of endoscopy. The current differences outlined in Table 14-2 are becoming blurred and hybrids are emerging.

The main pressure to reduce the component size will be to release space that could be used for other capsule functions for example biopsy, coagulation, or therapy. New engineering methods for constructing tiny moving parts and miniature actuators or even motors have been described. There are some engineering challenges to be solved. Transmission of sufficient power to medical devices in the body to allow extra functions is a major issue. Cleverly designed power management solutions to battery run devices may allow some new functions fairly soon. Controlling the orientation and movements of the capsule seems feasible. The development of external transmission systems which can beam power to devices in the human body needs more work but bio-engineers working in the cardiology area have shown that it is possible to induce currents in remote internal devices with externally applied systems.

Although semiconductor lasers exist which are small enough to swallow, the nature of lasers which have typical inefficiencies of 100–1000% make the idea of a remote laser in a capsule stopping bleeding or cutting out a tumor seem something of a pipe dream at present because of power requirements. The construction of an electrosurgical generator small enough to swallow and powered by small batteries is thinkable but currently difficult because of the limitations imposed by the internal resistance of batteries. Small motors are currently available to move components such as biopsy devices but need radio-controlled activators. One limitation is the low mass of the capsule endoscope. A force exerted on tissue for example by biopsy forceps may push the capsule away from the tissue.

Future diagnostic developments are likely to include capsule colonoscopy, attachment to the gut wall, ultrasound imaging, biopsy and cytology, propulsion methods, and therapy including tissue coagulation.

Challenge to Using Capsule Endoscopy for Colonoscopy

There are challenges to using wireless capsule endoscopy for colonoscopy (Fig. 14-3). Currently the capsule acquires images for 8 h and has usually reached the right side of the colon before the battery expires. The capsule would have to run for 24–48 h in order to perform a complete examination of the colon. The power problem could be addressed in several ways. Solutions to this difficulty might include: more batteries, batteries with a delay mode which are switched on when the capsule is in the ileum, external power transmission, or methods to move the capsule faster in the colon. Effective timed colon cleaning will be necessary. Deletion of identical frames would make it easier to examine the images since the capsule in the colon can remain stationary for prolonged periods. Wireless capsule colonoscopy has already generated images (Fig. 14-4) from all areas of the colon and has imaged pathology especially in the right side of the colon, but also in the rectum (Fig. 14-5).

Wireless laparoscopy is feasible (Figs. 14-6 and 14-7) but needs to develop and offer advantages over conventional laparoscopy. Wireless imaging of cardiac or vascular structures is possible but would require substantial development and control strategies. The manufacture of an autonomous video capsule the size of a red blood cell as described in Isaac Asimov's *The Fantastic Voyage* is some way in the future. Reduction in size by an order of magnitude is currently feasible with available components.

■ Table 14-2. Comparison of CMOS and CCD technology
CCD sensors create high-quality, low-noise images. CMOS sensors, traditionally, are more susceptible to noise.
Because each pixel on a CMOS sensor has several transistors located next to it, the light sensitivity of a CMOS chip tends to be lower. Many of the photons hitting the chip hit the transistors instead of the photodiode.
CCDs use a process that consumes lots of power. CCDs consume as much as 100 times more power than an equivalent CMOS sensor.
CMOS chips can be fabricated on just about any standard silicon production line, so they tend to be extremely inexpensive compared to CCD sensors.
CCD sensors have been mass-produced for a longer period of time, so they are maturer. They tend to have higher quality and more pixels.
CCD requires application of several clock signals, clock levels, and bias voltages, complicating system integration and increasing power consumption, overall system size, and cost.
CMOS architecture allows the signals from the entire array, from subsections, or even from a single pixel to be read out by a simple X-Y addressing technique – something a CCD can't do.

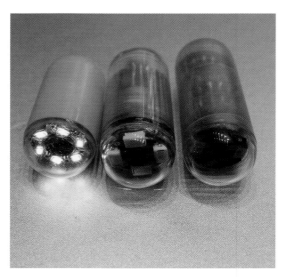

Fig. 14-3. Three capsule prototypes are shown. The one on the *right* side was the first prototype to be swallowed by a human. It is 3 mm longer than the current PillCam capsule. The capsule in the *middle* was a lightweight experimental capsule for colonoscopy

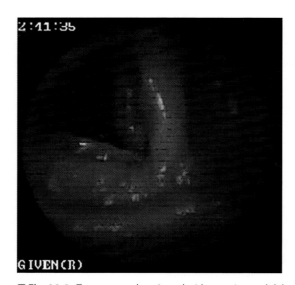

Fig. 14-4. Transverse colon viewed with experimental delay mode colonoscopy capsule

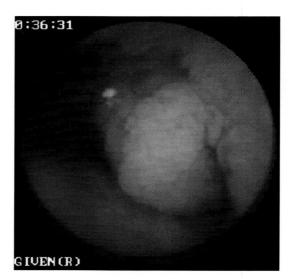

Fig. 14-5. Large rectal villous adenoma

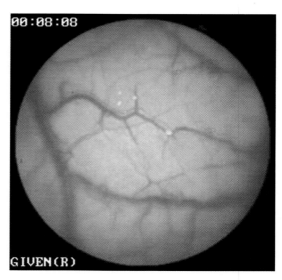

Fig. 14-6. Wireless laparoscopic capsule image of serosal surface of stomach

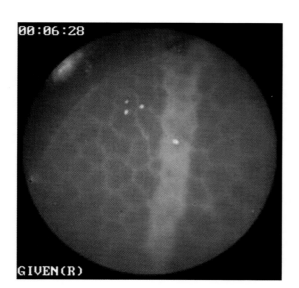

Fig. 14-7. Liver septum

Attachment of Capsule Endoscope to the GI Tract

The capsule might be stitched or clipped to the wall of the stomach so that prolonged examination of bleeding ulcers or varices becomes possible (◘ Fig. 14-8). An on/off radio-controlled command might be helpful to conserve power. Long-term endoscopy with wireless endoscopes attached to the wall of the gut could improve management of bleeding and other disorders.

Tissue Interactive Diagnostic Methods

At present the capsule does not take biopsies, aspirate fluid, or brush lesions for cytology. These common endoscopic maneuvers may be possible during capsule endoscopy. They require real-time viewing and will also require radio-controlled triggering and remote control capsule manipulation if they are to be used with precision. Biopsy using a spring loaded Crosby capsule-like device (◘ Fig. 14-9) with an evacuated chamber would be feasible with existing capsule technology and patients seem able to retrieve capsules from stool using a net and a magnet almost all the time in preliminary patient studies. Brush cytology (◘ Fig. 14-10) is another possibility and has been used in vivo.

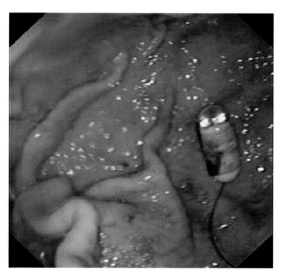

◘ **Fig. 14-8.** Capsule attached to stomach wall by thread

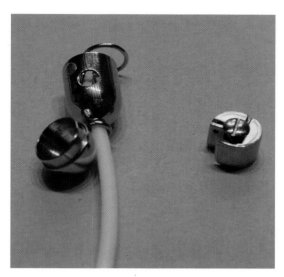

◘ **Fig. 14-9.** The components of a small bowel biopsy capsule (Watson)

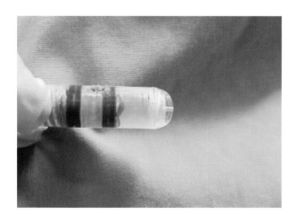

◘ **Fig. 14-10.** A capsule with a spring-loaded cytology brush

Electrostimulation for Propelling Capsule Endoscope

One way to manipulate a wireless capsule endoscope autonomously in the human GI tract is to use electrostimulation to propel the device for example with a pair of bipolar electrodes at either end of the capsule (■ Fig. 14-11). Electrodes attached to a PillCam have been used to propel this device in the human small intestine (■ Fig. 14-12). A dumbbell-shaped capsule allows the imaging capsule to view the traction capsule (■ Fig. 14-13). A radio-controlled electrostimulation capsule has been developed. Radio commands can be sent from a transmitter and aerial (■ Fig. 14-14) to the receiving traction capsule causing it to propel the video capsule (■ Fig. 14-15) forwards or backwards in the human GI tract (■ Fig. 14-16)

Waterjet propulsion has also been used to propel this very lightweight (3.7 g) capsule in the GI tract (■ Fig. 14-17).

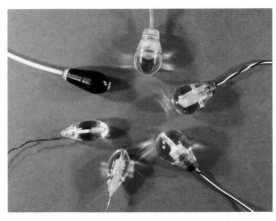

■ **Fig. 14-11.** Six wired prototype electrostimulation capsules with a pair of bipolar electrodes at either end of the capsule

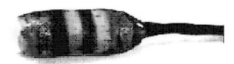

■ **Fig. 14-12.** Bipolar electrodes attached to PillCam capsule for first electrostimulation video capsule in a human volunteer

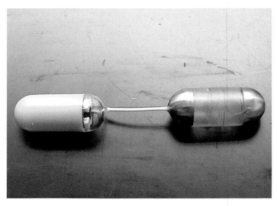

■ **Fig. 14-13.** A prototype dumbbell shape allows the imaging capsule to observe a capsule with a different function – in this case an electrostimulation capsule

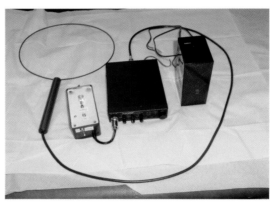

■ **Fig. 14-14.** This illustration shows a radio transmitter and aerial used to control capsule movement autonomously in the human small intestine

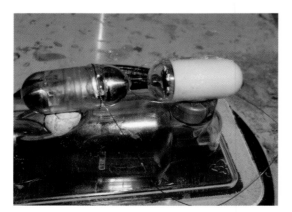

■ **Fig. 14-15.** The electrostimulation capsule tethered to a PillCam by threads is seen in the human intestine

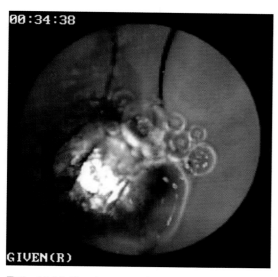

☐ Fig. 14-16. The electrostimulation capsule tethered to a PillCam by threads is seen in the human intesine

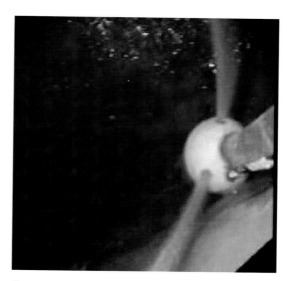

☐ Fig. 14-17. A waterjet is used to propel a wireless capsule using true jet propulsion

Capsule Coagulation

A prototype coagulation capsule has been built and tested which uses an exothermic chemical reaction to generate heat. It seems probable that other therapeutic applications will be added in the future.

Other future developments in capsule endoscopy are wireless power supply, capsule guidance system, drug delivery system, bodyfluid sampling technology, self-propelled capsule, and ultrasound capsule.

Conclusions

Video enteroscopy has opened up a new world of diagnoses and possibilities to the gastroenterologist. It is a privilege to see images of small intestinal abnormalities at video endoscopy such as an ulcerated Meckel's diverticulum or active bleeding from a tumor in the middle of the small intestine, which were not possible till recently. The development of wireless capsule endoscopy has changed video endoscopy of the small intestine into a much less invasive and more complete examination. The increasing use of these resources and the comfort and ease with which some of these examinations can be performed make it likely that wireless capsule video imaging will have a substantial impact on the management of small intestinal disease and other parts of the body.

Einstein who probably knew more than most about the potential impact of physics on the future of mankind was goaded during an interview in 1929 on Helgoland into saying »I never think about the future; it comes soon enough.«

References

Appleyard M, Glukhovsky A, Swain P (2001) Wireless capsule diagnostic endoscopy for recurrent small-bowel bleeding. N Engl J Med 34:232–233

Appleyard M, Fireman F, Glukhovsky A et al (2000) A randomized comparison of push enteroscopy and wireless capsule endoscopy in detecting small intestinal lesions in an animal model. Gastroenterology 119:1431–1438

Asimov I (1966) The Fantastic Voyage. Bantam, New York

Bardeen J. Brattain W, Shockley WB et al (1950) Semiconductor Amplifier »Three-Electrode Circuit Element Utilizing Semiconductive Materials«. U.S. Patent 2,524,035

Fossum ER (1993) Active pixel sensor: are CCD's dinosaurs? Proc SPIE 1900:2–14

Gong F, Swain P, Mills T (2000) Wireless endoscopy. Gastrointest Endosc 51:725–729

Hopkins H, Kapany NS (1954) A flexible fiberscope, using static scanning. Nature 173:39

Mackay RS (1957) Endoradiosonde. Nature 179:1239–1240

Noller HG (1960) Die Endoradiosonde. Dtsch Med Wochenschr 85:1707

Iddan G, Sturlesi D (1997) In vivo video camera. US patent issued 18 Feb 1997, filed 17 Jan 1995

Iddan G, Meron G, Glukovsky A et al (2000) Wireless capsule endoscopy. Nature 405:417

Mosse CA, Mills TN, Appleyard MN et al (2001) Electrical stimulation for propelling endoscopes. Gastrointest Endosc 54:79–83

Swain CP, Gong F, Mills TN (1996) Wireless transmission of a colour television moving image from the stomach using a miniature CCD camera, light source and microwave transmitter. Gut 39:A26

Zworkin VK (1957) Radio pill. Nature 179:898

Contributors of Illustrations

We thank the following colleagues for providing images for this book

Michael **Amthor**, M.D., Professor of Medicine, Department of Pathology, Diakonie Hospital Rotenburg/Wümme, Elise Averdick-Str. 17, 27342 Rotenburg/Wümme, Germany

Mark **Appleyard**, M.D., Department of Gastroenterology and Hepatology, Royal Brisbane and Women's Hospital, Butterfield Street, Herston Q 4029, Brisbane Australia

Martin **Bergmann**, M.D., Institute for Pathology, Ernst-Sievers-Str. 124, 49078 Osnabrück, Germany

Ruprecht **Botzler**, M.D., Gastroenterology Practice, Königstr. 81, 23552 Lübeck, Germany

Jörg **Caselitz**, M.D., Professor of Medicine, Department of Pathology, Asklepios Klinik Altona, Paul-Ehrlich-Str. 1, 22763 Hamburg, Germany

Wolfgang **Cordruwisch**, M.D., Medical Department III, Asklepios Klinik Barmbek, Rübenkamp 220, 22291 Hamburg, Germany

Åke **Danielsson**, M.D., Professor of Medicine, Department of Medicine, University Hospital Umeå, 901 87, Sweden

Henryk **Dancygier**, M.D., Professor of Medicine, Medical Clinic II, Klinikum Offenbach, Starkenburgring 66, 63069 Offenbach, Germany

Axel **de Rossi**, M.D., Gastroenterology Practice, Durlacher Allee 4, 76131 Karlsruhe, Germany

Michel **Delvaux**, M.D., Ph.D., Professor of Medicine, Department of Internal Medicine and Digestive Pathology, Centre Hospitalier Universitaire de Nancy, Hôpitaux de Brabois, Allée de Morvan, 54511 Vandoeuvre Les Nancy, France

Uwe Paul **Eggers**, M.D., Department of Diagnostic Radiology and Nuclear Medicine, Asklepios Klinik Altona, Paul-Ehrlich-Str. 1, 22763 Hamburg, Germany

Ursula **Engel**, M.D., Surgical Department I, Asklepios Klinik Altona, Paul-Ehrlich-Str. 1, 22763 Hamburg, Germany

Jann **Erdmann**, M.D., Medical Clinic, Klinikum Elmshorn, Agnes-Karll-Allee, 25337 Elmshorn, Germany

Siegbert **Faiss**, M.D., Professor of Medicine, Medical Department III, Asklepios Klinik Barmbek, Rübenkamp 220, 22291 Hamburg, Germany

Bernd **Falke**, M.D., Gastroenterology Practice, Hauptstr. 55, 28844 Weyhe, Germany

David E. **Fleischer**, M.D., Professor of Medicine, Mayo Clinic College of Medicine, Chair, Division of Gastroenterology and Hepatology, Mayo Clinic, 13400 East Shea Boulevard, Scottsdale, AZ 85259, USA

Christian **Florent**, M.D., Professor of Medicine, Fédération des Services d'Hépato-Gastro-Entérologie, Hôpital Saint-Antoine, 184 rue du Fg Saint-Antoine, 75571 Paris Cedex 12, France

Ingo **Franke**, M.D., Medical Clinic I, Klinikum Niederlausitz, Calauer Str. 8, 01968 Senftenberg, Germany

Wolfgang **Frier**, Photographic Department, Asklepios Klinik Altona, Paul-Ehrlich-Str. 1, 22763 Hamburg, Germany

Annette **Fritscher-Ravens,** M.D., Professor of Medicine, Department of Gastroenterology, St. Mary's Hospital, Imperial College, Praed Street, W2 1NY London, UK

Michaela **Garn**, M.D., Department of Diagnostic Radiology and Nuclear Medicine, Asklepios Klinik Altona, Paul-Ehrlich-Str. 1, 22763 Hamburg, Germany

Gérard **Gay**, M.D., Professor of Medicine, Department of Internal Medicine and Digestive Pathology, Centre Hospitalier Universitaire de Nancy, Hôpitaux de Brabois, Allée de Morvan, 54511 Vandoeuvre Les Nancy, France

Joachim **Gottschalk**, M.D., Professor of Medicine, Department of Pathology and Neuropathology, Asklepios Klinik Heidberg, Tangstedter Landstr. 400, 22417 Hamburg, Germany

Andreas **Gocht**, M.D., Professor of Medicine, Pathology Center, Pferdemarkt 12, 23552 Lübeck, Germany

Begoña **González-Suárez**, M.D., Department of Gastroenterology, Hospital Sant Pau, Sant Antoni Mª Claret 167, 08025 Barcelona, Spain

Dirk **Hartmann**, M.D., Department of Gastroenterology, Klinikum Ludwigshafen, Bremserstr. 79, 67063 Ludwigshafen, Germany

Patrick **Hein,** M.D., Department of Radiology, Charité Hospital, Campus Mitte, Schumannstr. 20/21, 10117 Berlin, Germany

Michael **Heine**, M.D., Professor of Medicine, Bremerhaven Pathology Institute, Postbrookstr. 101, 27574 Bremerhaven, Germany

Renate **Höhne**, M.D., Department of Pathology, Asklepios Klinik Altona, Paul-Ehrlich-Str. 1, 22763 Hamburg, Germany

Wilhelm-Wolfgang **Höpker**, M.D., Professor of Medicine, Department of Pathology, Asklepios Klinik Barmbek, Rübenkamp 220, 22291 Hamburg, Germany

Filip K. **Knop**, M.D., Department of Internal Medicine F, Gentofte Hospital, University of Copenhagen, Niels Andersensvej 65, 2900 Hellerup, Denmark

Johannes **Krüger**, M.D., Internal Department, Paracelsus Hospital, Wilstedter Str. 134, 24558 Henstedt-Ulzburg, Germany

Stefan **Krüger**, M.D., Professor of Medicine, Department of Pathology, Universitätsklinikum Schleswig-Holstein, Campus Lübeck, Ratzeburger Allee 160, 23538 Lübeck, Germany

Wilfred **Landry**, M.D., Gastroenterology Practice, Münchner Str. 64, 85221 Dachau, Germany

Wolfgang **Lehmann**, Visual Communication, Ihlandkoppel 31, 22337 Hamburg, Germany

Bernhard **Leisner**, M.D., Professor of Medicine, Department of Nuclear Medicine, Asklepios Klinik St. Georg, Lohmühlenstr. 5, 20099 Hamburg, Germany

Otto **Ljungberg**, M.D., Professor of Medicine, Department of Pathology, Malmö University Hospital, 20502 Malmö, Sweden

Michaela **Lürken**, M.D., Nuclear Medicine Practice, Universitätsklinikum Schleswig-Holstein, Campus Kiel, Arnold-Heller-Str. 9, 24105 Kiel, Germany

Brigitte **Mahn**, M.D., Department of Pathology, Asklepios Klinik St. Georg, Lohmühlenstr. 5, 20099 Hamburg, Germany

Christoph **Manegold**, M.D., Clinical Department, Bernhard-Nocht Institute of Tropical Medicine, Bernhard-Nocht-Str. 74, 20359 Hamburg, Germany

Ernst-Joachim **Malzfeldt**, M.D., Department of Diagnostic Radiology and Nuclear Medicine, Asklepios Klinik Altona, Paul-Ehrlich-Str. 1, 22763 Hamburg, Germany

Thomas **Mansfeld**, M.D., Surgical Department I, Asklepios Klinik Altona, Paul-Ehrlich-Str. 1, 22763 Hamburg, Germany

Sönke **Martens**, M.D., Medical Clinic, Klinikum Itzehoe, Robert-Koch-Str. 1, 25524 Itzehoe, Germany

Emese **Mihaly**, M.D., Ph.D., 2nd Department of Internal Medicine, Semmelweis University Medical School, 1088 Szentkirályi u. 46, Budapest, Hungary

Christian **Müller**, M.D., Radiology Department, Kreiskrankenhaus Husum, Erichsenweg 16, 25813 Husum, Germany

Bruno **Neu**, M.D., Medical Department II, Technical University of Munich, Klinkium rechts der Isar, Ismaningerstr. 22, 81675 Munich, Germany

Horst **Neuhaus**, M.D., Professor of Medicine, Medical Clinic, Evangelisches Krankenhaus Düsseldorf, Kirchfeldstr. 40, 40217 Düsseldorf, Germany

Markus **Oeyen,** M.D., Medical Department, Städtisches Krankenhaus St. Barbara Attendorn, Hohler Weg 9, 57439 Attendorn, Germany

Sybille **Othmar**, M.D., Radiology Practice, Schiessgrabenstr. 6, 21335 Lüneburg, Germany

Uwe **Peters**, M.D., Radiologist at Itzehoe Hospital, Robert-Koch-Str. 2, 25524 Itzehoe, Germany

Christopher **Pohland,** M.D., Surgical Department I, Asklepios Klinik Altona, Paul-Ehrlich-Str. 1, 22763 Hamburg, Germany

Rainer **Porschen**, M.D., Professor of Medicine, Department of Internal Medicine, Zentralkrankenhaus Bremen Ost, Züricher Str. 40, 28325 Bremen, Germany

Jürgen F. **Riemann**, M.D., Professor of Medicine, Department of Gastroenterology, Klinikum Ludwigshafen, Bremserstr. 79, 67063 Ludwigshafen, Germany

Patrick **Rogalla**, M.D., Professor, Department of Radiology, Charité Hospital, Campus Mitte, Schumannstr. 20/21, 10117 Berlin, Germany

Wolfgang **Saeger**, M.D., Professor of Medicine, Department of Pathology, Marienkrankenhaus, Angerstr. 6, 22087 Hamburg, Germany

Jürgen **Schmoll**, M.D., Bremerhaven Pathology Institute, Postbrookstr. 101, 27574 Bremerhaven, Germany

Hans-Michael **Schneider**, M.D., Professor of Medicine, Institute for Pathology, St. Vincentius-Kliniken, Südendstr. 37, 76137 Karlsruhe, Germany

Warwick A. **Selby,** M.D., Clinical Associate Professor of Medicine, University of Sydney, AW Morrow Gastroenterology and Liver Centre, Royal Prince Alfred Hospital, Camperdown, NSW 2050, Sydney, Australia

Virender K. **Sharma**, M.D., Associate Professor of Medicine, Mayo Clinic College of Medicine, Division of Gastroenterology and Hepatology, Mayo Clinic, 13400 East Shea Boulevard, Scottsdale, AZ 85259, USA

Erik **Skogestad,** M.D., Department of Internal Medicine, Sykehuset Innlandet Lillehammer, Anders Sandvigs Gate 17, 2624 Lillehammer, Norway

Florentin **Stachow,** M.D., Medical Department, Johanniter Krankenhaus Geesthacht–Lauenburg, Am Runden Berge 3, 21502 Geesthacht, Germany

Annette **Stelzer**, M.D., Department of Gastroenterology, Hepatology and Infectiology, University Hospital Düsseldorf, Moorenstr. 5, 40225 Düsseldorf, Germany

Frank **Stenschke**, M.D., 2nd Medical Clinic, Klinikum Offenbach, Starkenburgring 66, 63069 Offenbach, Germany

Wolfgang **Teichmann**, M.D., Professor of Medicine, Surgical Department I, Asklepios Klinik Altona, Paul-Ehrlich-Str. 1, 22763 Hamburg, Germany

Thomas **Thomsen**, M.D., Department of Gastroenterology, Friedrich-Ebert-Krankenhaus, Friesenstr. 11, 24531 Neumünster, Germany

Henrik **Thorlacius**, M.D., Professor of Medicine, Department of Medicine, Malmö University Hospital, 20502 Malmö, Sweden

Ervin **Tóth**, M.D., Ph.D., Professor of Medicine, Department of Medicine, Malmö University Hospital, 20502 Malmö, Sweden

André **Van Gossum**, M.D., Professor of Medicine, Department of Gastroenterology and Hepatopancreatology, Hôpital Erasme, Université Libre de Bruxelles, Route de Lennik 808, 1070 Brussels, Belgium

Winfried **Voderholzer**, M.D., Department of Hepatology and Gastroenterology, Charité Hospital, Campus Mitte, Schumannstr. 20/21, 10117 Berlin, Germany

Axel **von Herbay**, M.D., Professor of Medicine, Gastrointestinal Pathology, St. Mark's Hospital, Northwick Park, Watford Road, Harrow, HA1 3UJ, UK

Ullrich **Wahnschaffe**, M.D., Medical Clinic I, Charité Hospital, Campus Benjamin Franklin, Hindenburgdamm 30, 12200 Berlin, Germany

Andreas **Wandler**, M.D., Radiology Practice, Schäferkampsallee 5–7, 20357 Hamburg, Germany

Otto-Henning **Wegener**, M.D., Professor of Medicine, Department of Diagnostic Radiology and Nuclear Medicine, Asklepios Klinik Altona, Paul-Ehrlich-Str. 1, 22763 Hamburg, Germany

Doris **Welger**, M.D., Department of Diagnostic Radiology and Nuclear Medicine, Asklepios Klinik Altona, Paul-Ehrlich-Str. 1, 22763 Hamburg, Germany

Wilko **Weichert**, M.D., Pathology Institute, Charité Hospital, Campus Mitte, Schumannstr. 20/21, 10117 Berlin, Germany

Hanns-Olof **Wintzer**, M.D., Department of Pathology, Asklepios Klinik Harburg, Eissendorfer Pferdeweg 52, 21075 Hamburg, Germany

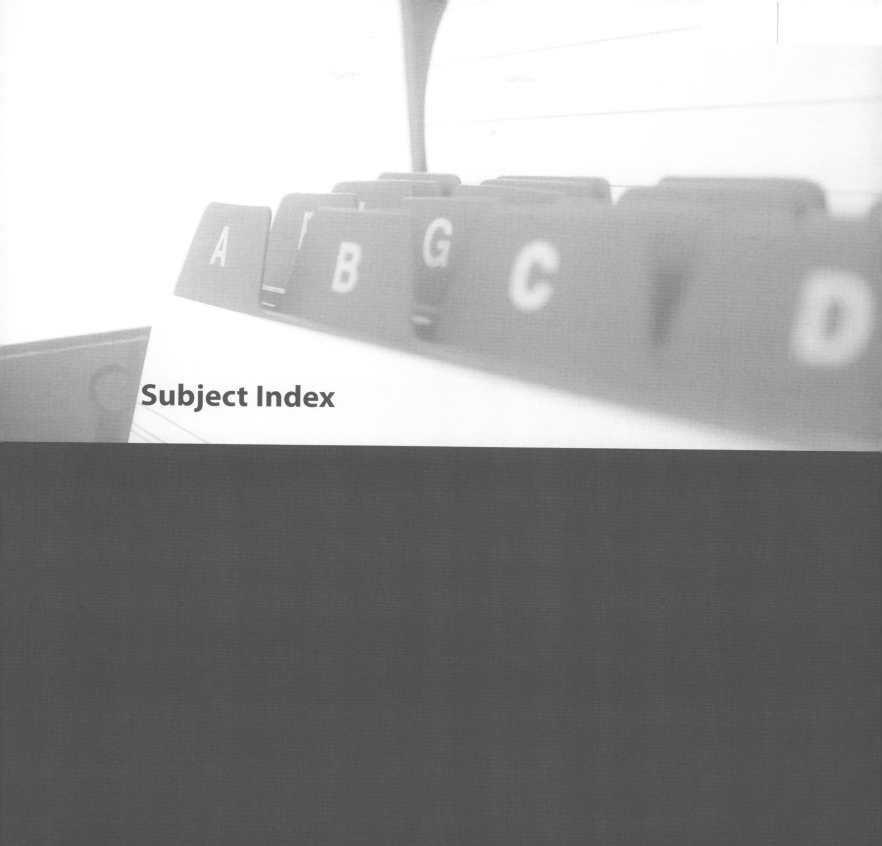

Subject Index